Organic Chemist's Desk Reference

Second Edition

Organic Chemist's Desk Reference

Second Edition

Caroline Cooper

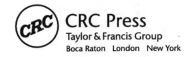

CRC Press
Taylor & Francis Group
Boca Raton   London   New York

CRC Press is an imprint of the
Taylor & Francis Group, an **informa** business

CRC Press
Taylor & Francis Group
6000 Broken Sound Parkway NW, Suite 300
Boca Raton, FL 33487-2742

© 2011 by Taylor and Francis Group, LLC
CRC Press is an imprint of Taylor & Francis Group, an Informa business

International Standard Book Number: 978-1-4398-1164-1 (Paperback)

Library of Congress Cataloging-in-Publication Data

Cooper, Caroline.
   Organic chemist's desk reference / Caroline Cooper. -- 2nd ed.
     p. cm.
   Rev. ed. of: The organic chemist's desk reference / P.H. Rhodes. 1995.
   Includes bibliographical references and indexes.
   ISBN 978-1-4398-1164-1 (pbk. : alk. paper)
   1. Chemistry, Organic--Handbooks, manuals, etc. I. Rhodes, P. H. Organic chemist's desk reference. II. Title.

QD257.7.R46 2010
547--dc22
                                         2010017181

Visit the Taylor & Francis Web site at
http://www.taylorandfrancis.com

and the CRC Press Web site at
http://www.crcpress.com

To Edward, Charles, and Sebastian

Contents

Preface

The *Organic Chemist's Desk Reference* first appeared in 1995. It was conceived as a companion volume to the sixth edition of the *Dictionary of Organic Compounds* (DOC6) but was also available separately. It was compiled by the members of the DOC team, coordinated by Peter Rhodes as principal author.

The first edition was widely welcomed, but such is the rate of development of the subject that nearly all the sections are now well out of date. The team that put together DOC6 in the 1990s is still largely together, and so the present volume consists of a major updating of the first edition, under the editorship of Caroline Cooper. After changes of ownership of the DOC database, this new edition appears under the imprint of CRC Press.

The preface to the first edition stated that "success in organic chemistry needs a lively appreciation of the other sciences—and not just other branches of chemistry ... in order to make a success of organic chemistry, the practitioner needs to know so many specialist facts and methods that the subject can be daunting to a nonspecialist." This statement is even truer now than it was then. The divisions between organic chemistry and other disciplines such as biochemistry and materials science have become further blurred, and the phenomenal changes in informatics since 1995 have impacted on many of the subject areas covered by this book. New associated subdisciplines—nanochemistry, assembly chemistry, "green" chemistry—have grown up. Whilst one or two of the subject areas covered by the first edition merely required some updating, the majority have been heavily revised, and some, notably the chapters on information resources and spectroscopic methods, are completely unrecognisable after a less than fifteen-year interval.

We hope therefore that the new edition will be welcomed not just by mainstream organic chemists, but by anyone working in one or more of these overlap areas, by anyone else who has to make occasional use of organic chemistry techniques as part of their daily work, or who needs to interpret the results of others.

John Buckingham

Acknowledgments

I should like to thank the following people for their contributions:

Gerald Pattenden (University of Nottingham) gave valuable help at the planning stage.
John Buckingham and Rupert Purchase (Consultants, CRC Press) wrote many of the updated
   sections of the book.

The following kindly contributed chapters:

Ross Denton (University of Nottingham)
Matt Griffiths (CRC Press)
Nelu Grinberg (Boehringer Ingelheim Pharmaceuticals, Ridgefield, CT, USA)
Maureen Julian (Virginia Polytechnic Institute, Blacksburg, USA)
James McCullagh (University of Oxford)

Additional sections were written by:

Keith Baggaley and Terry Ward (Consultants, CRC Press)
Janice Shackleton in the London office of CRC Press, organised the typescript and diagrams.
   The diagrams were drawn by Trupti Desai and Jenny Francis retyped the material from
   the first edition.
Finally, Fiona Macdonald at CRC Press in Boca Raton, commissioned and supervised the
   project.

1 The Organic Chemistry Literature

1.1 ABSTRACTING AND OTHER CURRENT AWARENESS SERVICES

There has been a strong trend in recent years toward the merging of previously separate information products, both in terms of ownership (Chemical Abstracts Service (CAS) being an exception) and technically (standardisation of search engines so as to facilitate searching across the previously distinct products). As with primary journals, the situation concerning what is free access and what is subscription only remains complex. The boundary between abstracting services and other information products has also become progressively blurred as (1) many journal publishers, e.g., Elsevier, have introduced searchable contents files, and (2) products formerly regarded as fulfilling only an abstracting function have enhanced their features to include substructure search, spectroscopic files, physical property prediction, etc.

Some of these files are accessible through more than one portal, with different search engines and charging protocols. For example, *Current Contents Search* is available on DIALOG charged on a per-search, per-hit, per-print basis.

Backfiles available in print only (e.g., *Index Chemicus* pre-1993) are now of very limited use and likely to be difficult to obtain.

1.1.1 CHEMICAL ABSTRACTS

First published in 1907, *Chemical Abstracts* (CA) justly claims to be the "key to the world's chemical literature." The history and evolution of *Chemical Abstracts* are described in R. E. Maizell, *How to Find Chemical Information: A Guide for Practicing Chemists, Educators, and Students* (New York, Wiley, 1998, pp. 60–106, 107–39).

Until 2009, Chemical Abstracts Service (CAS; www.cas.org; a division of the American Chemical Society) produced and marketed *Chemical Abstracts* in a number of different *printed* and *electronic* formats. In 2010 CA print products (with the exception of CA *Selects*) ceased to be published and access to CA was restricted to subscribers to the electronic versions: Chemical Abstracts Web Edition, SciFinder®, and the CAS databases available from STN.

1.1.1.1 Printed Products
For the organic chemist, knowledge of, and access to, the more familiar components of the *printed products* of *Chemical Abstracts* is still desirable: CA abstracts; CA Volume Indexes and CA Collective Indexes; CA Index Guide; *CAS Source Index* (CASSI); *Registry Handbook: Number Section*; the *Ring Systems Handbook*; and *CA Selects*.

1.1.1.1.1 Publication Schedule and Content
Until the end of 2009, the printed edition of *Chemical Abstracts* was published weekly. The abstracts part of CA categorises the chemical literature into six basic types of entries: (1) serial publications, (2) proceedings and edited collections, (3) technical reports, (4) dissertations, (5) new book and audio-visual materials announcements, and (6) patent documents. The abstracts are classified in

eighty sections arranged into five broad groupings: *Biochemistry* (Sections 1–20), *Organic Chemistry* (Sections 21–34), *Macromolecular Chemistry* (Sections 35–46), *Applied Chemistry and Chemical Engineering* (Sections 47–64), and *Physical, Inorganic and Analytical Chemistry* (Sections 65–80). Each printed weekly issue also contained a Keyword Index, a Patent Index, and an Author Index. Within any one section, serial publication abstracts, proceedings, edited collection abstracts, and dissertation abstracts come first; new book and audio-visual materials announcements second; and patent document abstracts third.

In the early years of publication, CA provided full and complete abstracts (but inferior to *Chemische Zentralblatt*; see Section 1.1.2). For the organic chemist, these abstracts contain useful experimental details and physical properties of chemical substances. With the usual reservations concerning accuracy, the early abstracts can be a partial substitute for the original literature when in relatively obscure journals and patents. Around 1950–1970, abstracts became progressively more findings orientated and did not attempt to abstract all the new data contained in original documents. Abstracts are now more concise, with text averaging about one hundred words. The first sentence of a CA abstract highlights the primary findings and conclusions reported in the original document. The text that follows the first sentence elaborates upon these highlighted findings and emphasises the following significant data: (1) purpose and scope of the reported work; (2) new reactions, compounds, materials, techniques, procedures, apparatus, properties, and theories; (3) new applications of established knowledge; and (4) results of the investigation together with the authors' interpretation and conclusions. The terminology used in the CA abstract reflects that used by the author(s) in the original document. Abstracts are suitable for the evaluation of reported research, but the original documents are consulted for the compilation of the *Chemical Abstracts* Volume Indexes.

For the patent literature, an abstract is published in CA for the first patent received. Subsequent patents covering the same invention are not abstracted but entered into the Patent Concordance organised alphabetically by country (or group of countries) of issue. The abstraction of all new and existing chemical substances reported in complete patent specifications has been a particularly useful feature of *Chemical Abstracts* since its inception. Further details of the patent literature and patent abstracts are given in Section 1.4.

1.1.1.1.2   CA Abstract Numbers

Since 1967, CA abstracts have been numbered sequentially in each (semiannual) volume of *Chemical Abstracts*; the abstract number includes a computer-generated check letter. Before the introduction of computer-assisted production in 1967, abstracts were located in CA indexes by the sequentially numbered columns on each page in each issue. The letters *a* to *i* were also assigned to every column to assist in the location of the abstract. Before 1947, a superscript number was used instead of a letter. These older methods did not give each abstract a unique identifier. In SciFinder, all pre-1967 abstracts have been assigned a unique abstract number. These new CA abstract numbers cannot be used to find abstracts in printed (non-electronic) pre-1967 *Chemical Abstracts*, and are a potential source of confusion if this distinction between the procedures for locating pre- and post-1967 abstracts is not appreciated.

The symbol *pr* in printed CA Chemical Subject Indexes denotes "preparation," and was first introduced in July–December 1994 (Volume 121). Abstracts are assigned *pr* on an intellectual basis by CAS document analysts if the original source material provides information on preparation or related concepts such as manufacture, purification, recovery, synthesis, extraction, generation, isolation, and secretion.

1.1.1.2   CA Volume Indexes and CA Collective Indexes

CA Volume Indexes are in-depth compilations, whose entries are selected by the CAS indexer from original documents and not just from the abstracts. Printed editions of the CA Volume Indexes were published annually until 1962 and, thereafter semiannually (every six months) until 2009.

Volume Indexes to CA are based on a controlled vocabulary developed by CAS. To provide chemists with more rapid indexing of the contents of individual CA issues, a form of quick indexing (designated as the *Keyword Index*) was published with each issue from 1963 to 2009. Keyword Indexes use a more informal vocabulary than the concise terms in Volume Indexes and are not a substitute for them.

CA Collective Indexes (CIs) combine into single, organised listings the contents of individual Volume Indexes. Printed ten-year (decennial) CA Collective Indexes were published for abstracts issued from 1907 to 1956 (1st CI to 5th CI); five-year (quinquennial) Collective Indexes were published in a print format for abstracts issued from 1957 to 2001 (6th CI to 14th CI). The 15th CI (2002 to 2006) was published in a CD-ROM format only. Table 1.1 gives details of the publication dates and constituent volume numbers for the decennial and quinquennial CA Collective Indexes.

The contents of CA Volume Indexes and CA Collective Indexes are a *General Subject Index*, a *Chemical Substance Index*, a *Formula Index*, an *Author Index*, and a *Patent Index*. The development of these indexes from 1907 to 2006 is traced in Table 1.1. Although the convenience of online and CD-ROM searching has relegated the usage of printed CA Indexes; nevertheless, for some searches they retain an advantage, for example, in scanning for the known salts and simple derivatives of pharmacologically active substances, searching for stereoisomers and their derivatives, and checking variants in authors' names.

1.1.1.2.1   General Subject Index
- The General Subject Index links subject terms, such as reactions, processes and equipment, classes of substances, and biochemical and biological subjects, including plant and animal species, with their corresponding CA abstract numbers.
- Most entries include a text modification phrase, which further describes aspects of the topic covered in the original document.
- Before using the General Subject Index, the *Chemical Abstracts* Index Guide (see Section 1.1.1.3) should be consulted in order to obtain the correct index headings.
- Prior to 1972, general subjects and chemical substances appeared together in a Subject Index.

1.1.1.2.2   Chemical Substance Index
- *The Chemical Substance Index* was initiated during the ninth Collective Index period (1972 to 1976); before 1972, chemical substances and general subjects were in a single Subject Index.
- This index consists of an alphabetical listing of CA Index Names, each of which identifies a specific chemical substance linked to the appropriate CA abstract number. Chemical *Substance Indexes* (and the earlier Subject Indexes) reflect changes in chemical nomenclature, and in particular the revision of nomenclature implemented for the ninth Collective Index period. (See Section 3.2 and Chapter 7 for a description of the changes to CA Index Names and stereochemical descriptors.)
- During the eighth Collective Index period (1967 to 1971), the CAS Chemical Registry System was introduced (see Section 9.1), and chemical substances were further identified by their *CAS Registry Numbers* in the eighth and subsequent printed Collective Indexes and in Volume Indexes from Volume 71 (July to December 1969) onward.

1.1.1.2.3   Formula Index
- The Formula Index links the molecular formulae of chemical substances with their CA Index Names, CAS registry numbers, and CA abstract numbers. Molecular formulae are arranged according to the Hill system order (see Section 10.1).

TABLE 1.1
CA Collective Indexes Content

Collective Index	15th[a]	14th[a]	13th[a]	12th[a]	11th[a]	10th[a]	9th	8th	7th	6th	5th	4th	3rd	2nd	1st
Years covered	2002–2006	1997–2001	1992–1996	1987–1991	1982–1986	1977–1981	1972–1976	1967–1971	1962–1966	1957–1961	1947–1956	1937–1946	1927–1936	1917–1926	1907–1916
Volumes	136–145	126–135	116–125	106–115	96–105	86–95	76–85	66–75	56–65	51–55[b]	41–50	31–40	21–30	11–20	1–10
Author Index	•	•	•	•	•	•	•	•	•	•	•	•	•	•	•
Subject Index							c	•	•	•	•	•	•	•	•
General Subject Index	•	•	•	•	•	•	•								
Chemical Substance Index	•	•	•	•	•	•	•								
Formula Index	•	•	•	•	•	•	•	•	•	•	•	d	d	d	
Numerical Patent Index						•	•	•	•	•	•	•	f	f	f
Patent Concordance						•	•	•	•						
Patent Index	•	•	•	•	•[e]										
Index of Ring Systems			g	•	•	•	•	•	•	g	g	g	g	g	g
Index Guide	•	•	•	•	•	•	•	•							

Source: Table 1.1 is reproduced with the permission of Chemical Abstracts Service, Columbus, Ohio, and the American Chemical Society (CACS). Copyright © 2010. All rights reserved.

a   The 15th Collective Index was published in a CD-ROM format only. The 10th to 14th Collective Indexes, respectively, were published both in print and in CD-ROM formats. Beyond the 15th Collective Index, CA content continues to be available in electronic format through the CAS search tools SciFinder® and STN.®

b   In 1957, the indexing period was changed from ten years (Decennial Index) to five years (Collective Index).

c   The Subject Index was subdivided into the General Subject and Chemical Substance Indexes beginning with the ninth Collective Index period.

d   27-year Collective Formula Index (1920–1946).

e   In 1981, the Numerical Patent Index and Patent Concordance were merged into the Patent Index.

f   Thirty-year Numerical Patent Index (1907–1936), compiled by the Science-Technology Group, Special Libraries Association (Ann Arbor, MI: J. W. Edwards, 1944).

g   The Index of Ring Systems was discontinued after the twelfth Collective Index period. For the 1st to the 6th Collective Indexes, Ring System Information was included in the introduction to the Subject Index; for the 7th to the 12th Collective Indexes, the Index of Ring Systems was bound with the Formula Index.

- Volumes 1–13 of *Chemical Abstracts* had no Formula Index. Formula Indexes, listing formulae in the Hill order, were produced annually from Volume 14 (1920), and there is a Collective Formula Index that covers Volumes 14–40 (1920–1946).

1.1.1.2.4   Author Index
- The Author Index is an alphabetical listing of names of authors, coauthors, inventors, and patent assignees linked to the CA abstract number.
- Both personal and corporate names are included. The name of the first author is linked with the title of the original document or patent. Coauthors are cross-referred to the name of the first author.
- A system for the alphabetization and ordering of personal names in CA has evolved, and is explained in the introduction to the Author Indexes in the Volume Indexes and the Collective Indexes.

1.1.1.2.5   Patent Index
- The Patent Index is an alphabetical listing of national and international patent offices using a standardised two-letter code for the country of issue (AD, Andorra, to ZW, Zimbabwe). Within the listing for each country (or group of countries), patents are arranged in ascending patent number order.
- Each patent number is followed by either a CA abstract number and a complete history of all equivalent documents, or a cross-reference to the patent number of the first abstracted patent in the patent family. This feature of the index, detailing a patent family, is the CA Patent Concordance.
- Separate Numerical Patent Indexes with CA abstract numbers were published for the periods 1907 to 1936 (CA Volumes 1–30) (by the Special Libraries Association) and 1937 to 1946 (CA Volumes 31–40) and 1947 to 1956 (CA Volumes 41–50) (by the American Chemical Society), respectively. Numerical Patent Indexes became part of CA Collective Indexes from the sixth CI onward (1957 to 1961). The CA Patent Concordance was started in 1963, and merged with the Numerical Patent Index in 1981 to form the Patent Index.

1.1.1.3   *Chemical Abstracts* Index Guide
CA Index Guides explain CA indexing policy and provide cross-references from chemical substance names and general subject terms used in the scientific literature to the equivalent names and terminology found in *Chemical Abstracts*. Index Guides are therefore a useful bridge between the scientific literature and CA General Subject and Chemical Substance Indexes. The first Index Guide was published with the 8th CI in 1968. Starting in 1992, new editions were issued after the first, fifth, and tenth volumes of a five-year Collective Index period. Successive editions of the Index Guide reflect changes in CA policy, content, vocabulary, and nomenclature, and therefore always replace the immediate preceding edition. The last printed edition of the Index Guide covered the fifteenth Collective Index period, 2002–2006.

A CA Index Guide contains the following parts:

- The introduction describes cross-references, parenthetical terms, and the indexing policy notes listed in the main part of the Index Guide.
- The *Index Guide*, the main part of the publication, is an alphabetical sequence of chemical substance names selected from the literature (including trivial names used for natural products, International Nonproprietary Names (INN), trade names, and code names) with cross-references to the chemical substance names used in CA Chemical Substance Indexes. CAS registry numbers are provided as part of the cross-reference entry. Also in this part of the Index Guide (beginning in 1985) are the CA General Subject Index headings (excluding Latinised genus and species names) and diagrams for stereoparents.

- Appendix I: *Hierarchies of General Subject Headings* lists the general and specific headings that have been developed by CAS for the General Subject Index and the hierarchies employed for these headings.
- Appendix II: *Indexes to Chemical Abstracts: Organisation and Use* is a comprehensive account of the organisation, and relationships, of the CA Chemical Substance Index, CA General Subject Index, CA Formula Index, and CA Index of Ring Systems. This appendix also describes the CAS Chemical Registry System and the criteria applied in selecting CA index entries.
- Appendix III: *Selection of General Subject Headings* discusses the content of the CA General Subject Index.
- Appendix IV: *Chemical Substance Index Names* describes the CAS rules for naming substances entered in the CA Chemical Substance Indexes and given CAS registry numbers. For the organic chemist especially, this appendix is a detailed explanation of CAS rules for naming organic chemical substances and the CAS convention for stereochemical descriptors. CAS revised its rules for naming chemical substances during the ninth and fifteenth Collective Index periods, respectively, and adopted new rules for stereochemical descriptors during 1997–1998. These changes are explained in Chapters 3 and 7.

1.1.1.4 *CAS Source Index* (CASSI)

The *Chemical Abstracts Service Source Index*, commonly referred to as CASSI, gives details of the journals and related literature cited in *Chemical Abstracts* since 1907. In addition, CASSI contains entries for those publications covered by *Chemische Zentralblatt* and its predecessors from 1830–1969 and the publications cited by Beilstein prior to 1907. The most recent printed cumulative edition of CASSI spanned the period 1907–2004. Printed supplements to CASSI were published quarterly from 2005 to 2009. The fourth quarterly supplement each year cumulated and replaced the preceding three supplements, and was effectively an annual update. Publication of the printed edition of CASSI ceased in 2009, but CASSI remains available and updated in a searchable CD-ROM format (CASSI on CD, first produced in the 1990s).

Entries in CASSI include the following information: complete title for a serial or a nonserial publication, abbreviated title, variant title, ISSN, ISBN, translation of the title (for some foreign language titles only), name and address of the publisher or sales agency where the publications may be obtained, and a history of the serial publication, such as predecessor and successor titles. Entries in CASSI are arranged alphabetically according to the abbreviated form of the serial or nonserial title.

For the organic chemist, CASSI is particularly useful for providing:

- The recognised and authoritative abbreviations of journals and other publications in the chemistry literature.
- The complete journal titles for abbreviations used for serials and nonserials in *Chemical Abstracts* from 1907 to 2002. (Starting with Volume 136 (2002), *Chemical Abstracts* began to quote the full journal or publication title as part of the abstract instead of the CASSI abbreviation.)

CASSI abbreviations for about fifteen hundred leading journals are listed on a free website (*CAplus Core Journal Coverage List*). Also on the web is the *CAS Source Index (CASSI) Search Tool* (http://cassi.cas.org/search.jsp).

1.1.1.5 Registry Handbook: Number Section

Following the introduction of the system of CAS registry numbers in 1965 (see Chapter 9), CAS published the *Registry Handbook—Number: Section*. The initial handbook covered the period 1965–1971 (registry numbers 35-66-5 to 33913-68-7). Annual supplements of registry numbers were published from 1972 to 2001 (registry numbers 33913-69-8 to 380148-63-0), when publication of the printed version ceased. There was also a series of *Registry Handbook: Registry Number Updates* published from 1965 to 2001, which gave details of discontinued registry numbers and any updates.

Entries in the *Registry Handbook* list CAS registry numbers in numerical sequence, and their associated CA Index Names and molecular formulae. Concomitantly with the printed edition, CAS developed an online searchable database of registry numbers, *CAS Registry*. By April 2010, this database contained the details of over 53,000,000 organic and inorganic substances and 61,722,079 sequences, and the most recent CAS registry number was 1217435-73-8.

1.1.1.6 Ring Systems Handbook

See Section 1.3 and Chapter 4 for more information.

1.1.1.7 Electronic Products

1.1.1.7.1 *Chemical Abstracts on CD-ROM*

The tenth to fifteenth CA Collective Indexes and Abstracts (1977–2006) were produced in a CD-ROM format, and annual updates were issued from 2007. These CD-ROM versions of *Chemical Abstracts* incorporate a number of useful and browsable search indexes with Boolean functionality, some of which are not in the printed product:

- Word Index
- CAS Registry Number Index
- Author Index
- General Subject Index
- Patent Index
- Formula Index
- Compound Index
- Chemical Abstract Number Index
- Organisation
- Journal Title Index
- Language Index
- Year of Publication Index
- Document Type Index

1.1.1.7.2 *Chemical Abstracts Web Edition*

Chemical Abstracts web edition was introduced in 2008 and is an alternative web-based product for accessing *Chemical Abstracts*. The web edition has the following features:

- Electronic access to fully indexed records in CAS databases corresponding to the customer's subscription period to *Chemical Abstracts* from 1996 to the present
- Multiple ways to browse information, including:
  - Bibliographic indexes
  - Subject indexes
  - Substance indexes
- Basic and advanced search capabilities with refine options
- Capability to search across multiple years
- Option to save answers locally or on the CAS server
- Modern, browser-based interface

1.1.1.7.3 *SciFinder*

SciFinder is the preferred portal to access chemical information from the CAS databases and is designed for use by chemists in commercial organisations. *SciFinder Scholar* is a version for universities and academic institutions that lacks some supplementary features. Both can be searched by substructure in addition to other methods.

In 2009, there were two ways to access: from a client version installed on a computer or via web access. The client version is being phased out as the web version is being developed. Both versions have the same functionality. Advantages of SciFinder include the ability to combine answer sets and the ability to see all the substances linked to an abstract in a grid layout. Clicking on a substance structure or registry number allows the user to modify the structure for future searches or to explore reactions. SciFinder also provides access to the full text of the article through the ChemPort Connection. This allows the user to directly access the article when permissions for access are enabled or to purchase the article when they are not enabled.

Table 1.2 shows the databases and information available from SciFinder.

1.1.1.7.4   CAS Databases Available on STN

STN is an online database service jointly owned by CAS and FIZ Karlsruhe. Chemical Abstracts Service provides a range of online databases covering chemistry and related sciences (see also Table 1.2):

CAplus[SM] covers the literature from 1907 to the present, plus more than 133,000 pre-1907 journal records and more than 1,250 records for U.S. patents issued from 1808 to 1859. Includes article references from more than ten thousand major scientific worldwide journals, conference proceedings, technical reports, books, patents, dissertations, and meeting abstracts.

CAS Registry is a structure and text-searchable database containing information on approximately 46 million organic and inorganic substances and over 60 million sequences with associated CAS registry numbers.

CASREACT® is a structure and text-searchable organic chemical reaction database containing more than 17 million single- and multistep reactions with more than six hundred thousand records from journal articles and patents with reaction information. Coverage is from 1840 to the present.

CHEMCATS® is a database of more than 34 million commercially available chemicals from more than nine hundred suppliers and one thousand catalogues.

CHEMLIST® is a regulated chemicals listing. Regulated substances listed on the Environmental Protection Agency Toxic Substances Control Act Inventory, the European Inventory of Existing Commercial Chemical Substances, and the Domestic and Nondomestic Substances List from Canada are well covered, as well as other lists of hazardous substances. More than 249,000 substances are listed.

CIN® (Chemical Industry Notes) contains bibliographic and abstract information from journals, trade magazines, and newspapers.

1.1.1.7.5   CA Selects

Issued biweekly, CA Selects Plus, CA Selects, and CA Selects on the Web are current awareness bulletins, in print and electronic format, comprising the CA abstracts of all papers on a particular topic covered in *Chemical Abstracts*. No indexes are provided. There are over two hundred topics available. Those of interest to organic chemists include:

- Amino acids, peptides, and proteins
- Asymmetric synthesis and induction
- Beta-lactam antibiotics
- Carbohydrates (chemical aspects)
- Natural product synthesis
- New antibiotics

TABLE 1.2
SciFinder Content

Database	Content
	Reference Databases
CAplus^SM	Literature from 1907 to the present plus selected pre-1907 references. Sources include journals, patents, conference proceedings, dissertations, technical reports, books, and more.
	CAplus covers a wide spectrum of science-related information, including chemistry, biochemistry, chemical engineering, and related sciences.
MEDLINE®	Biomedical literature from more than 4,780 journals and 70 countries, covering literature from 1950 to the present.
	Structure Database
CAS REGISTRY^SM	Specific chemical substances, including organic and inorganic compounds, sequences, coordination compounds, polymers, and alloys covering 1957 to the present, with some classes going back to the early 1900s.
	Reaction Database
CASREACT®	Reaction information for single- and multiple-step reactions from 1840 to the present.
	Commercial Source Database
CHEMCATS®	Chemical source information, including supplier addresses and pricing information derived from current chemical catalogues and libraries, retrieved for individual substances.
	Regulatory Database
CHEMLIST®	Regulatory information records from 1979 to the present, including substance identity information, inventory status, sources, and compliance information.

Information available from SciFinder includes:

Content Area	Information Available
References	• Title
	• Author/editor/inventor
	• Company name/corporate source/patent assignee
	• Publication year
	• Source, publication, date, publisher, volume, issue, pagination, CODEN, ISSN
	• Patent identification, including patent, application, priority, and patent family information
	• Abstract of the article or patent
	• Indexing
	• Supplementary terms
	• Citations
	• Substances, sequences, and reactions discussed within the document
Substances	• Chemical name
	• CAS Registry Number®
	• Molecular formula
	• Structure diagram
	• Sequence information, including GenBank® and patent annotations
	• Property data, including spectral diagrams
	• Commercial source information from chemical supplier catalogs
	• Regulatory information
	• Editor notes
	• Documents in which the substance is referenced
	• Reactions in which the substance participates

(continued on next page)

TABLE 1.2 (continued)
SciFinder Content

Content Area	Information Available
Reactions	• Reaction diagrams, including reactants, products, reagents, catalysts, solvents, and step notes • Document in which the reaction is referenced • Additional substance details, reactions, references, regulatory information, and commercial source information for all reaction participants • Notes

Source: Table 1.2 is reproduced from the Chemical Abstracts Service, Columbus, Ohio, and the American Chemical Society (CACS). Copyright © 2010. All rights reserved..

Note: SciFinder retrieves information contained in databases produced by Chemical Abstracts Service (CAS) as well as in the MEDLINE® database of the National Library of Medicine (NLM).

- Novel natural products
- Novel sulfur heterocycles
- Organic stereochemistry
- Organofluorine chemistry
- Organophosphorus chemistry
- Organosulfur chemistry (journals)
- Porphyrins
- Prostaglandins
- Synthetic macrocyclic compounds
- Steroids (chemical aspects)

Detailed information about CAS products can be found at www.cas.org.

1.1.2 CHEMISCHES ZENTRALBLATT

A German-language abstracting publication that ran from 1830 to 1969. For the period 1907–1969 its coverage and quality of abstracts were usually superior to CAS, and it may still be useful occasionally. An electronic file with advanced search capabilities is available from FIZ CHEMIE Berlin on a subscription basis (www.fiz-chemie.de/zentralblatt).

Review: Weiske, C., *Chem. Ber.*, 106, I–XVI, 1973.

1.1.3 INDEX CHEMICUS

Founded by the Institute for Scientific Information (ISI), now owned by Thomson-Reuters, Index Chemicus is now part of the Web of Science service, which is in turn part of the Web of Knowledge^SM (www.thomsonreuters.com/products_services/scientific/Web_of_Science). The electronic file goes back to 1993 and contains data on 2.6 million compounds. The Web of Science abstracts over 10,000 journals; separate figures are not available for chemistry, but the coverage can be browsed free online.

1.1.4 CURRENT CONTENTS

Also now part of the Web of Science (formerly an ISI product; the electronic version is called Current Contents Search®, which is updated weekly. Gives contents and bibliographic data for papers published in 7,600 scientific journals (chemistry titles not separately counted). Includes prepublication access to some electronic journals.

1.1.5 CHEMISTRY CITATION INDEX

Also part of the Web of Science, this is the successor to the ISI Citation Index and uniquely allows forward searching from a given paper to all subsequent papers that have cited it. The electronic version is called Science Citation Index Expanded. It covers 6,400 journals across all of science, mostly English language. It is possible to subscribe to the Citation Reports service, which sends automatic reports of citation activity relevant to a particular paper or papers.

1.1.6 METHODS IN ORGANIC SYNTHESIS AND NATURAL PRODUCTS UPDATE

These two bulletins are issued monthly by the Royal Society of Chemistry, and each contain about 250 items per issue. Methods in Organic Synthesis (MOS) gives reaction schemes for new synthetic methods reported in the current literature, while Natural Products Update (NPU) covers papers dealing with the isolation, structure determination, and synthesis of natural products. In each case, subscribers have access to the searchable web version.

1.1.7 CURRENT CHEMICAL REACTIONS

Also part of the Web of Science. Abstracts 1 million reactions back to 1986.
See also synthesis databases listed below, e.g., Science of Synthesis.

1.2 PRINCIPAL ELECTRONIC DICTIONARIES

This heading covers tertiary databases that are highly edited and which contain assessed data on compound properties, reactions, etc. Clearly there are trade-offs between breadth of coverage, degree of editing, and currency. However, modern electronic methods make it possible to update a large data set within a reasonable period of the appearance of new information in the primary literature, and allow its reconciliation with existing data.

1.2.1 THE CHAPMAN & HALL/CRC CHEMICAL DATABASE

This database was set up in 1979 to produce the fifth edition of the *Dictionary of Organic Compounds* (DOC), a printed dictionary founded by I. M. Heilbron in 1934. It was subsequently published in electronic form and considerably expanded, especially into natural products and organometallic and inorganic compounds. The sixth edition of DOC (1995) was the last in printed form. Database segments are now available in DVD (formerly CD-ROM) format, as a web version, and for in-house loading by arrangement.

The two principal electronic subsets of the database now available are the following:

The Dictionary of Natural Products (DNP) is a comprehensive resource, now containing approximately 200,000 compounds organised into approximately 80,000 entries. DNP contains highly edited taxonomic information, and a recently introduced feature is hyperlinking to the *Catalogue of Life,* the most authoritative taxonomic resource.

The Combined Chemical Dictionary (CCD) contains every compound on the database (approximately 500,000), including natural products, inorganics, and organometallics, but without some of the specialist features of DNP, such as the *Catalogue of Life* link.

The coverage of CCD in respect to general organics consists of the following:

- The basic fundamental organic compounds of simple structure that are frequently required as starting materials, and which have usually been the subject of extensive physicochemical study
- Compounds with a well-established use, e.g., pesticides and drugs in current use

- Laboratory reagents and solvents
- Other compounds with interesting chemical, structural, or biological properties, including intriguing molecules that have been specially synthesised in order to investigate their chemical and physical properties

CCD is very easy to use and especially valuable for getting an overview of particular compounds or types of compounds, and in teaching applications. The careful selection of references (labelled to show their relevance) and user-friendly nomenclature (with extensive synonym range) takes the user straight to the best literature, and the whole database is kept topical. It is not intended as a comprehensive resource but is often the best place to start the search process. Particularly valuable features are the extensive coverage of CAS numbers and hazard/toxicity information.

The following subset dictionaries have been published in recent years from the Chapman & Hall/CRC database, and are intended as desktop references for the specialist worker. Now published by CRC Press each (except the older titles) consists of a large, single-volume printed dictionary accompanied by a fully searchable CD-ROM uniform in format and search capabilities (including substructure searching) with the main database. A new interface for text and structure searching by ChemAxon was released in 2009.

Dictionary of Alkaloids with CD-ROM, 2nd ed., ed. J. Buckingham et al., CRC Press, 2010. Contains enhanced entries for all alkaloids from the Chapman & Hall database (20,000+ alkaloids, comprehensive record).
Dictionary of Carbohydrates with CD-ROM, 2nd Ed. ed. P. M. Collins, Chapman & Hall/CRC Press, 2005. Contains all the carbohydrates from the Chapman & Hall database.
Dictionary of Food Compounds with CD-ROM, ed. S. Yannai, Chapman & Hall/CRC Press, 2003. Provides information on natural food constituents, additives, and contaminants.
Dictionary of Marine Natural Products with CD-ROM, ed. J. W. Blunt and M. H. G. Munro, Chapman & Hall/CRC, 2007. Comprehensive coverage of marine natural products known to 2006.
Dictionary of Organophosphorus Compounds, ed. R. S. Edmundson, Chapman & Hall, 1988. Structures, properties, and bibliographic data for 20,000 organophosphorus compounds (print only, no CD-ROM).
Dictionary of Steroids, ed. D. N. Kirk et al., 2 vols., Chapman & Hall, 1991. Covers over 15,000 steroids in 6,000 entries (print only, no CD-ROM).

(See also the *Lipid Handbook* in Sections 1.3 and 5.6.)

For more information about subscriptions/prices or to ask for a trial of *Dictionary of Natural Products, Combined Chemical Dictionary,* or other chemistry products, contact e-reference@taylorandfrancis.com.

1.2.2 BEILSTEIN, CROSSFIRE, AND REAXYS

1.2.2.1 Beilsteins Handbuch der Organischen Chemie

Beilsteins Handbuch der Organischen Chemie evolved from the original two-volume first edition compiled by Friedrich Konrad Beilstein (1838–1906) and published between 1881 and 1883 to a multi-volume behemoth, which, when publication of the printed version was terminated in 1998, spanned the literature of organic chemistry in 503 volumes and contained 440,814 pages.

The fourth edition and its supplements, published from 1918 onward, is the definitive (and last) printed edition and is the record of all organic compounds synthesised before December 31, 1979.

TABLE 1.3
The Series of the Beilstein Handbook

Series	Abbreviation	Years Covered	Colour[a]
Basic Series (Hauptwerk)	H	Up to 1910	Green
Supplementary Series I	E I	1910–1919	Dark red
Supplementary Series II	E II	1920–1929	White
Supplementary Series III	E III	1930–1949	Blue
Supplementary Series III/IV	E III/IV[b]	1930–1959	Blue/black
Supplementary Series IV	E IV	1950–1959	Black
Supplementary Series V	E V	1960–1979	Red

[a] The colour refers to the colour of the label on the spine of the books. Series H to E IV are bound in brown. Series E V is bound in blue.

[b] Volumes 17–27 of Supplementary Series III and IV covering the heterocyclic compounds are combined in a joint issue.

(It does not cover natural products that have not been synthesized.) In addition to the main work (literature 1771–1910), there are five supplementary series, as shown in Table 1.3.

E V is in English, previous series are in German. The property data included for the common and frequently handled chemicals are exhaustive, carefully edited, and extremely valuable.

In the printed version, each series comprises twenty-seven volumes (or groups of volumes) known as Bands 1–27 according to functional group seniority. Bands 1–4 cover alicyclic compounds, 5–16 alicyclic, and 17–27 heterocyclic. Groups of compounds are allocated a Beilstein system number that allows forward searching for the same and related compounds in earlier or later supplementary series. However, knowledge of how to use printed Beilstein in this way is largely redundant in the electronic version, and in any case most users of the printed version would now use the Formula Indexes. (The Name Indexes are not recommended because of many complex nomenclature changes since 1918). There is a three-volume index covering the Hauptwerk and Supplements E I and E II that is still valuable for locating information from the pre-1920 literature that is not covered by CAS. In later supplements the bands are separately indexed, but there is also the Centennial Index published in 1991 and 1992 in thirteen volumes, which covers the Hauptwerk and Supplements E I to E IV inclusive. These indexes use the Hill system (see Chapter 10), although it should be noted that earlier individual volumes use the Richter system (e.g., O precedes N). The indexes also refer to the page numbers, not to the Beilstein system numbers.

Printed Beilstein can also be tricky to use because compounds are often treated as derivatives of an unexpected parent, so that, for example, 2-methylfuran and 3-methylfuran do not occur together; 2-methylfuran is first followed by numerous halogeno-, azido-, etc., 2-methylfurans. Various user guides to the printed Beilstein have been published at different times.

Although the later editions of the Handbuch were far larger than Beilstein's own versions, they remained true to his vision of a comprehensive, reliable coverage of the organic literature for many decades. Eventually, however, the sheer enormity of the chemical literature rendered such perfection impossible, and the Handbuch began to lag behind the literature, especially during and after the disruptions caused by World War II. The fourth supplement covering the literature through 1959 was not fully completed until 1987. The fifth supplement, now in English, essentially abandoned the idea of comprehensiveness and settled for a selective coverage of the heterocyclic literature between 1960 and 1979. It finally ceased publication in print in 1998, nearly twenty years after its literature closing date.

Beilstein's work was resurrected by conversion of the printed work into an electronic format, the Beilstein Database. Details of this transition and the earlier marketed electronic formats of the

Beilstein Database are described in *The Beilstein System: Strategies for Effective Searching*, ed. S. R. Heller (Washington, DC: American Chemical Society, 1997). In the 1990s, the Beilstein Institute together with MDL produced an Internet-based client-server system of the Beilstein Database, *CrossFire Beilstein*, which is now owned and updated by Elsevier Information Systems, Frankfurt.

1.2.2.2 CrossFire Beilstein and Reaxys

CrossFire Beilstein is available to subscribers as part of the CrossFire Database Suite. This package consists of *CrossFire Beilstein*, *CrossFire Gmelin*, and *Patent Chemistry Database*. Since January 2009, the contents of these three databases have been merged and are accessible through a new web-based interface, *Reaxys* (Table 1.4).

For organic chemists, the core of the information available through CrossFire Beilstein and Reaxys is the data from *Beilsteins Handbuch der Organischen Chemie* from the Basic Series to Supplementary Series IV covering the literature from 1779 to 1959. The complete *Handbuch* information is available for more than 1.1 million compounds. In addition, for the primary literature from 1960 to 1979, there are data on about 3 million more compounds.

Searching CrossFire Beilstein is fairly intuitive. Predefined search forms allow for searches on the following information:

- Bibliographic data
- Substance identification data
- Molecular formula search
- Reaction data
- Physical data (including melting and boiling point, density, refractive index)
- Spectroscopic data
- Pharmacological data
- Ecotoxicological data
- Solubility data

In addition there is a Structure/Reaction search option. Guides and a "Help" button provide detailed information for searching CrossFire Beilstein.

To avoid obtaining multiple hits, either a combination of search terms is recommended or, preferably, a search using structure or substructure.

TABLE 1.4
Content Information of Reaxys

	Beilstein	**Gmelin**	**Patent Chemistry Database**
Origins	*Beilstein Handbook of Organic Chemistry*, 4th edition	*Gmelin Handbook of Inorganic and Organometallic Chemistry*	U.S. Patent and Trademark Office and esp@cenet
Subject scope	Organic chemistry	Inorganic and organometallic chemistry	Organic chemistry and life sciences
Time span	Journals since 1771, and patent publications from 1869 to 1980	Journals from 1772 to 1995	U.S. patents from 1976, and WIPO and European patents from 1978
Special notes	At present (2009) updates limited to abstracting ~200 organic synthesis journals	Limited to ~100 inorganic journals	Created by Elsevier to expand patent coverage of Beilstein with the same literature selection and extraction criteria

Source: Reproduced from N. Xiao, *Issues in Science & Technology Librarianship*, No. 59 (Summer 2009). With permission.

Additional tools in Reaxys enhance the structure searching options and include:

- A synthesis planner to design the optimum synthesis route (see below)
- Generation of structure from names, InChI (see Section 9.2) keys, or CAS registry numbers
- Linkage to Scopus and eMolecules (a free website for commercially available compounds)
- Search result filters by key properties, synthesis yield, or other ranking criteria
- Multistep reactions to identify precursor reactions underlying synthesis of target compounds

Each chemical reaction has a Reaxys Rx-ID, which is a unique registry number in this database, and is fully searchable. The table view of the records listed also presents possible synthesis route(s) of reactions with possible yield, conditions, and references. Results can be sorted, and redefined by filters.

Similar to a chemical reaction and its Rx-ID, a substance also has its unique Reaxys registry number (Rx-RN), which is assigned to each substance when it is registered for the first time in the database. If a CAS registry number is available for the compound, it will be displayed as a part of the property data. The availability of a substance's CAS registry number enables users to easily identify specific compounds between Reaxys and CAS databases (e.g., SciFinder Scholar, STN, SciFinder web), which are now e-linked.

One of the special features of Reaxys is "Synthesis Plans," which integrates reactions and substances, as well as providing literature search results within one interface. Users can take advantage of this feature to develop better search synthesis strategies.

After selecting a specific substance or reaction, users can:

- Transfer the search result (e.g., a substance or a reaction) to the "Synthesis Plans" tab
- Follow "quick hits" to search for optimum or alternative synthesis routes
- "Synthesise" to get all relevant synthetic routes for desired product
- "Modify" to get all alternative synthetic routes for desired product
- Further refine results by applying analytical filters

With its additional functionalities compared with CrossFire Beilstein, Reaxys allows users to identify specific chemicals more easily, and optimise synthesis routes with detailed reaction information. Selected reactions and substances can be exported into different file formats, and selected references can be exported into reference management software.

(The historical information in this section is reproduced, with permission, from the University of Texas at Austin Library website.)

1.2.3 ELSEVIER'S ENCYCLOPEDIA OF ORGANIC CHEMISTRY

Edited by F. Radt (Elsevier, 1940–1956; Springer, 1959–1969) and with similar coverage and style to Beilstein. It is in English but only Volumes 12–14, condensed carboisocyclic compounds, were published. Publication was suspended in 1956, but further supplements were published by Springer until the steroid sections in Beilstein appeared. It provides a good entry to the old literature on naphthalenes, anthracenes, etc., but is now difficult to find and is not available electronically.

1.2.4 PUBCHEM

A free-access database of small molecules (fewer than one thousand atoms and one thousand bonds), compiled by the U.S. National Center for Biotechnology Information (NCBI), a component of the National Institutes of Health (NIH) (pubchem.ncbi.nlm.nih.gov).

To date it includes data on 37 million fully characterised compounds as well as mixtures, complexes, and uncharacterised substances. It provides information on chemical properties, structures (including InChI and SMILES (see Section 9.3) strings), synonyms, and bioactivity.

1.3   USEFUL REFERENCE WORKS AND REVIEW SERIES

This list comprises some of the more important reference books and review series dealing with organic chemistry. For major abstracting services, such as *Chemical Abstracts*, and dictionaries, such as the *Dictionary of Natural Products*, see the preceding sections.

Many of the larger reference works given here have made, or are making, the transition to electronic access. In assessing the worth of the latest available electronic version, which may not carry a definite edition number, it is important to check the thoroughness of the updating process and ensure that a reputation founded on a large backfile continues to be justified in terms of currency.

Accounts of Chemical Research, American Chemical Society. Wide-ranging review journal with a bias toward interdisciplinary methods and techniques.

ACS Symposium Series, American Chemical Society, produced and marketed by OUP America. Ongoing series of books developed from the ACS technical divisions symposia. Topics tend toward industrial chemistry but include some organic topics.

Advanced Organic Chemistry, 5th ed., ed. F. A. Carey and R. J. Sundberg, 2 vols., Springer, 2008.

Advances in Heterocyclic Chemistry, ed. A. Katritzky, Academic Press. A review series that reached vol. 96 by 2008.

Alkaloids, Chemistry and Biology, ed. R. H. F. Manske, then A. Brossi, then G. A. Cordell; Academic Press, then Wiley, then Elsevier; 1949–. The leading review series devoted to alkaloids.

Atlas of Stereochemistry, 2nd ed., ed. W. Klyne and J. Buckingham, 2 vols. Supplement by J. Buckingham and R. A. Hill, 1986. The standard reference on absolute configurations, though now rather out of date.

CAS Ring Systems Handbook. The last edition of this major reference work was published by CAS in 2003 with semiannual supplements until it was discontinued in 2008. The first part of the handbook, the Ring Systems File, contains structural diagrams and related data for 133,326 unique representative CA index ring systems and 4,492 caged systems (polyboranes, metallocenes, etc.). Information accompanying each ring system includes a Ring File number, the CAS registry number, a structural diagram illustrating the numbering system, the current CA name, and the molecular formula. The ring systems are arranged by their ring analysis, which is given before each group of ring systems having a common ring analysis. The handbook also includes the Ring Formula Index and the Ring Name Index, which are designed to provide access to the contents of the Ring System File. This handbook is particularly useful for accessing the numbering systems used in complex molecules. (See Section 4.1 for details of the use of the handbook.)

Chemical Reviews, American Chemical Society. Monthly authoritative reviews across the whole of chemistry.

Chemical Society Reviews, Royal Society of Chemistry. Monthly reviews across the whole of chemistry.

Chemistry of Functional Groups, ed. S. Patai, Z. Rappoport, and others, Wiley, 1964–. An extensive multivolume series. Each volume covers all aspects of a particular class of compound defined by functional group. Recent volumes are now available online and the titles of the complete series are at http://eu.wiley.com and http://www3.interscience.wiley.com.

A summary of the content of the series may be found in Patai, S., *Patai's 1992 Guide to the Chemistry of Functional Groups*, New York, Wiley, 1992.

Chemistry of Heterocyclic Compounds ("Weissberger"), published by Wiley. An extensive series covering heterocyclic compounds class by class with supplementary volumes as desirable. Each volume covers one or more ring systems. Titles of the complete series 1950–2008 may be found at http://www3.interscience.wiley.com.

Comprehensive Heterocyclic Chemistry III, 15 vols., Elsevier, 2008. Several authors. Large but gives a faster and more general survey than the Weissberger series. Available electronically at www.sciencedirect.com.

Comprehensive Medicinal Chemistry II, ed. D. Triggle and J. Taylor, 8 vols., Elsevier, 2006.

Comprehensive Organic Chemistry, ed. D. H. R. Barton and W. D. Ollis, 6 vols. Pergamon, 1979.

Comprehensive Organic Functional Group Transformations, ed. A. R. Katritzky, O. Meth-Cohn, and C. W. Rees, 7 vols., Pergamon, 1995; *Comprehensive Organic Functional Group Transformations II,* ed. A. R. Katritzky and R. J. K. Taylor, 7 vols., Elsevier, 2004.

Comprehensive Organic Synthesis, ed. B. M. Trost and I. Fleming, 9 vols., Pergamon/Elsevier, 1992.

CRC Handbook of Chemistry and Physics, 90th ed., ed. D. R. Lide, 2009. Well-known convenient one-volume reference, updated annually. Extensive tables of physicochemical properties across the whole of chemistry and physics, including common organic compounds.

Encyclopedia of Reagents for Organic Synthesis, ed. L. A. Paquette and others, 8 vols., Wiley, 1995. The second edition was published in February 2009. The original printed publication reviewed ca. 3,500 reagents and the new edition 4,111 reagents and 50,000 reactions; figures for the current electronic version are not available. Available online as e-EROS at www3.interscience.wiley.com. There is also *Handbook of Reagents for Organic Synthesis* by the same authors.

Fieser's Reagents for Organic Synthesis, Wiley. An alphabetical listing of reagents used in syntheis. Began with a single volume in 1967 by Louis and Mary Fieser, followed by updates. Vol. 24, ed. T. Ho, 2008. Available as a set of volumes (1–23) with cumulative index. Not available online.

Greene's Protective Groups in Organic Synthesis, 4th ed., ed. T. W. Greene and P. G. M. Wuts, Wiley-Interscience, 2006.

Kirk-Othmer Encyclopedia of Chemical Technology, 5th ed., 26 vols., Wiley, 2004–2007, and *Ullmanns Encyclopedia of Industrial Chemistry*, 6th ed., 40 vols., Wiley, 2003. These two major compcting/complementary encyclopedias are now owned by the same publisher, and a merger would seem likely in due course. *Ullmanns* was originally published in German (now English) and has a European/Japanese focus; *Kirk-Othmer* is published in English with a North American bias. Despite their titles, they contain much pure chemistry. They are available online from www.interscience.wiley.com. For a short review comparing and contrasting them, see C. Craig, www.istl.org/06-spring/databases4.

The Lipid Handbook with CD-ROM, 3rd ed., ed. F. D. Gunstone, J. L. Harwood, and A. J. Dijkstra, CRC Press, 2007. A large one-volume reference work in two parts; a 780-page monograph on lipid chemistry, followed by a 617-page dictionary that is a reprint of all lipid entries from the CRC database (see Section 1.2.1), also searchable on the CD-ROM version in a format uniform with the main database.

March's Advanced Organic Chemistry, 6th ed., ed. M. B. Smith and J. March, Wiley, 2007.

Martindale, The Complete Drug Reference, 36th ed., ed. S. Sweetman, 2 vols., Pharmaceutical Press, 2009. Monographs on drugs and ancillary substances, 5,820 described. Also available on CD-ROM, and online at www.medicinescomplete.com.

The Merck Index, 14th ed., ed. M. J. O'Neil, Wiley, 2006. A useful one-volume work containing ten thousand brief monographs on drugs and simple laboratory chemicals. Includes a CD-ROM; also available online through, among others, Dialog at www.library.dialog.com/bluesheets and Cambridgesoft at http://the merckindex.cambridgesoft.com.

Methods in Enzymology, Elsevier, 1955–. An ongoing series with over three hundred volumes, each devoted to a specific topic in biochemistry. Earlier volumes contain useful properties/procedures for small molecules of biochemical interest.

Natural Product Reports, Royal Society of Chemistry. 1984–. Review series with timely updates on different classes of natural products, though the coverage depends on the availability of a suitable specialist reviewer at any one time. Each issue starts with a very useful current awareness section, "Hot off the Press."

Organic Reactions, Wiley, 1942–. Contains review chapters, each devoted to a single reaction of wide applicability. Vol. 70, ed. L. E. Overman, published in 2008.

Organic Syntheses, 1921–. Formerly published by Wiley but now independent under the editorial board (Organic Syntheses, Inc.). Series giving checked and edited procedures for particular compounds or groups of compounds of interest. Collective volumes were issued containing revised versions of annual parts. Available free at www.orgsyn.org. Articles from recent volumes that have not yet been incorporated in the searchable database can be seen at Org.Syn Express.

The Pesticide Manual, 15th ed., British Crop Protection Council, 2009. One-volume publication containing monographs on several hundred pesticides and agrochemicals, current and obsolete. Also available as a CD-ROM.

Progress in the Chemistry of Organic Natural Products (formerly *Fortschritte der Chemie Organischer Naturstoffe*) ("Zechmeister"), Springer, 1938–. Review series on various classes of natural products, with one or more topics covered in each volume. Had reached vol. 89 by 2008.

Progress in Heterocyclic Chemistry. Elsevier. Review series. Vol. 19, ed. G. W. Gribble and J. A. Joule, published in 2008, consists of a critical review of the 2006 literature preceded by two chapters on current heterocyclic topics. Individual chapters can be purchased as PDF files.

Rodds's Chemistry of Carbon Compounds, 2nd ed., ed. S. Coffey, 1964–1989. Supplementary volumes, ed. M. F. Ansell, 1973–1990; 2nd supplement, ed. M. Sainsbury, Elsevier, 1991–2002. A monograph covering the whole of organic chemistry in five volumes plus supplements: Vol. I, aliphatic compounds; II, alicyclic compounds; III, aromatic compounds; IV, heterocyclic compounds; and V, indexes and miscellaneous update volumes (e.g., *Electrochemistry*, 2002). A good source for getting a rapid overview of an unfamiliar class of compounds, for example, but now showing its age. There is a cumulative index to the whole second edition and supplements. It is available online at ScienceDirect.com. It is not known if a new edition is planned.

Science of Synthesis, multi-authored, Thieme Verlag. The subscription electronic version of Houben-Weyl, originally an exhaustive multivolume German language encyclopedia of synthetic methods. The printed version eventually contained 146,000 procedures, 580,000 structures, and 700,000 references. SoS retains the readable-text format of the original, with extensive HTML and structure markup for searchability. The current version (3.6) consists of 38 volumes and 215,000 reactions (www.science-of-synthesis.com).

Specialist Periodical Reports, RSC. A series of one-volume updates on developments in particular areas of research. Approximately ten titles remain current. The more popular appear annually; other titles are sporadic or discontinued. Those of most interest to organic chemists are *Amino Acids, Peptides and Proteins* (Vol. 36, literature coverage to 2003, published 2007), *Carbohydrates* (Vol. 34, literature coverage to 2002, published 2003), and *Organophosphorus Chemistry* (Vol. 37, literature coverage to 2007, published 2008).

Other titles cover NMR, catalysis, etc. Some chapters are available on free access, but the
majority are on a payment basis by licence agreement.

Theilheimer's Synthetic Methods of Organic Chemistry, Karger, 1948–. Most recent: Vol. 72,
ed. G. Tozer-Hotchkiss, 2008. Another large synthetic methods compendium, less electronically available than *Science of Synthesis*, although the latest volumes have an ActiveBook
electronic search facility.

1.4 PATENTS, INCLUDING PATENT AWARENESS SERVICES
Terry Ward

A patent is an exclusive right granted by a state to an inventor or its assignee to make use of an
invention or process for a fixed period of time in exchange for its public disclosure. Formerly the
terms under which patents were granted varied considerably between countries, but in recent years
attempts have been made to standardise international rules, and all technology patents (including
chemical patents) by members of the World Trade Organisation (WTO) are now granted for a period
of twenty years from the date of filing.

Each country issues its own patents valid only in that country, so the same invention is usually
patented in several countries. These patent duplications are known as equivalents. Equivalents may
be filed in different languages, which can be useful if the original is in a language unfamiliar to the
researcher. Abstracting services will generally abstract the first published application with a cross-
index to their equivalents in other countries.

Before a patent is granted, the patent application is examined by the relevant national patent
office for novelty, invention, and utility. Since this process is lengthy, most authorities publish the
unexamined application eighteen months after the patent is filed. Although information present in
patents may subsequently be reported in the open literature, the original patent application will
always be the earliest publication of its chemical content. These are of particular interest to organic
chemists because of the large number of newly synthesised compounds that are reported particularly by the pharmaceutical and agrochemical industries.

Apart from applications to national authorities, patent applications may also be made through
the European Patent Office (EPO) and the International Bureau of the World Intellectual Property
Organisation (WIPO) under the Patent Cooperation Treaty (PCT).

The EPO was set up by the European Patent Convention of 1973, and its first patents were granted
in 1980. At the end of 2008, contracting states to the EPO comprised the twenty-seven member
states of the European Union plus Croatia, Iceland, Liechtenstein, Monaco, Norway, Switzerland,
Turkey, and Macedonia. The EPO grants patents in whichever of these countries are designated on
the specification, and the patent documents are published in English, French, or German.

The PCT came into force in 1978 and by November of 2008 provided for filing in 139 countries.
Submission of a PCT application to a single patent office of a PCT contracting state automatically
designates all other member states. A centralised novelty search report is then passed on to member
states, each of which decide whether to grant a patent. The WIPO does not grant the patents. The
PCT applications themselves are published eighteen months after filing in one of eight languages,
at present (end of 2008) Arabic, Chinese, English, French, German, Japanese, Russian, or Spanish.
An abstract is published in English.

1.4.1 MARKUSH STRUCTURES

Chemical patents often contain Markush structures, named after Eugene Markush, who was the
first inventor to win a claim allowing such structures in 1925. These generic structures allow large
numbers of compounds to be claimed even though few of these will actually have been synthesised.

An example is shown below where X, Y, Z, and R can refer to a wide range of atoms or chemical groups specified by the inventor.

Markush Structure

1.4.2 PATENT NUMBERING

When searching for patents a basic understanding of patent documentation and numbering systems is helpful. Published patent documents comprise two types: patent applications and granted patents. It is important to note that these two documents may have different serial numbers. A patent application is the initial document submitted to a patent office describing the invention. This application will be subject to examination by the patent office for compliance with relevant patent laws and may or may not lead to a granted patent. Published applications and granted patents are assigned a unique publication number comprising a two-letter country code (see http://www.wipo.org/ for a full list) followed by a serial number of up to twelve digits (varies with country) followed by a type code comprising a letter, usually A, B, or C. These type codes distinguish between different publication stages of the same patent and originally corresponded to the unexamined application, examined application, or granted patent documents, respectively. However, over the years considerable variation has developed between different jurisdictions in their use. For example, the EPO only publishes at two stages: A for applications and B for granted patents. Again, prior to 2001, U.S. patents were only published as the granted A patent, but since January 2001, they follow the same two-stage publication and A, B designation as the EPO. These letter codes may also be followed by a numerical suffix indicating the number of times the specification has been published with modifications, e.g., A1 (patent application with search report) or A2 (patent application without search report), etc. A full list of type codes used by CAS may be found at http://www.cas.org/expertise/cascontent/ caplus/patcoverage/patkind.html. In the case of patent applications, but not granted patents, the serial number may begin with a year code. These year codes may vary with time, leading to some confusion. For example, PCT applications from 1978 to the end of 2003 begin with the last two digits of the Western year; however, from the beginning of 2004 PCT applications begin with all four-year digits. Postmillennium Japanese application numbers also begin with a four-digit Western year code, but prior to the millennium the year code corresponded to the year of the Japanese emperor's reign (Yoen year). The present emperor, Akihito, ascended the throne in 1989, which is year 1 of the current cycle (Heisei period). Therefore, the Heisei year equals the last two numbers of the Western year minus 88. The previous emperor, Hirohito, reigned from 1926 to 1989 (Showa period). Accordingly, the Showa year equals the last two numbers of the Western year minus 25. Obviously, there is an overlapping period in 1989 at the interregnum. Heisei and Showa periods are often abbreviated as H and S. Some examples of patent number formats are given below:

WO2005021545 A1 (2005 PCT application with four-digit year code)
WO9640757 A2 (1996 PCT application with two-digit year code)
US5096901 A (U.S. granted patent, issued prior to 2001, no year code)
US7189852 B2 (U.S. granted patent issued after January 1, 2001, with pregrant publication, no year code; note, if no pregrant publication, then B1)
US20050054561 A1 (2005 U.S. patent application with four-digit year code)
JP5019556 B1 (1993 Japanese examined application, Yoen year 5)

1.4.3 PATENT AWARENESS SERVICES

Since patents are not normally held in research libraries, most researchers obtain their initial information on patents from abstracting services. The foremost of these, *Chemical Abstracts* (CA), has covered chemical, biochemical, and chemical engineering patents from 1907 to the present. CAS abstracts over one hundred thousand patents annually from fifty-seven patent authorities. These abstracts are based on the earliest published patent or patent application, and where an invention is patented in more than one country, the equivalent patents are cross-referenced. In the print version this is done through the Patent Indexes, but for the electronic versions equivalent patents are listed in one entry based on a common priority date. Cross-indexing allows an equivalent patent in an alternative language to be identified if required. Only real chemical substances are indexed by CA; virtual compounds exemplified only within a generic Markush structure are not indexed. However, Markush structures can be searched on the CAS Markush database (MARPAT) containing more than 750,000 Markush structures from patents covered by CAS from 1961 to present.

Most patents are now available free online from one or more patent authorities. The most useful of these are the EPO, U.S., and Japanese patent office sites.

The EPO esp@cenet (ep.espacenet.com) database contains more than 60 million patents from 85 countries worldwide (not just European Convention countries). The database is searchable by application number, assignee, inventor, or keywords from the title or abstract. Chemical structure searches are not possible. Patents can be viewed as images of the original document in PDF format one page at a time, or the whole patent can be viewed as a text document. Instantaneous translation from French or German into English is available for the latter document type if required. Equivalent published patents, if any, are also listed and are available in PDF format. The text documents do not show chemical structures or diagrams, but these can be viewed in PDF format if required.

The U.S. Patent and Trade Mark Office (USPTO) database (http://patft.uspto.gov/) provides access to granted U.S. patents from 1976 and patent applications from March 2001. Patents can be viewed as text documents (without structures or diagrams) or as single-page images of the original document in TIFF format. Patents prior to 1976 and back to 1790 are available as TIFF images only.

The Industrial Property Digital Library of the Japanese Patent Office (JPO's IPDL; http://www.ipdl.inpit.go.jp/homepg_e.ipdl) provides access to Japanese patent document in Japanese text. However, for non-Japanese readers, instantaneous machine translations from Japanese to English of the full documents are available over the Internet from 1974 onwards. English abstracts are also available for recent patents.

Free patent information is provided by the website http://www.freepatentsonline.com/, covering U.S., EP, and PCT patents/applications and Japanese patent abstracts. In addition to the usual text-based searches in various search fields, this site also enables graphically input chemical structure searches to be performed on over 9 million compounds (including prophetic compounds) using exact structure, substructure, or chemical similarity searches. Chemistry searches using SMILES strings or chemical names are also possible. Full patent documents may be viewed in text or PDF format.

Chemical patent abstracts can be found in the *Chemical Patent Index* (published by Thompson Scientific). This is derived from the *Derwent World Patent Index* and provides abstracts of chemical patents from at least thirty-nine countries, including the EPO and PCT, and is updated weekly. All chemical patents are covered from 1970 to date, with additional coverage of pharmaceutical patents from 1963, agricultural patents from 1965, and polymers from 1966. Searching is based on the full patent specification, not just the abstract. In addition to text searching, the use of Derwent's structural fragment codes allows structure searching on both specifically disclosed compounds and Markush structures. Polymers may also be searched using structural polymer codes.

1.5 CHEMINFORMATICS COMPANIES

The development of algorithms for the handling of chemical structures and data, and the application of artificial intelligence to property prediction, etc., led to the emergence of companies specialising in chemical software applications, now known as chem(o)informatics. Ideally such enterprises should couple with large dictionary databases.

The pioneer in this area was Molecular Design, later MDL Systems, which after a period of ownership by Elsevier was acquired by Symyx in 2007. The company now serves drug design R&D within the corporate client sector.

Symyx also runs the *Available Chemicals Directory,* launched originally by ACD Labs as a merged database of chemical supplier catalogues with structure search capability. The database provides access to over 1 million commercially available chemical compounds. The original concept has been extensively developed with the addition of other freely available software packages.

ChemAxon (www.chemaxon.com/marvin) provides services such as MarvinSketch (structure and reaction query editor), MarvinSpace (3D structure visualisation), and several others.

ChemSpider was launched in 2007. It is an open-access service in which constituent databases, the largest of which is Web of Science, are linked on a free-access basis, and which uses algorithms to identify and extract chemical names from documents and web pages and convert them to structures and InChI and SMILES identifiers. Access to the core service is free, but the user may be routed to charging component databases. At launch, ChemSpider contained 21 million compounds. At the time of writing, it was too early to assess the success of the service. It was bought by the Royal Society of Chemistry in 2009.

Registration is free at www.chemspider.com. For a description of ChemSpider, see Williams, A., *Chemistry International*, 30 (1), 2008, available online at www.iupac.org/publications.

2 Primary Journals

This chapter gives details of the principal journals in organic chemistry plus some of the more important journals in other areas of chemistry and biochemistry that may contain important information on organic chemistry. The following items of information are given:

- Full journal title.
- CASSI abbreviated title. CASSI (the *Chemical Abstracts Service Source Index*) includes details on all journals cited in *Chemical Abstracts* since 1907, together with some cited in *Beilstein* and *Chemisches Zentralblatt* back to 1830. CASSI gives an abbreviated title for each journal, and these are widely used and recognised.[1]
- Years of publication.
- A statement, if applicable, that a journal does not have volume numbers, together with details of when volume numbers were introduced or discontinued. Volume numbers are given for some of the longer-established journals that have seen several changes of title.
- Some indication of subject matter where it is not obvious from the title, or where a journal is published in two or more parts.
- Changes of journal and superseded titles.
- Translation journals.
- Name of the publisher of the current title (2009) and online (web) archive, or of the publisher of the online (web) archive for a former title.[2]
- Information on free online access to the full text of chemistry journals on the web (as of 2009).[3]

Accounts of Chemical Research [*Acc. Chem. Res.*] (1968–). Review journal. Publisher: ACS.

Acta Chemica Scandinavica [*Acta Chem. Scand.*] (1947–1973, 1989–1999). From 1974–1988 (Vols. 29–42) divided into Series A [*Acta Chem. Scand., Ser. A*] (physical and inorganic chemistry) and Series B [*Acta Chem. Scand., Ser. B*] (organic chemistry and biochemistry). In 1999, absorbed in part by *Journal of the Chemical Society, Dalton Transactions*, *Journal of the Chemical Society, Perkin Transactions 1*, and *Journal of the Chemical Society, Perkin Transactions 2*. See *Journal of the Chemical Society*. Free online full-text archive at http://actachemscand.dk/.

Acta Chimica Sinica. See *Chinese Journal of Chemistry* and *Huaxue Xuebao*.

Acta Chimica Slovenica [*Acta Chim. Slov.*] (1993–). Formerly *Vestnik Slovenskega Kemijskega Drustva* [*Vestn. Slov. Kem. Drus.*] (1954–1992). Free online full-text archive from 1998. Publisher: Slovenian Chemical Society.

Acta Crystallographica [*Acta Crystallogr.*] (1948–1967). In 1968, divided into Section A [*Acta Crystallogr., Sect. A*] (1968–) (current subtitle: foundations of crystallography) and Section B [*Acta Crystallogr., Sect. B*] (1968–) (current subtitle: structural science). Later sections added are Section C [*Acta Crystallogr., Sect. C*] (1983–) (crystal structure communications), formerly *Crystal Structure Communications* [*Cryst. Struct. Commun.*] (1972–82); Section D [*Acta Crystallogr., Sect. D*] (1993–) (biological crystallography); Section E [*Acta Crystallogr., Sect. E*] (2001–) (structure reports online); and Section F [*Acta Crystallogr., Sect. F*] (2005–) (structural biology and crystallisation communications). (Additional CASSI abbreviated subtitles are omitted.) Some online free access to recent archives for Sections A–F. Publisher: International Union of Crystallography. http://journals.iucr.org/.

Acta Pharmaceutica [*Acta Pharm. (Zagreb, Croatia)*] (1992–). Formerly *Acta Pharmaceutica Jugoslavia* [*Acta Pharm. Jugosl.*] (1951–91). Publisher: Croatian Pharmaceutical Society.

Acta Pharmaceutica Fennica. See *European Journal of Pharmaceutical Sciences*.

Acta Pharmaceutica Nordica. See *European Journal of Pharmaceutical Sciences*.

Acta Pharmaceutica Suecica. See *European Journal of Pharmaceutical Sciences*.

Advanced Synthesis & Catalysis [*Adv. Synth. Catal.*] (Vol. 343–, 2001–). Formerly *Journal für Praktische Chemie* [*J. Prakt. Chem.*] (Vols. 1–270, 1834–1943; Vols. 273–333, 1954–1991; Vols. 341–342, 1999–2000) and *Journal für Praktische Chemie—Chemiker-Zeitung* [*J. Prakt. Chem./Chem. Ztg.*] (Vols. 334–340, 1992–1998) (following a merger with *Chemiker-Zeitung* [*Chem.-Ztg.*] (1879–1991)). Between 1943 and 1944, the journal was briefly titled *Journal für Makromolekulare Chemie* [*J. Makromol. Chem.*] (Vols. 271–272, 1943–1944). Alternative volume numbers are also used: Vols. 109–270 (1870–1943) are numbered Vols. 1–162 (the second series); Vols. 271–272 (1943–1944) are numbered Vols. 1–2 (the third series); and Vols. 273–310 (1954–1968) are numbered Vols. 1–38 (the fourth series). Free online full-text archive 1870–1938 from Gallica (Bibliothèque nationale de France): http:// gallica.bnf.fr/. Publisher (current title and online archive from 1834): Wiley.

Agricultural and Biological Chemistry. See *Bioscience, Biotechnology, and Biochemistry*.

Aldrichimica Acta [*Aldrichim. Acta*] (1968–). Free online full-text archive. Publisher: Sigma-Aldrich.

American Chemical Journal. See *Journal of the American Chemical Society*.

Anales de Quimica [*An. Quim.*] (1968–1979, 1990–1995). From 1980 to 1989, divided into Series A [*An. Quim., Ser. A*] (physical and technical), Series B [*An. Quim., Ser. B*] (inorganic and analytical), and Series C [*An. Quim., Ser. C*] (organic and biochemical). Became *Anales de Quimica International Edition* [*An. Quim. Int. Ed.*] (1996–1998). No longer published.

Angewandte Chemie [*Angew. Chem.*] (1988–). From 1888 to 1941, the title was *Zeitschrift fur Angewandte Chemie* [*Z. Angew. Chem.*]. In German, but in 1962 an International Edition in English [*Angew. Chem., Int. Ed. Engl.*] (1962–) was launched, which in 1998 became *Angewandte Chemie, International Edition* [*Angew. Chem., Int. Ed.*] (1998–). The German and English editions have different volume and page numbers. Vol. 1 of the international edition corresponds to Vol. 74 of the German edition. In 1982 and 1983, miniprint supplements were issued. In 1991, *Angewandte Chemie* absorbed *Zeitschrift für Chemie* [*Z. Chem.*] (1961–90). Publisher: Wiley.

Annalen. See *Liebigs Annalen*.

Annalen der Chemie und Pharmazie. See *Liebigs Annalen*.

Annales de Chimie [*Ann. Chim. (Cachan, Fr.)*] (2004–). Previous CASSI abbreviation *Ann. Chim. (Paris)* (1789–1815, 1914–2003). From 1816 to 1913, the title was *Annales de Chimie et de Physique* [*Ann. Chim. Phys.*]. There have been various series of volume numbers; the fifteenth series, Vol. 1 appeared in 1976. From 1978 (Vol. 3) series designations ceased. Since 1973 this journal has specialised in solid-state chemistry; in 1978 *Science de Matériaux* became a subtitle. Free online full-text archive 1841–1913 from Gallica (Bibliothèque nationale de France): http://gallica.bnf.fr/. Publisher: Lavoisier.

Annales Pharmaceutiques Français [*Ann. Pharm. Fr.*] (1943–). Formed by a merger of *Journal de Pharmacie et de Chemie* [*J. Pharm. Chim.*] (1842–1942) and *Bulletin des Sciences Pharmacologiques* [*Bull. Sci. Pharmacol*] (1899–1942). Free online full-text archive 1842–1894 from Gallica (Bibliothèque nationale de France): http://gallica.bnf.fr/. Publisher: Elsevier.

Annali di Chimica [*Ann. Chim. (Rome)*] (1950–2007). Formerly *Annali di Chimica Applicata* [*Ann. Chim. Appl.*] (1914–1918, 1924–1949). Superseded by *ChemSusChem* [*ChemSusChem*] (2008–). Online archive publisher (2004–2007): Wiley.

Annals of the New York Academy of Science [*Ann. N.Y. Acad. Sci.*] (1877–). Irregular. No issue numbers. Publishers: The New York Academy of Sciences and Wiley.

Antibiotiki i Khimioterapiya [*Antibiot. Khimioter.*] (1988–). Formerly *Antibiotiki* [*Antibiotiki (Moscow)*] (1956–1984) and *Antibiotiki i Meditsinskaya Bioteknologiya* [*Antibiot. Med. Biotekhnol.*] (1985–1987). Publisher: Media Sphera, Moscow.

Applied Organometallic Chemistry [*Appl. Organomet. Chem.*] (1987–). Publisher: Wiley.

Archiv der Pharmazie [*Arch. Pharm. (Weinheim, Ger.)*] (1835–). From 1924–1971 known as *Archiv der Pharmazie und Berichte der Deutschen Pharmazeutischen Gesellschaft* [*Arch. Pharm. Ber. Dtsch. Pharm. Ges.*]. Publisher: Wiley.

Archives of Biochemistry and Biophysics [*Arch. Biochem. Biophys.*] (1951–). Formerly *Archives of Biochemistry* [*Arch. Biochem.*] (1942–1951). Publisher: Elsevier.

Arhiv za Kemiju. See *Croatica Chemica Acta.*

Arkiv foer Kemi. See *Chemica Scripta.*

ARKIVOC [*ARKIVOC*] (2000–). Electronic journal. Open access. Free online full-text archive from 2000. Publisher: ARKAT USA, Inc.

Arzneimittel-Forschung [*Arzneim.-Forsch.*] (1951–). Drug research. Publisher: Editio Cantor Verlag, Aulendorf, Germany

Asian Journal of Chemistry [*Asian J. Chem.*] (1989–). Absorbed *Asian Journal of Chemistry Reviews* [*Asian. J. Chem. Rev.*] (1990–95). Publisher: Asian Journal of Chemistry, Sahibabad, Ghaziabad, Uttar Pradesh, India.

Australian Journal of Chemistry [*Aust. J. Chem.*] (1953–). Superseded *Australian Journal of Scientific Research, Series A* [*Aust. J. Sci. Res., Ser. A*] (1948–52). Publisher: CSIRO Publishing.

Beilstein Journal of Organic Chemistry [*Beilstein J. Org. Chem.*] (2005–). Electronic journal. Open access. Free online full-text archive from 2005. Publisher: Beilstein-Institut, Frankfurt am Main, Germany.

Berichte. See *Chemische Berichte.*

Berichte der Bunsen-Gesellschaft [*Ber. Bunsen-Ges.*] (1963–1998). Formerly *Zeitschrift für Elektrochemie und Angewandte Physikalische Chemie* [*Z. Elektrochem. Angew. Phys. Chem.*] (1894–1951) (publication suspended 1945 to 1947) and *Zeitschrift für Elektrochemie* [*Z. Elektrochem.*] (1951–1962). Merged with *Journal of the Chemical Society, Faraday Transactions* to form *Physical Chemistry Chemical Physics.*

Berichte der Deutschen Chemischen Gesellschaft. See *Chemische Berichte.*

Biochemical and Biophysical Research Communications [*Biochem. Biophys. Res. Commun.*] (1959–). Publisher: Elsevier.

Biochemical Journal [*Biochem. J.*] (1906–). From 1973 to 1983, alternate issues subtitled *Molecular Aspects* and *Cellular Aspects.* Free online full-text archive. Publisher: Portland Press Ltd. Essex.

Biochemical Society Transactions [*Biochem. Soc. Trans.*] (1973–). Replaced a proceedings section formerly included in *Biochemical Journal.* Publisher: Portland Press Ltd., Essex.

Biochemical Systematics and Ecology [*Biochem. Syst. Ecol.*] (1974–). Formerly *Biochemical Systematics* [*Biochem. Syst.*] (1973). Publisher: Elsevier.

Biochemistry [*Biochemistry*] (1962–). Publisher: ACS.

Biochimica et Biophysica Acta [*Biochim. Biophys. Acta*] (1947–). Issued in different sections. Publisher: Elsevier.

Biochimie [*Biochimie*] (1971–). Formerly *Bulletin de la Société de Chimie Biologique* [*Bull. Soc. Chim. Biol.*] (1914–70). Publisher: Elsevier.

Biological and Pharmaceutical Bulletin. See *Chemical and Pharmaceutical Bulletin.*

Biological Chemistry [*Biol. Chem.*] (Vol. 377, 1996–). Superseded *Biological Chemistry Hoppe-Seyler* [*Biol. Chem. Hoppe-Seyler*] (Vols. 366–377, 1985–1996). Formerly *Zeitschrift für Physiologische Chemie* [*Z. Physiol. Chem.*] (1877–1895) and *Hoppe-Seyler's Zeitschrift für Physiologische Chemie* [*Hoppe-Seyler's Z. Physiol. Chem.*] (1895–1984). Publisher: Walter de Gruyter, New York and Berlin.

Biological Mass Spectrometry. See *Journal of Mass Spectrometry.*

Biomedical and Environmental Mass Spectrometry. See *Journal of Mass Spectrometry.*

Biomedical Mass Spectrometry. See *Journal of Mass Spectrometry.*

Bioorganic and Medicinal Chemistry [*Bioorg. Med. Chem.*] (1993–). Publisher: Elsevier.

Bioorganic and Medicinal Chemistry Letters [*Bioorg. Med. Chem. Lett.*] (1991–). Publisher: Elsevier.

Bioorganic Chemistry [*Bioorg. Chem.*] (1971–). Publisher: Elsevier.

Bioorganicheskaya Khimiya [*Bioorg. Khim.*] (1975–). In Russian. *Bioorganicheskaia Khimiya* is an alternative spelling. There is an English language translation called *Russian Journal of Bioorganic Chemistry* [*Russ. J. Bioorg. Chem.*] (1993–). Formerly *Soviet Journal of Bioorganic Chemistry* [*Sov. J. Bioorg. Chem. (Engl. Transl.)*] (1975–1992). Publisher: Springer/MAIK Nauka/Interperiodica.

Bioscience, Biotechnology, and Biochemistry [*Biosci., Biotechnol., Biochem.*] (Vol. 56–, 1992–). Formerly *Bulletin of the Agricultural Chemical Society of Japan* [*Bull. Agric. Chem. Soc. Jpn.*] (1924–1960) and *Agricultural and Biological Chemistry* [*Agric. Biol. Chem.*] (1961–1991). Free online full-text archive. Publisher: Japan Society for Bioscience, Biotechnology and Agrochemistry.

Bulletin de la Société de Chimie Biologique. See *Biochimie.*

Bulletin de la Société Chimique de France [*Bull. Soc. Chim. Fr.*] (1858–1997). Five series of volume numbers were assigned between 1858 and 1954. No volume numbers issued from 1955 to 1991; 1992 is Vol. 129; 1997 is Vol. 134. From 1933 to 1945, published as *Bulletin de la Société Chimique de France, Documentation* (abstracts, obituaries, etc.) and *Bulletin de la Société Chimique de France, Memoires* (research papers). From 1978 to 1984, each issue was split into two parts (la première partie: chimie analytique, minérale et physico-chimie; la deuxième partie: chimie moléculaire). In order to distinguish the two parts for these years, the page number is prefixed by the part number, e.g., Es-Seddiki, S., et al., *Bull. Soc. Chim. Fr.*, 1984, II-241. No longer published. Superseded by *European Journal of Inorganic Chemistry* and *European Journal of Organic Chemistry.*

Bulletin des Sciences Pharmacologiques. See *Annales Pharmaceutiques Français.*

Bulletin des Sociétés Chimiques Belges [*Bull. Soc. Chim. Belg.*] (1904–1997). Formerly *Bulletin de l'Association Belge des Chimistes* (1887–1903). No longer published. Superseded by *European Journal of Inorganic Chemistry* and *European Journal of Organic Chemistry.*

Bulletin of the Academy of Sciences of the USSR, Division of Chemical Sciences. See *Izvestiya Akademii Nauk, Seriya Khimicheskaya.*

Bulletin of the Chemical Society of Japan [*Bull. Chem. Soc. Jpn.*] (1926–). Free online full-text archive. Publisher: The Chemical Society of Japan.

Bulletin of the Korean Chemical Society [*Bull. Korean Chem. Soc.*] (1980–). Free online full-text archive from 1980. Publisher: Korean Chemical Society.

Bulletin of the Polish Academy of Sciences, Chemistry [*Bull. Pol. Acad. Sci., Chem.*] (1983–). Formerly *Bulletin de l'Academie Polonaise des Sciences, Serie des Sciences Chimiques* [*Bull. Acad. Pol. Sci., Ser. Sci. Chim.*] (1960–1982). Publisher: Polish Academy of Sciences, Warsaw.

Bulletin of the Research Council of Israel. See *Israel Journal of Chemistry.*

Canadian Journal of Chemistry [*Can. J. Chem.*] (1951–). Continuation of *Canadian Journal of Research* [*Can. J. Res.*] (1929–1935) and its subsequent Section B [*Can. J. Res., Sect. B*] (1935–1950) (chemical sciences). Free online full-text archive 1951–1997. Publisher: NRC Research Press.

Carbohydrate Letters [*Carbohydr. Lett.*] (1994–2001). No longer published.

Carbohydrate Polymers [*Carbohydr. Polym.*] (1981–). Publisher: Elsevier.

Carbohydrate Research [*Carbohydr. Res.*] (1965–). Publisher: Elsevier.

Cellular and Molecular Life Sciences [*Cell. Mol. Life Sci.*] (1997–). Formerly *Experientia* [*Experientia*] (1945–1996). Publisher: Springer.

Central European Journal of Chemistry [*Cent. Eur. J. Chem.*] (2003–). Publisher: Versita, Warsaw, Poland, and Springer.

ChemBioChem [*ChemBioChem*] (2000–). Publisher: Wiley.

Chemica Scripta [*Chem. Scr.*] (1971–1989). Successor to *Arkiv foer Kemi* [*Ark. Kemi*] (1949–1971). No longer published.

Chemical Biology & Drug Design [*Chem. Biol. Drug Des.*] (2006–). Formerly *Journal of Peptide Research.* Publisher: Wiley.

Chemical & Pharmaceutical Bulletin [*Chem. Pharm. Bull.*] (1958–). Formerly *Pharmaceutical Bulletin* [*Pharm. Bull.*] (1953–1957). In 1993 biologically oriented papers were transferred to *Biological & Pharmaceutical Bulletin* [*Biol. Pharm. Bull.*] (1993–). Free online full-text archive. Publisher: The Pharmaceutical Society of Japan.

Chemical Communications (Cambridge) [*Chem. Commun. (Cambridge)*] (1996–). Formerly *Chemical Communications* [*Chem. Commun.*] (1965–1968); *Journal of the Chemical Society* [Part] *D* [*J. Chem. Soc. D*] (1969–1971); and *Journal of the Chemical Society, Chemical Communications* [*J. Chem. Soc., Chem. Commun.*] (1972–1995). No volume numbers. See also *Journal of the Chemical Society* and *Proceedings of the Chemical Society, London.* Publisher: RSC.

Chemical Papers [*Chem. Pap.*] (1985–). Formerly *Chemické Zvesti* [*Chem. Zvesti*] (1947–1984). Publisher: Versita, Warsaw, Poland, and Springer.

Chemical Record [*Chem. Rec.*] (2001–). A review journal. Publisher: Wiley.

Chemical Reviews [*Chem. Rev.*] (1924–). Publisher: ACS.

Chemical Society Reviews [*Chem. Soc. Rev.*] (1972–). Successor to *Quarterly Reviews of the Chemical Society* [*Q. Rev., Chem. Soc.*] (1947–1971) and *RIC Reviews* [*RIC Rev.*] (1968–1971). Publisher: RSC.

Chemické Listy [*Chem. Listy*] (1951–). Formerly *Chemické Listy pro Vedu a Prumysl* [*Chem. Listy Vedu Prum.*] (1907–1950). Publisher: Czech Chemical Society.

Chemické Zvesti. See *Chemical Papers.*

Chemiker-Zeitung. See *Advanced Synthesis & Catalysis.*

Chemische Berichte [*Chem. Ber*] (1947–96). Formerly *Berichte der Deutschen Chemischen Gesellschaft* [*Ber. Dtsch. Chem. Ges.*] (1868–1945), which from 1919 to 1945 was divided into Abteilung A [*Ber. Dtsch. Chem. Ges. A*] (Vereinsnachrichten) and Abteilung B [*Ber. Dtsch. Chem. Ges. B*] (Abhandlungen). Early volumes are often cited colloquially as *Berichte*. In 1997, merged with *Recueil des Travaux Chimiques des Pays-Bas* to form *Chemische Berichte/Recueil* [*Chem. Ber./Recl.*] (1997). No longer published. In 1998, superseded by *European Journal of Inorganic Chemistry.* Free online full-text archive 1868–1901 from Gallica (Bibliothèque nationale de France): http://gallica.bnf.fr/. Online archive publisher: Wiley.

Chemische Berichte/Recueil. See *Chemische Berichte.*

Chemistry—An Asian Journal [*Chem.—Asian J.*] (2006–). Publisher: Wiley.

Chemistry—A European Journal [*Chem.—Eur. J.*] (1995–). Publisher: Wiley.

Chemistry & Biodiversity [*Chem. Biodiversity*] (2004–). Publisher: Verlag Helvetica Chimica Acta AG, Zürich/Wiley.

Chemistry & Industry [*Chem. Ind. (London)*] (1923–). Formerly *Journal of the Society of Chemical Industry, London, Review Section* [*J. Soc. Chem. Ind., London, Rev. Sect.*] (1918–22). No volume numbers. Publisher: The Society of Chemical Industry.

Chemistry and Physics of Lipids [*Chem. Phys. Lipids*] (1966–). Publisher: Elsevier.

Chemistry Express [*Chem. Express*] (1986–1993) (Journal of Kinki Chemical Society, Japan). No longer published.

Chemistry Letters [*Chem. Lett.*] (1972–). No volume numbers. Some free online full-text issues from 2002. Publisher: The Chemical Society of Japan.

Chemistry of Heterocyclic Compounds. See *Khimiya Geterotsiklicheskikh Soedinenii*.

Chemistry of Natural Compounds. See *Khimiya Prirodnykh Soedinenii*.

ChemMedChem [*ChemMedChem*] (2006–). See also *Farmaco*. Publisher: Wiley.

Chimia [*Chimia*] (1947–). No volume numbers. Publisher: Swiss Chemical Society.

Chimica Therapeutica. See *European Journal of Medicinal Chemistry*.

Chinese Chemical Letters [*Chin. Chem. Lett.*] (1991–). Free online full-text archive 1999–2006. Publisher: Elsevier.

Chinese Journal of Chemistry [*Chin. J. Chem.*] (1990–). Formerly *Acta Chimica Sinica* [*Acta Chim. Sin. (Engl. Ed.)*] (1983–1989). *Chin. J. Chem.* and *Huaxue Xuebao* are two separate journals, and *Chin. J. Chem.* does not contain translations from *Huaxue Xuebao*. Publisher: Shanghai Institute of Organic Chemistry (Chinese Academy of Sciences) and Wiley-VCH on behalf of the Chinese Chemical Society.

Chirality [*Chirality*] (1989–). Publisher: Wiley.

Collection of Czechoslovak Chemical Communications [*Collect. Czech. Chem. Commun.*] (1929–). Publisher: Institute of Organic Chemistry and Biochemistry, Czech Republic.

Comptes Rendus Chimie [*C. R. Chim.*] (Vol. 5, 2002–). See also *Comptes Rendus Hebdomadaires des Seances de l'Academie des Sciences*. Publisher: French Academy of Sciences/Elsevier.

Comptes Rendus Hebdomadaires des Seances de l'Academie des Sciences [*C. R. Hebd. Seances Acad. Sci.*] (Vols. 1–261, 1835–1965). In 1966, divided into Series A: *Comptes Rendus des Seances de l'Academie des Sciences, Serie A* [*C. R. Seances Acad. Sci., Ser. A*] (Vols. 262–291, 1966–1980) (mathematical sciences); Series B [*C. R. Seances Acad. Sci., Ser. B*] (Vols. 262–291, 1966–1980) (physical sciences); Series C [*C. R. Seances Acad. Sci., Ser. C*] (Vols. 262–291, 1966–1980) (chemical sciences); and Series D [*C. R. Seances Acad. Sci., Ser. D*] (Vols. 262–291, 1966–1980) (life sciences). Series B–D were superseded by Series 2 [*C. R. Seances Acad. Sci., Ser. 2*] (physics, chemistry, astronomy, earth, and planetary sciences; formerly Series B + C) (Vols. 292–297, 1981–1983) and Series 3 [*C. R. Seances Acad. Sci., Ser. 3*] (life sciences; formerly series D) (Vols. 292–297, 1981–1983). Series 2 was superseded by *Comptes Rendus de l'Academie des Sciences, Serie II: Mecanique, Physique, Chimie, Sciences de la Terre et de l'Univers* [*C. R. Acad. Sci., Ser. II: Mec., Phys., Chim., Sci. Terre Univers.*] (Vols. 298–317, 1984–1993). Series II was replaced, in part, by Series IIb [*C. R. Acad. Sci., Ser. IIb: Mec., Phys., Chim., Astron.*] (Vols. 318–325, 1994–1997), and Series IIb was superseded, in part, by Series IIc [*C. R. Acad. Sci., Ser. IIc: Chim.*] (Vols. 1–4, 1998–2001). Series IIc was replaced by *Comptes Rendus Chimie* [*C. R. Chim.*] (Vol. 5–, 2002–). Free online full-text archive 1835–1965 from Gallica (Bibliothèque nationale de France): http://gallica.bnf.fr/. Publisher: French Academy of Sciences/Elsevier.

Contemporary Organic Synthesis [*Contemp. Org. Synth.*] (1994–1997). Review journal. No longer published. Online archive publisher: RSC.

Croatica Chemica Acta [*Croat. Chem. Acta*] (1956–). Formerly *Arhiv za Kemiju* [*Arh. Kem.*] (1927–1955). Free online full-text issues from 1998. Publisher: Croatica Chemica Acta, Zagreb, Croatia.

Crystal Structure Communications. See *Acta Crystallographia*.

Current Organic Chemistry [*Curr. Org. Chem.*] (1997–). Publisher: Bentham Science Publishers Ltd.

Current Organic Synthesis [*Curr. Org. Synth.*] (2004–). Publisher: Bentham Science Publishers Ltd.

Current Protein & Peptide Science [*Curr. Protein Pept. Sci.*] (2000–). Publisher: Bentham Science Publishers Ltd.

Dalton Transactions [*Dalton Trans.*] (2003–). No volume numbers. Formerly *Journal of the Chemical Society, Dalton Transactions* [*J. Chem. Soc., Dalton Trans.*] (1972–2002). See also *Journal of the Chemical Society*. Publisher: RSC.

Doklady Akademii Nauk [*Dokl. Akad. Nauk*] (1933–). In Russian. Until 1992, the title was *Doklady Akademii Nauk SSSR* [*Dokl. Akad. Nauk SSSR*]. There is an English language translation of the chemistry section called *Doklady Chemistry* [*Dokl. Chem.*] (1956–). Publisher: Springer/MAIK Nauka/Interperiodica.

Egyptian Journal of Chemistry [*Egypt. J. Chem.*] (1958–). From 1960 to 1969, the title was *Journal of Chemistry of the United Arab Republic* [*J. Chem. U.A.R.*]. From 1970 to 1971, the title was *United Arab Republic Journal of Chemistry* [*U.A.R. J. Chem.*]. Publisher: National Information and Documentation Centre, Cairo, Egypt.

European Journal of Inorganic Chemistry [*Eur. J. Inorg. Chem.*] (1998–). Formed by the merger of *Bulletin de la Société Chimique de France*, *Bulletin des Sociétés Chimique Belges*, *Chemische Berichte/Recueil*, and *Gazzetta Chimica Italiana*. No volume numbers. Publisher: Wiley.

European Journal of Medicinal Chemistry [*Eur. J. Med. Chem.*] (1974–). Formerly *Chimica Therapeutica* [*Chim. Ther.*] (1965–1973). Publisher: Elsevier.

European Journal of Organic Chemistry [*Eur. J. Org. Chem.*] (1998–). Formed by the merger of *Bulletin de la Société Chimique de France*, *Bulletin des Sociétés Chimique Belges*, *Liebigs Annalen/Recueil*, and *Gazzetta Chimica Italiana*. No volume numbers. Publisher: Wiley.

European Journal of Pharmaceutical Sciences [*Eur. J. Pharm. Sci.*] (1993–). Formed by a merger of *Acta Pharmaceutica Fennica* [*Acta Pharm. Fenn.*] (1977–1992) with *Acta Pharmaceutica Nordica* [*Acta Pharm. Nord.*] (1989–1992). *Acta Pharmaceutica Nordica* was formed by a merger of *Acta Pharmaceutica Suecica* [*Acta Pharm. Suec.*] (1964–1988) and *Norvegica Pharmaceutica Acta* [*Norv. Pharm. Acta*] (1983–1986). Publisher: Elsevier.

Farmaco [*Farmaco*] (1989–2005) (Drugs). Incorporates *Farmaco, Edizione Scientifica* [*Farmaco, Ed. Sci.*] (1953–1988) and *Farmaco, Edizione Pratica* [*Farmaco, Ed. Prat.*] (1953–1988). No longer published. Replaced by *ChemMedChem*.

Finnish Chemical Letters [*Finn. Chem. Lett.*] (1974–1989). No longer published.

Fitoterapia [*Fitoterapia*] (1947–). The Journal for the Study of Medicinal Plants. Formerly *Estratti Fluidi Titolati*. Publisher: Elsevier.

Gazzetta Chimica Italiana [*Gazz. Chim. Ital.*] (1871–1997). From 1891 to 1922, published in two parts. No longer published. Superseded by *European Journal of Inorganic Chemistry* and *European Journal of Organic Chemistry*.

Green Chemistry [*Green Chem.*] (1999–). Publisher: RSC.

Helvetica Chimica Acta [*Helv. Chim. Acta*] (1918–). Publisher: Verlag Helvetica Chimica Acta AG, Zürich/Wiley.

Heteroatom Chemistry [*Heteroat. Chem.*] (1990–). Publisher: Wiley.

Heterocycles [*Heterocycles*] (1973–). Publisher: The Japan Institute of Heterocyclic Chemistry/Elsevier.

Heterocyclic Communications [*Heterocycl. Commun.*] (1994–). Publisher: Freund Publishing House Ltd., Tel Aviv, Israel.

Hoppe-Seylers Zeitschrift für Physiologische Chemie. See *Biological Chemistry*.

Huaxue Xuebao [*Huaxue Xuebao*] (Journal of Chemistry) (1953–; suspended 1966–1975). In Chinese. Continues, in part, *Journal of the Chinese Chemical Society (Peking)* [*J. Chin. Chem. Soc. (Peking)*] (1933–1952; suspended 1937–1939). Has been called *Acta Chimica Sinica (Chinese Edition)* [*Acta Chim. Sin. (Chin. Ed.)*]. Until 1981, *Chemical Abstracts* named *Huaxue Xuebao* as *Hua Hsueh Hsueh Pao*. Publisher: China International Book Trading Corp., Beijing.

Indian Journal of Chemistry [*Indian J. Chem.*] (1963–1975). In 1976, divided into Section A [*Indian J. Chem., Sect. A*] (1976–) (inorganic, bioinorganic, physical, theoretical, and analytical) and Section B [*Indian J. Chem., Sect. B*] (1976–) (organic and medicinal). (Additional CASSI abbreviated subtitles omitted.) *Indian Journal of Chemistry* was a successor to *Journal of Scientific and Industrial Research* [*J. Sci. Ind. Res.*] (1942–1962), which from 1946 to 1962 was divided into Section A [*J. Sci. Ind. Res., Sect. A*] (general), Section B [*J. Sci. Ind. Res., Sect. B*] (physical sciences), and Section C [*J. Sci. Ind. Res., Sect. C*] (biological sciences). Free online full-text issues from 2007. Publisher: National Institute of Science Communication and Information Resources, New Delhi, India.

Indian Journal of Heterocyclic Chemistry [*Indian J. Heterocycl. Chem.*] (1991–). Publisher: Indian Journal of Heterocyclic Chemistry, Lucknow, India.

Inorganica Chimica Acta [*Inorg. Chim. Acta*] (1967–). Publisher: Elsevier.

Inorganic and Nuclear Chemical Letters. See *Polyhedron*.

Inorganic Chemistry [*Inorg. Chem.*] (1962–). Publisher: ACS.

Inorganic Chemistry Communications [*Inorg. Chem. Commun.*] (1998–). Publisher: Elsevier.

International Journal of Peptide and Protein Research [*Int. J. Pept. Protein Res.*] (1972–96). Formerly *International Journal of Protein Research* [*Int. J. Protein Res.*] (1969–1971). Merged with *Peptide Research* [*Pept. Res.*] (1988–1996) to form *Journal of Peptide Research*. Online archive publisher: Wiley.

International Journal of Peptide Research and Therapeutics [*Int. J. Pept. Res. Ther.*] (2005–). Formerly *Letters in Peptide Science* [*Lett. Pept. Sci.*] (1994–2003). (Not published in 2004.) Publisher: Springer.

International Journal of Sulfur Chemistry. See *Phosphorus, Sulfur and Silicon and the Related Elements*.

Israel Journal of Chemistry [*Isr. J. Chem.*] (1963–). Successor to *Bulletin of the Research Council of Israel* [*Bull. Res. Counc. Isr.*] (1951–1955) and its subsequent Section A [*Bull. Res. Counc. Isr., Sect. A*] (1955–1963) (1955–1957, maths, physics, and chemistry; 1957–1963, chemistry). Publisher: Laser Pages Publishing Ltd., Jerusalem.

International Journal of Sulfur Chemistry. See *Phosphorus, Sulfur and Silicon and the Related Elements*.

IUBMB Life [*IUBMB Life*] (1999–). Formerly *Biochemistry International* [*Biochem. Int.*] (1980–) and *Biochemistry and Molecular Biology International* [*Biochem. Mol. Biol. Int.*] (1993–1999). Publisher: Wiley.

Izvestiya Akademii Nauk, Seriya Khimicheskaya [*Izv. Akad. Nauk, Ser Khim.*] (1993–). In Russian. Formerly *Izvestiya Akademii Nauk SSSR, Seriya Khimicheskaya* [*Izv. Akad. Nauk SSSR, Ser. Khim.*] (1936–1992). *Izvestiya Akademii Nauk SSSR, Otdelenie Khimicheskikh Nauk* [*Izv. Akad. Nauk SSSR, Otd. Khim. Nauk*] was an alternative title from 1940 to 1963. There is an English language translation called *Russian Chemical Bulletin* [*Russ. Chem. Bull.*] (1993–); from July 2000, also called *Russian Chemical Bulletin, International Edition*. Formerly *Bulletin of the Academy of Sciences of the USSR, Division of Chemical Sciences* [*Bull. Acad. Sci. USSR, Div. Chem. Sci. (Engl. Transl.)*]. The Russian language version has no volume numbers; volume numbers were assigned to the translation from 1971 (Vol. 20). Publisher: Russian Academy of Sciences/Springer.

Japanese Journal of Antibiotics. See *Journal of Antibiotics*.

Japanese Journal of Chemistry. See *Nippon Kagaku Kaishi*.

Journal de Pharmacie et de Chimie. See *Annales Pharmaceutiques Français*.

Journal für Praktische Chemie. See *Advanced Synthesis & Catalysis*.

Journal of Agricultural and Food Chemistry [*J. Agric. Food Chem.*] (1953–). Publisher: ACS.

Journal of Antibiotics [*J. Antibiot.*] (1948–). English language translation of the Japanese language journal *Japanese Journal of Antibiotics* [*Jpn. J. Antibiot.*]. From 1953 to 1967 published as Series A [*J. Antibiot., Ser. A*] (English language) and Series B [*J. Antibiot., Ser. B*] (Japanese language). Publisher: Japan Antibiotics Research Association, Tokyo.

Journal of Asian Natural Products Research [*J. Asian Nat. Prod. Res.*] (1998–). Publisher: Taylor & Francis.

Journal of Biochemistry [*J. Biochem. (Tokyo)*] (1922–). Publisher: The Japanese Biochemical Society/Oxford University Press.

Journal of Biological Chemistry [*J. Biol. Chem.*] (1905–). Free online full-text archive. Publisher: The American Society for Biochemistry and Molecular Biology.

Journal of Carbohydrate Chemistry [*J. Carbohydr. Chem.*] (1982–). Successor to *Journal of Carbohydrates, Nucleosides, Nucleotides* [*J. Carbohydr., Nucleosides, Nucleotides*] (1974–1981), which was divided into *Journal of Carbohydrate Chemistry* and *Nucleosides & Nucleotides* [*Nucleosides Nucleotides*] (1982–1999), later *Nucleosides, Nucleotides & Nucleic Acids* [*Nucleosides, Nucleotides Nucleic Acids*]. Publisher: Taylor & Francis.

Journal of Chemical Crystallography [*J. Chem. Crystallogr.*] (1994–). Formerly *Journal of Crystal and Molecular Structure* [*J. Cryst. Mol. Struct.*] (1971–1981) and *Journal of Crystallographic and Spectroscopic Research* [*J. Crystallogr. Spectrosc. Res.*] (1982–1993). Publisher: Springer.

Journal of Chemical Ecology [*J. Chem. Ecol.*] (1975–). Publisher: Springer.

Journal of Chemical Education [*J. Chem. Educ.*] (1924–). Publisher: ACS Division of Chemical Education.

Journal of Chemical Research [*J. Chem. Res.*] (2004–). Formerly *Journal of Chemical Research, Miniprint* [*J. Chem. Res., Miniprint*] (1977–2003) (a miniprint/microfiche, full-text version) and *Journal of Chemical Research, Synopsis* [*J. Chem. Res., Synop.*] (1977–2003) (a synopsis version). No volume numbers. Publisher: Science Reviews 2000 Ltd., UK.

Journal of Chemical Sciences [*J. Chem. Sci. (Bangalore, India)*] (2004–). Formerly *Proceedings—Indian Academy of Sciences, Section A* [*Proc.—Indian Acad. Sci., Sect. A*] (1934–1979) and *Proceedings—Indian Academy of Sciences, Chemical Sciences* [*Proc.—Indian Acad. Sci., Chem. Sci.*] (1980–2003). Free online full-text archive from 1977. Publisher: Indian Academy of Sciences/Springer.

Journal of Chemistry of the United Arab Republic. See *Egyptian Journal of Chemistry*.

Journal of Fluorine Chemistry [*J. Fluorine Chem.*] (1971–). Publisher: Elsevier.

Journal of General Chemistry of the USSR. See *Zhurnal Obshchei Khimii*.

Journal of Heterocyclic Chemistry [*J. Heterocycl. Chem.*] (1964–). Publisher: HeteroCorporation, USA/Wiley.

Journal of Labelled Compounds and Radiopharmaceuticals [*J. Labelled Compd. Radiopharm.*] (1976–). Formerly *Journal of Labelled Compounds* [*J. Labelled Compd.*] (1965–1975). Publisher: Wiley.

Journal of Lipid Mediators and Cell Signalling [*J. Lipid Mediators Cell Signalling*] (1994–1997). Formerly *Journal of Lipid Mediators* [*J. Lipid Mediators*] (1989–1993). Merged with *Prostaglandins* [*Prostaglandins*] (1972–1997) to become *Prostaglandins & Other Lipid Mediators*.

Journal of Lipid Research [*J. Lipid Res.*] (1959–). Free online full-text archive. Publisher: The American Society for Biochemistry and Molecular Biology.

Journal of Magnetic Resonance [*J. Magn. Reson.*] (1969–1992, 1997–). Formerly divided into Series A [*J. Magn. Reson., Ser. A*] (1993–1996) and Series B [*J. Magn. Reson., Ser. B*] (1993–1996). Publisher: Elsevier.

Journal of Mass Spectrometry [*J. Mass Spectrom.*] (1995–). Formerly *Organic Mass Spectrometry* [*Org. Mass Spectrom.*] (1968–1994). Incorporates *Biological Mass Spectrometry* [*Biol. Mass Spectrom.*] [1991–1994], formerly *Biomedical Mass Spectrometry*

[*Biomed. Mass Spectrom.*] (1974–85) and *Biomedical and Environmental Mass Spectrometry* [*Biomed. Environ. Mass Spectrom.*] (1986–). Publisher: Wiley.

Journal of Medicinal Chemistry [*J. Med. Chem.*] (1963–). Formerly *Journal of Medicinal and Pharmaceutical Chemistry* [*J. Med. Pharm. Chem.*] (1959–1962). Publisher: ACS.

Journal of Medicinal Plant Research. See *Planta Medica*.

Journal of Molecular Structure [*J. Mol. Struct.*] (1967–). From 1981 onward, some volumes have been published as *THEOCHEM* [*THEOCHEM*]; each of these volumes has a *Journal of Molecular Structure* volume number and a different *THEOCHEM* volume number. Publisher: Elsevier.

Journal of Natural Medicines [*J. Nat. Med.*] (2006–). Formerly *Shoyakugaku Zasshi* [*Shoyakugaku Zasshi*], Journal of Pharmacognosy (1952–1993) and *Natural Medicines* [*Nat. Med., Tokyo, Jpn.*] (1994–2005). Publisher: Springer, Japan.

Journal of Natural Products [*J. Nat. Prod.*] (1979–). Formerly *Lloydia* [*Lloydia*] (1938–1978). Publisher: ACS.

Journal of Natural Products [*J. Nat. Prod. (Gorakhpur, India)*] (2008–). Electronic journal. Open access. Free online full-text issues at www.JournalOfNaturalProducts.com. Not related to the *Journal of Natural Products* published by ACS.

Journal of Organic Chemistry [*J. Org. Chem.*] (1936–). Publisher: ACS.

Journal of Organic Chemistry of the USSR. See *Zhurnal Organicheskoi Khimii*.

Journal of Organometallic Chemistry [*J. Organomet. Chem.*] (1963–). Publisher: Elsevier.

Journal of Peptide Research [*J. Pept. Res.*] (1997–2005). Formed by the merger of *International Journal of Peptide and Protein Research* and *Peptide Research*. Superseded by *Chemical Biology & Drug Design*. Online archive publisher: Wiley.

Journal of Peptide Science [*J. Pept. Sci.*] (1995–). Publisher: European Peptide Society and Wiley.

Journal of Pharmaceutical Sciences [*J. Pharm. Sci.*] (1961–). Publisher: American Pharmacists Association/Wiley.

Journal of Pharmacy and Pharmacology [*J. Pharm. Pharmacol.*] (1929–). From 1929 to 1948, the title was *Quarterly Journal of Pharmacy and Pharmacology* [*Q. J. Pharm. Pharmacol.*]. Publisher: Pharmaceutical Press.

Journal of Physical Organic Chemistry [*J. Phys. Org. Chem.*] (1988–). Publisher: Wiley.

Journal of Scientific and Industrial Research. See *Indian Journal of Chemistry*.

Journal of Steroid Biochemistry and Molecular Biology [*J. Steroid Biochem. Mol. Biol.*] (1990–). Formerly *Journal of Steroid Biochemistry* [*J. Steroid Biochem.*] (1969–90). Publisher: Elsevier.

Journal of Sulfur Chemistry [*J. Sulfur Chem.*] (Vol. 25–, 2004–). Formed by the merger of *Sulfur Letters* [*Sulfur Lett.*] (Vols. 1–26, 1982–2003) and *Sulfur Reports* [*Sulfur Rep.*] (Vols. 1–24, 1980–2003). Publisher: Taylor & Francis.

Journal of Synthetic Organic Chemistry. See *Yuki Gosei Kagaku Kyokaishi*.

Journal of the American Chemical Society [*J. Am. Chem. Soc.*] (1879–). Absorbed *American Chemical Journal* [*Am. Chem. J.*] (1879–1913). Publisher: ACS.

Journal of the Brazilian Chemical Society [*J. Braz. Chem. Soc.*] (1990–). Free online full-text archive. Publisher: Brazilian Chemical Society.

Journal of the Chemical Society [*J. Chem. Soc.*] (Vols. 1–32, 1849–1877, 1926–1965). Vol. 1 also assigned to the year 1848. Volume numbers were discontinued in 1925. From 1849 to 1862, an alternative title was *Quarterly Journal, Chemical Society* [*Q. J., Chem. Soc.*] (1849–1862). From 1878 to 1925, issued as *Journal of the Chemical Society, Transactions* [*J. Chem. Soc., Trans.*] (Vols. 33–127, 1878–1925) and *Journal of the Chemical Society, Abstracts* [*J. Chem. Soc., Abstr.*] (Vols. 34–128, 1878–1925). (Odd-numbered volume numbers only used for the *Transactions*; even-numbered volume numbers only used for the *Abstracts*). In 1966, divided into Part A [*J. Chem. Soc. A*] (1966–1971) (inorganic),

Part B [*J. Chem. Soc. B*] (1966–1971) (physical organic), and Part C [*J. Chem. Soc. C*] (1966–1971) (organic). *Chemical Communications* [*Chem. Commun.*] (1965–1969) became Part D [*J. Chem. Soc. D*] (1970–1971). In 1972, Parts A–D were superseded by *Journal of the Chemical Society, Dalton Transactions* [*J. Chem. Soc., Dalton Trans.*] (1972–2002) (inorganic); *Journal of the Chemical Society, Perkin Transactions 1* [*J. Chem. Soc., Perkin Trans. 1*] (1972–2002) (organic and bioorganic); *Journal of the Chemical Society, Perkin Transactions 2* [*J. Chem. Soc., Perkin Trans. 2*] (1972–2002) (physical organic); and *Journal of the Chemical Society, Chemical Communications* [*J. Chem. Soc., Chem. Commun.*] (1972–1995) (preliminary communications), respectively. In 1996, *Journal of the Chemical Society, Chemical Communications* became *Chemical Communications (Cambridge)*. In 2003, *Journal of the Chemical Society, Dalton Transactions* became *Dalton Transactions*, and *Journal of the Chemical Society, Perkin Transactions 1* and *Journal of the Chemical Society, Perkin Transactions 2* merged to become *Organic & Biomolecular Chemistry*. Online archive publisher: RSC.

Journal of the Chemical Society, Faraday Transactions [*J. Chem. Soc., Faraday Trans.*] (Vols. 86–94, 1990–1998). Formerly *Transactions of the Faraday Society* [*Trans. Faraday Soc.*] (Vols. 1–67, 1905–1971). In 1972, divided into two parts: *Journal of the Chemical Society, Faraday Transactions 1* [*J. Chem. Soc., Faraday Trans. 1*] (Vols. 68–85, 1972–1989) and *Journal of the Chemical Society, Faraday Transactions 2* [*J. Chem. Soc., Faraday Trans. 2*] (Vols. 68–85, 1972–1989). In 1999, merged with *Berichte der Bunsen-Gesellschaft* to form *Physical Chemistry Chemical Physics*. Online archive publisher: RSC.

Journal of the Chemical Society of Japan. See *Nippon Kagaku Kaishi*.

Journal of the Chemical Society of Pakistan [*J. Chem. Soc. Pak.*] (1979–). Publisher: Chemical Society of Pakistan.

Journal of the Chinese Chemical Society *(Peking)*. See *Huaxue Xuebao*.

Journal of the Chinese Chemical Society *(Taipei)* [*J. Chin. Chem. Soc. (Taipei)*] (1954–). In English. Free online full-text issues from 1988. Publisher: The Chemical Society, Taipei, Taiwan.

Journal of the Indian Chemical Society [*J. Indian Chem. Soc.*] (Vol. 5–, 1928–). Formerly *Quarterly Journal of the Indian Chemical Society* [*Q. J. Indian Chem. Soc.*] (Vols. 1–4, 1924–1927). Publisher: The Indian Chemical Society.

Journal of the Pharmaceutical Society of Japan. See *Yakugaku Zasshi*.

Journal of the Royal Netherlands Chemical Society. See *Recueil des Travaux Chimiques des Pays-Bas*.

Journal of the Science of Food and Agriculture [*J. Sci. Food Agric.*] (1950–). Publisher: The Society of Chemical Industry/Wiley.

Journal of the Society of Chemical Industry. See *Chemistry & Industry*.

Journal of the South African Chemical Institute. See *South African Journal of Chemistry*.

Justus Liebigs Annalen der Chemie. See *Liebigs Annalen*.

Khimiko-Farmatsevticheskii Zhurnal *(Khim.-Farm. Zh.)* (1967–). In Russian. There is an English language translation called *Pharmaceutical Chemistry Journal* [*Pharm. Chem. J. (Engl. Transl.)*] (1967–). Translation published by Springer.

Khimiya Geterotsiklicheskikh Soedinenii [*Khim. Geterotsikl. Soedin.*] (1965–). In Russian. There is an English language translation called *Chemistry of Heterocyclic Compounds* [*Chem. Heterocycl. Compd.*] (1965–). The translation has volume numbers; the Russian language version has no volume numbers. Translation published by Springer.

Khimiya Prirodnykh Soedinenii [*Khim. Prir. Soedin.*] (1965–). In Russian. There is an English language translation called *Chemistry of Natural Compounds* [*Chem. Nat. Compd.*] (1965–). Translation published by Springer.

Kogyo Kagaku Zasshi [*Kogyo Kagaku Zasshi*] (1898–1971) (Journal of Industrial Chemistry). In Japanese. No longer published. Merged with *Nippon Kagaku Zasshi* to form *Nippon Kagaku Kaishi*.

Liebigs Annalen [*Liebigs Ann.*] (1995–1996). Formerly *Annalen der Pharmacie* [*Ann. Pharm. (Lemgo, Ger.)*] (Vols. 1–32, 1832–1839) and *Justus Liebigs Annalen der Chemie* [*Justus Liebigs Ann. Chem.*] (1840–1978). Sometimes referred to colloquially as *Annalen*. Other former titles, not adopted by CASSI, are *Annalen der Chemie und Pharmacie* [*Ann. Chem. Pharm.*] (1840–1873) and *Justus Liebigs Annalen der Chemie und Pharmacie* [*Justus Liebigs Ann. Chem. Pharm.*] (1873–1874). In 1979, became *Liebigs Annalen der Chemie* [*Liebigs Ann. Chem.*] (1979–1994), which was superseded by *Liebigs Annalen* [*Liebigs Ann.*] (1995–1996). Volume numbers were used until 1972 (Vol. 766). In 1997, merged with *Recueil des Travaux Chimiques des Pays-Bas* to form *Liebigs Annalen/Recueil* [*Liebigs Ann./Recl.*] (1997). No longer published. In 1998, superseded by *European Journal of Organic Chemistry*. Online archive publisher: Wiley.

Letters in Organic Chemistry [*Lett. Org. Chem.*] (2004–). Publisher: Bentham Science Publishers Ltd.

Letters in Peptide Science. See *International Journal of Peptide Research and Therapeutics*.

Liebigs Annalen/Recueil. See *Liebigs Annalen*.

Lipids [*Lipids*] (1966–). Publisher: American Oil Chemists' Society/Springer.

Lloydia. See *Journal of Natural Products*.

Magnetic Resonance in Chemistry [*Magn. Reson. Chem.*] (Vol. 23–, 1985–). Formerly *Organic Magnetic Resonance* [*Org. Magn. Reson.*] (1969–1984). Publisher: Wiley.

Magyar Kemiai Folyoirat [*Magy. Kem. Foly.*] (1895–) (Hungarian Journal of Chemistry). Until 1949, the title was *Magyar Chemiai Folyoirat* [*Magy. Chem. Foly.*]. Free online full-text issues (in English and in Hungarian) from 2004. Publisher: Kultura, Budapest, Hungary.

Marine Drugs [*Mar. Drugs*] (2003–). Free online full-text archive from 2003. Publisher: Molecular Diversity Preservation International (MDPI), Basel, Switzerland.

Mendeleev Communications [*Mendeleev Commun.*] (1991–). Publisher: Russian Academy of Sciences/Elsevier.

Molbank [*Molbank*] (2002–). Formerly a section of *Molecules*. Electronic journal. Open access. Free online full-text archive from 2002. Publisher: Molecular Diversity Preservation International (MDPI), Basel, Switzerland.

Molecules [*Molecules*] (1996–). Electronic journal. Open access. Free online full-text archive from 1996. Publisher: Molecular Diversity Preservation International (MDPI), Basel, Switzerland.

Monatshefte für Chemie [*Monatsh. Chem.*] (1880–). From 1880 to 1967, the title, which was not adopted by CASSI, was *Monatshefte für Chemie und Verwandte Teile Anderer Wissenschaften* [*Monatsh. Chem. Verw. Teile Anderer Wiss.*]. Publisher: Springer.

Natural Product Communications [*Nat. Prod. Commun.*] (2006–). Publisher: Natural Product, Inc., Westerville, Ohio.

Natural Product Letters. See *Natural Product Research*.

Natural Product Reports [*Nat. Prod. Rep.*] (1984–). Review journal. Publisher: RSC.

Natural Product Research [*Nat. Prod. Res.*] (2003–2006). From 2006, issued as Part A [*Nat. Prod. Res., Part A*] and Part B [*Nat. Prod. Res., Part B*]. Formerly *Natural Product Letters* [*Nat. Prod. Lett.*] (1992–2002). Publisher: Taylor & Francis.

Natural Product Sciences [*Nat. Prod. Sci.*] (1995–). Publisher: Korean Society of Pharmacognosy, Seoul, South Korea.

Nature [*Nature (London)*] (1869–). Publisher: Nature Publishing Group/Macmillan Publishers Ltd.

Nature Chemical Biology [*Nat. Chem. Biol.*] (2005–). Publisher: Nature Publishing Group/ Macmillan Publishers Ltd.

Nature Chemistry [*Nat. Chem.*] (2009–). Publisher: Nature Publishing Group/Macmillan Publishers Ltd.

Naturwissenschaften [*Naturwissenschaften*] (1913–). Publisher: Springer.

New Journal of Chemistry [*New J. Chem.*] (1987–). Formerly *Nouveau Journal de Chimie* [*Nouv. J. Chim.*] (1977–1986). Publisher: RSC.

Nippon Kagaku Kaishi [*Nippon Kagaku Kaishi*] (1972–2002) (Journal of the Chemical Society of Japan). In Japanese. No English language translation is available. Formed by the merger of *Nippon Kagaku Zasshi* [*Nippon Kagaku Zasshi*] (Japanese Journal of Chemistry) (1948–1971) and *Kogyo Kagaku Zasshi*. Formerly *Tokyo Kagaku Kaishi* [*Tokyo Kagaku Kaishi*] (1880–1920) (Journal of the Tokyo Chemical Society) and *Nippon Kagaku Kaishi (1921–47)* [*Nippon Kagaku Kaishi (1921–47)*] (1921–1947). In pre-1960s issues of *Chemical Abstracts*, called *Journal of the Chemical Society of Japan* [*J. Chem. Soc. Jpn.*]. No longer published. Free online full-text archive 1880–2002 from J-Stage at http://www.jstage.jst.go.jp/browse/.

Norvegica Pharmaceutica Acta. See *European Journal of Pharmaceutical Sciences*.

Nouveau Journal de Chimie. See *New Journal of Chemistry*.

Nucleosides, Nucleotides & Nucleic Acids [*Nucleosides, Nucleotides Nucleic Acids*] (Vol. 19–, 2000–). Formerly *Journal of Carbohydrates, Nucleosides, Nucleotides* [*J. Carbohydr., Nucleosides, Nucleotides*] (1974–1981), which was divided into *Nucleosides & Nucleotides* [*Nucleosides Nucleotides*] (Vols. 1–18, 1982–1999) and *Journal of Carbohydrate Chemistry* [*J. Carbohydr. Chem.*]. Publisher: Taylor & Francis.

Open Medicinal Chemistry Journal [*Open Med. Chem. J.*] (2007–). Electronic journal. Open access. Free online full-text archive from 2007. Publisher: Bentham Open.

Open Natural Products Journal [*Open Nat. Prod. J.*] (2008–). Electronic journal. Open access. Free online full-text archive from 2008. Publisher: Bentham Open.

Open Organic Chemistry Journal [*Open Org. Chem. J.*] (2007–). Electronic journal. Open access. Free online full-text archive from 2007. Publisher: Bentham Open.

Organic & Biomolecular Chemistry [*Org. Biomol. Chem.*] (Vol. 1–, 2003–). Formed by a merger of *Journal of the Chemical Society, Perkin Transactions 1* and *Journal of the Chemical Society, Perkin Transactions 2*. See also *Journal of the Chemical Society*. Publisher: RSC.

Organic Magnetic Resonance. See *Magnetic Resonance in Chemistry*.

Organic Mass Spectrometry. See *Journal of Mass Spectrometry*.

Organic Preparations and Procedures International [*Org. Prep. Proced. Int.*] (1971–). Formerly *Organic Preparations and Procedures* [*Org. Prep. Proced.*] (1969–70). Publisher: Taylor & Francis.

Organic Communications [*Org. Commun.*] (2007–). Electronic journal. Open access. Free online full-text archive from 2008. Publisher: Academy of Chemistry of Globe, Turkey.

Organic Letters [*Org. Lett.*] (1999–). Publisher: ACS.

Organic Process Research & Development [*Org. Process Res. Dev.*] (1997–). Publisher: ACS.

Organometallics [*Organometallics*] (1982–). Publisher: ACS.

Oriental Journal of Chemistry [*Orient. J. Chem.*] (1985–). Publisher: Oriental Scientific Publishing Company, Bhopal, Madhya Pradesh, India.

Peptide Research. See *International Journal of Peptide and Protein Research*.

Peptides [*Peptides (Amsterdam, Neth.)*] (2007–). Previous CASSI abbreviations include *Peptides (N. Y.)* (1980–2006). Publisher: Elsevier.

Pharmaceutical Bulletin. See *Chemical and Pharmaceutical Bulletin*.

Pharmazie [*Pharmazie*] (1946–). Publisher: Govi-Verlag Pharmazeutischer Verlag, Eschborn, Germany.

Phosphorus, Sulfur and Silicon and the Related Elements [*Phosphorus, Sulfur Silicon Relat. Elem.*] (1989–). Formerly *Phosphorus and Sulfur and the Related Elements* [*Phosphorus Sulfur Relat. Elem.*] (1976–1988), which was formed by a merger of *Phosphorus and the Related Group V Elements* [*Phosphorus Relat. Group V Elem.*] (1971–1976) and *International Journal of Sulfur Chemistry* [*Int. J. Sulfur Chem.*] (1973–1976). *International*

Journal of Sulfur Chemistry was previously divided into Part A [*Int. J. Sulfur Chem., Part A*] (1971–1972) (original experimental and theoretical studies); Part B [*Int. J. Sulfur Chem., Part B*] (1971–1972), previously *Quarterly Reports on Sulfur Chemistry* [*Q. Rep. Sulfur Chem.*] (1966–1970); and Part C [*Int. J. Sulfur Chem., Part C*] (1971–1972), previously *Mechanisms of Reactions of Sulfur Compounds* [*Mech. React. Sulfur Compd.*] (1966–1970). Publisher: Taylor & Francis.

Physical Chemistry Chemical Physics [*Phys. Chem. Chem. Phys.*] (Vol. 1–, 1999–). Formed by the merger of *Berichte der Bunsen-Gesellschaft* and *Journal of the Chemical Society, Faraday Transactions*. Publisher: RSC (in cooperation with other scientific societies).

Phytochemistry [*Phytochemistry*] (1961–). Publisher: Elsevier.

Phytochemistry Letters [*Phytochem. Lett.*] (2008–). Publisher: Phytochemical Society of Europe/Elsevier.

Planta Medica [*Planta Med.*] (1953–). Sometimes referred to as *Journal of Medicinal Plant Research: Planta Medica* [*J. Med. Plant Res.: Planta Med.*]. Publisher: Thieme.

Polish Journal of Chemistry [*Pol. J. Chem.*] (1978–2009). Formerly *Roczniki Chemii* [*Rocz. Chem.*] (1921–77). Publisher: Polish Chemical Society. No longer published. Superseded by *European Journal of Inorganic Chemistry* and *European Journal of Organic Chemistry*.

Polyhedron [*Polyhedron*] (1982–). Successor to *Journal of Inorganic and Nuclear Chemistry* [*J. Inorg. Nucl. Chem.*] (1955–81) and *Inorganic and Nuclear Chemistry Letters* [*Inorg. Nucl. Chem. Lett.*] (1965–81). Publisher: Elsevier.

Proceedings of the Chemical Society, London [*Proc. Chem. Soc, London*] (1885–1914, 1957–1964). Superseded by *Chemical Communications* [*Chem. Commun.*] (1965–1969). From 1915 to 1956 there was a proceedings section in *Journal of the Chemical Society*. See also *Chemical Communications (Cambridge)*.

Proceedings of the National Academy of Sciences of the United States of America [*Proc. Natl. Acad. Sci. U.S.A.*] (1863–). Free online full-text archive (online issues available six months after the print publication; some current full-text content also free online). Publisher: National Academy of Sciences, United States.

Prostaglandins & Other Lipid Mediators [*Prostaglandins Other Lipid Mediators*] (1998–). Formed by a merger of *Prostaglandins* [*Prostaglandins*] (1972–1997) and *Journal of Lipid Mediators and Cell Signalling* [*J. Lipid Mediators Cell Signalling*] (1994–97). Publisher: Elsevier.

Protein & Peptide Letters [*Protein Pept. Lett.*] (1994–). Publisher: Bentham Science Publishers Ltd.

Pure and Applied Chemistry [*Pure Appl. Chem.*] (1960–). Free online full-text archive. Publisher: IUPAC.

Quarterly Reviews of the Chemical Society. See *Chemical Society Reviews*.

Records of Natural Products [*Rec. Nat. Prod.*] (2007–). Electronic journal. Open access. Free online full-text archive from 2007. Publisher: Academy of Chemistry of Globe, Turkey.

Recueil des Travaux Chimiques des Pays-Bas [*Recl. Trav. Chim. Pays-Bas*] (1882–1996). Also known as *Journal of the Royal Netherlands Chemical Society* [*J. R. Neth. Chem. Soc.*]. From 1897 to 1919, the title was *Recueil des Travaux Chimiques des Pays-Bas et de la Belgique* [*Recl. Trav. Chim. Pays-Bas Belg.*], and from 1980 to 1984, the title was *Recueil: Journal of the Royal Netherlands Chemical Society* [*Recl.: J. R. Neth. Chem. Soc.*]. No longer published. Merged with *Chemische Berichte* [*Chem. Ber.*] to form *Chemische Berichte/Recueil* and with *Liebigs Annalen* [*Liebigs Ann.*] to form *Liebigs Annalen/Recueil*.

Regulatory Peptides [*Regul. Pept.*] (1980–). Publisher: Elsevier.

Revue Roumaine de Chimie [*Rev. Roum. Chem.*] (1964–). Formerly *Revue de Chimie, Academie de la Republique Populaire Roumaine* [*Rev. Chim. Acad. Repub. Pop. Roum.*] (1954–1963). Also known as *Roumanian Journal of Chemistry*. Publisher: Romanian Academy.

Roczniki Chemii. See *Polish Journal of Chemistry*.

Rossiiskii Khimicheskii Zhurnal [*Ross. Khim. Zh.*] (Russian Chemical Journal) (1993–). In Russian. Formerly *Zhurnal Vsesoyuznogo Khimicheskogo Obshchestva im. D. I. Mendeleeva* [*Zh. Vses. Khim. O–va. im. D. I. Mendeleeva*] (1960–1991) (Journal of the D. I. Mendeleev All-Union Chemical Society). In Russian. There is an English language translation entitled *Mendeleev Chemistry Journal* [*Mendeleev Chem. J.*] (1966–). Translation published by Allerton Press, Inc., New York.

Russian Chemical Bulletin. See *Izvestiya Akademii Nauk, Seriya Khimicheskaya*.

Russian Chemical Reviews. See *Uspekhi Khimii*.

Russian Journal of Applied Chemistry. See *Zhurnal Prikladnoi Khimii*.

Russian Journal of Bioorganic Chemistry. See *Bioorganicheskaya Khimiya*.

Russian Journal of General Chemistry. See *Zhurnal Obshchei Khimii*.

Russian Journal of Inorganic Chemistry. See *Zhurnal Neorganicheskoi Khimii*.

Russian Journal of Organic Chemistry. See *Zhurnal Organicheskoi Khimii*.

Science [*Science (Washington, D.C.)*] (1883–). Publisher: American Association for the Advancement of Science. http://www.sciencemag.org/.

Scientia Pharmaceutica [*Sci. Pharm.*] (1930–). Free online full-text archive from 2006. Publisher: The Austrian Journal of Pharmaceutical Sciences.

South African Journal of Chemistry [*S. Afr. J. Chem.*] (1977–). Formerly *Journal of the South African Chemical Institute* [*J. S. Afr. Chem. Inst.*] (1922–1976). Free online full-text archive from 2001. Publisher: South African Bureau for Scientific Publications.

Soviet Journal of Bioorganic Chemistry. See *Bioorganicheskaya Khimiya*.

Spectrochimica Acta [*Spectrochim. Acta*] (1939–1966). From Vol. 23, divided into Part A [*Spectrochim. Acta, Part A*] (1967–) (molecular spectroscopy; from 1995, subtitle is *Molecular and Biomolecular Spectroscopy*) and Part B [*Spectrochim. Acta, Part B*] (1967–) (atomic spectroscopy). Publisher: Elsevier.

Steroids [*Steroids*] (1963–). Publisher: Elsevier.

Synfacts [*Synfacts*] (2005–). Publisher: Thieme.

Synlett [*Synlett*] (1989–). No volume numbers. Publisher: Thieme.

Synthesis [*Synthesis*] (1969–). No volume numbers. Publisher: Thieme.

Synthesis and Reactivity in Inorganic, Metal-Organic, and Nano-Metal Chemistry [*Synth. React. Inorg., Met.-Org., Nano-Met. Chem.*] (2005–). Formerly *Synthesis in Inorganic and Metal-Organic Chemistry* [*Synth. Inorg. Met.-Org. Chem.*] (1971–1973) and *Synthesis and Reactivity in Inorganic and Metal-Organic Chemistry* [*Synth. React. Inorg. Met.-Org. Chem.*] (1974–2004). Publisher: Taylor & Francis.

Synthetic Communications [*Synth. Commun.*] (1971–). Publisher: Taylor & Francis.

Tetrahedron [*Tetrahedron*] (1957–). From 1958 to 1962, more than one volume number was issued each year: 1957, Vol. 1; 1958, Vols. 2–4; 1959, Vols. 5–7; 1960, Vols. 8–11; 1961, Vols. 12–16; 1962, Vols. 17–18; 1963, Vol. 19 et seq.; 2009, Vol. 65. Publisher: Elsevier.

Tetrahedron: Asymmetry [*Tetrahedron: Asymmetry*] (1990–). Publisher: Elsevier.

Tetrahedron Letters [*Tetrahedron Lett.*] (1959–). In the print edition, volume numbers were first used in 1980 (Vol. 21). In the online edition, volume numbers were assigned from 1959–1960 (called Vol. 1). The forty-eight issues for 1959–1960 were paginated separately, and the issue numbering differs between the print and online editions: print edition, Issues 1–21 (1959); Issues 1–27 (1960); online edition, Issues 1–21 (1959); Issues 22–48 (1960). Publisher: Elsevier.

Tetrahedron, Supplement [*Tetrahedron, Suppl.*] (1958–1981). Irregular. No volume numbers. No longer published.

THEOCHEM. See *Journal of Molecular Structure*.

Turkish Journal of Chemistry [*Turk. J. Chem.*] (1992–). Formerly *Doga: Turk Kimya Dergisi* (and related titles). Free online full-text archive from 1996. Publisher: The Scientific and Technological Research Council of Turkey.

United Arab Republic Journal of Chemistry. See *Egyptian Journal of Chemistry*.

Uspekhi Khimii [*Usp. Khim.*] (1932–). In Russian. There is an English language translation entitled *Russian Chemical Reviews* [*Russ. Chem. Rev.*] (1960–). Publisher: Russian Academy of Sciences/Turpion Ltd., London.

Yakugaku Zasshi [*Yakugaku Zasshi*] (1881–) (Journal of Pharmacy). Also known as *Journal of the Pharmaceutical Society of Japan*. In Japanese. No English language translation is available. Free online full-text archive from 1881. Publisher: The Pharmaceutical Society of Japan, Tokyo.

Yuki Gosei Kagaku Kyokaishi [*Yuki Gosei Kagaku Kyokaishi*] (1943–). Also known as *Journal of Synthetic Organic Chemistry* [*J. Synth. Org. Chem. Jpn.*]. In Japanese. No English language translation of the full text is available, but tables of contents in English from 2000 are on the publisher's website. Publisher: The Society of Synthetic Organic Chemistry, Japan.

Zeitschrift für Angewandte Chemie. See *Angewandte Chemie*.

Zeitschrift für Anorganische und Allgemeine Chemie [*Z. Anorg. Allg. Chem.*] (1892–). From 1892 to 1915 and 1943 to 1950, the title was *Zeitschrift für Anorganische Chemie* [*Z. Anorg. Chem.*]. Publisher: Wiley.

Zeitschrift für Chemie. See *Angewandte Chemie*.

Zeitschrift für Kristallographie [*Z. Kristallogr.*] (1978–). Formerly titled *Zeitschrift für Kristallographie und Mineralogie* [*Z. Kristallogr. Mineral.*] (1877–1915) and *Zeitschrift für Kristallographie, Kristallgeometrie, Kristallphysik, Kristallchemie* [*Z. Kristallogr., Kristallgeom., Kristallphys., Kristallchem.*] (1921–1977; not published 1945–1954). Also called *Zeitschrift für Kristallographie, Mineralogie und Petrographie, Abteilung A* [*Z. Kristallogr. Mineral. Petrogr, Abt. A*] (1930–1945). Publisher: Oldenbourg Verlagsgruppe.

Zeitschrift für Kristallographie: New Crystal Structures [*Z. Kristallogr. New Cryst. Struct.*] (1997–). Publisher: Oldenbourg Verlagsgruppe.

Zeitschrift für Naturforschung [*Z. Naturforsch.*] (1946). In 1947, divided into Teil A [*Z. Naturforsch., A*] (1947–) (physical sciences) and Teil B [*Z. Naturforsch., B*] (1947–) (chemical sciences), to which was later added Teil C [*Z. Naturforsch., C*] (1973–) (biosciences—previously included in Teil B). (Additional CASSI abbreviated subtitles omitted.) Publisher: Verlag der Zeitschrift für Naturforschung, Tübingen, Germany.

Zhurnal Neorganicheskoi Khimii [*Zh. Neorg. Khim.*] (1956–). In Russian. There is an English language translation called *Russian Journal of Inorganic Chemistry* [*Russ. J. Inorg. Chem.*] (1959–). Formerly *Journal of Inorganic Chemistry (USSR)* [*J. Inorg. Chem. (USSR)*] (1956–1958). Publisher: MAIK Nauka/Interperiodica.

Zhurnal Obshchei Khimii [*Zh. Obshch. Khim.*] (1931–). In Russian. There is an English language translation called *Russian Journal of General Chemistry* [*Russ. J. Gen. Chem.*] (1993–). Formerly *Journal of General Chemistry of the USSR* [*J. Gen. Chem. USSR (Engl. Transl.)*] (1949–1992). Publisher: Springer/MAIK Nauka/Interperiodica. The antecedence of this title is *Zhurnal Russkago Khimicheskago Obshchestva* [*Zh. Russ. Khim. O–va.*] (Vols. 1–4, 1869–1872); *Zhurnal Russkago Khimicheskago Obshchestva i Fizicheskago Obshchestva* [*Zh. Russ. Khim. O–va. Fiz. O–va.*] (Vols. 5–10, 1873–1878); *Zhurnal Russkago Fiziko-Khimicheskago Obshchestva* [*Zh. Russ. Fiz.-Khim. O–va.*] (Vols. 11–38, 1879–1906); *Zhurnal Russkogo Fiziko-Khimicheskago Obshchestva, Chast Khimicheskaya* [*Zh. Russ. Fiz.-Khim. O–va., Chast Khim.*] (Vols. 39–62, 1907–1930); and *Zhurnal Russkogo Fiziko-Khimicheskago Obshchestva, Chast Fizicheskaya* [*Zh. Russ. Fiz.-Khim. O–va., Chast Fiz.*] (Vols. 39–62, 1907–1930). *Zhurnal Russkogo Fiziko-Khimicheskago Obshchestva, Chast Khimicheskaya* was superseded by *Zhurnal Obshchei Khimii*. Early volumes of *Chemical Abstracts* used an anglicized version for *Zh. Russ. Fiz.-Khim. O–va.: J. Russ. Phys.-Chem. Soc.* or *J. Russ. Phys. Chem. Soc.* CASSI interchanges *Russkogo* and *Russkago* in the transliteration of these Russian titles.

Zhurnal Organicheskoi Khimii [*Zh. Org. Khim.*] (1965–). In Russian. There is an English language translation called *Russian Journal of Organic Chemistry* [*Russ. J. Org. Chem.*] (1993–). Formerly *Journal of Organic Chemistry of the USSR* [*J. Org. Chem. USSR (Engl. Transl.)*] (1965–92). Publisher: Springer/MAIK Nauka/Interperiodica.

Zhurnal Prikladnoi Khimii [*Zh. Prikl. Khim. (St Petersburg)*]. Formerly *Zh. Prikl. Khim. (Leningrad)* (1928–). In Russian. There is an English language translation called *Russian Journal of Applied Chemistry* [*Russ. J. Appl. Chem.*] (1993–). Formerly *Journal of Applied Chemistry of the USSR* [*J. Appl. Chem. USSR (Engl. Transl.)*] (1950–1992). Publisher: Springer/MAIK Nauka/Interperiodica.

ENDNOTES

1. *CAS Source Index* (CASSI) abbreviations. The most recent printed cumulative compendium of CASSI abbreviated titles is for the period 1907–2004. Annual printed updates are also issued, and a CD version is available, in which the cumulative titles and the annual updates are combined (currently CASSI on CD covers the period 1907–2008). From 2010, only the CD version of CASSI is published. CASSI abbreviations for about 1,500 leading journals are listed on a free website (*CAplus Core Journal Coverage List*).

   Augmenting the CD version of CASSI is the *CAS Source Index* (CASSI) Search Tool (http://cassi. cas.org/search.jsp). Available from January 2010, the CASSI search tool is a free, web-based resource that can be used to quickly identify or confirm journal titles and abbreviations for publications indexed by CAS since 1907, including serial and non-serial scientific and technical publications.

   CASSI abbreviations sometimes include the geographical location of the publisher of a journal and the subtitles of those journals, which are divided into named parts or sections. The details are omitted here, apart from a few exceptions.

2. Some leading publishers of chemistry journals:

Publisher	Abbreviated Name	Internet Address
American Chemical Society, Washington D.C.	ACS	http://pubs.acs.org/
Elsevier, Oxford (and elsewhere)	Elsevier	http://www.sciencedirect.com/science
John Wiley & Sons, Inc., Hoboken, NJ (includes Wiley-Blackwell, Wiley InterScience, Wiley-VCH)	Wiley	http://eu.wiley.com/WileyCDA/ Section/index.html
MAIK Nauka/Interperiodica	...	http://www.maik.rssi.ru/
Royal Society of Chemistry, Cambridge	RSC	http://www.rsc.org/
Springer Publishing Company, New York and Berlin	Springer	http://www.springerpub.com/
Taylor & Francis Group, London	Taylor & Francis	http://www.taylorandfrancisgroup.com/
Thieme Publishing Group, Stuttgart, Germany	Thieme	http://www.thieme-chemistry.com/

3. Electronic sources for chemistry journals. With very few exceptions, all the current printed chemistry journals are available online, and some recent additions to the chemistry literature are *only* available electronically. For the majority of titles, access to the online full text of a journal and its archive is by paid subscription, but for an increasing number of chemistry journals, free online open access to current issues and full-text archives, either partial or complete, is now allowed. For some authors, open access of published papers on the web may be a condition of funding of their research.

   Tables of contents for the current and archival issues of chemistry journals are free online, and usually abstracts are also provided by the publisher. Search engines give details of the Internet addresses (URLs) for chemistry journals, and there are also websites that provide hyperlinks to most of the chemistry journals currently online, for example, Cambridge University's Department of Chemistry website: http://www.ch.cam.ac.uk/c2k/. Free full-text chemistry journals on the web are listed on the Belarusian State University website: http://www.abc.chemistry.bsu.by/current/fulltext.htm. (The content and permanence of any website cannot be guaranteed, and Internet addresses are subject to modification.)

3 Nomenclature Fundamentals

Currently the best book available is Fox, R. B., and Powell, W. H., *Nomenclature of Organic Compounds, Principles and Practice*, 2nd ed. New York (ACS/OUP, 2001).

This and the following chapters are intended as a quick reference guide, and should not replace the International Union of Pure and Applied Chemistry (IUPAC) publications for definitive guidance nor the CAS 2007 documentation for a full description of the current CAS nomenclature system.

The indexing and location of substances is now largely done by substructure, and the function of nomenclature is much more to provide an acceptable name for a given compound in a particular context. A given compound may have several equally valid names, and a name intelligible to a fellow organic chemist may not be appropriate for publication in, for example, fire regulations. For many purposes it is sufficient to be able to recognise from the name that the correct compound has been tracked down as a result of searching by substructure, molecular formula, etc.

- Do not needlessly proliferate systematic names.
- Make sure that you have checked all available information products to ensure that a compound you are reporting is in fact new. For synthetic compounds carry out a structure search against *Chemical Abstracts* and Beilstein; for newly isolated natural products, the *Dictionary of Natural Products* (see Section 1.2.1) is the best source.
- When reporting new natural products, avoid duplicating trivial names. Check against the *Dictionary of Natural Products* and CAS.

3.1 IUPAC NOMENCLATURE

IUPAC (www.iupac.org) promulgates general nomenclature recommendations. The IUPAC website is particularly useful for classes of compounds where the nomenclature has its own specialised rules, e.g., carbohydrates and organophosphorus compounds. IUPAC nomenclature is a series of protocols, not a precise recipe, so it is often possible to arrive at two or more systematic names that each accord with IUPAC recommendations.

The following IUPAC recommendations of principal interest to organic chemists are available at www.iupac.org/publications:

> *Nomenclature of Organic Compounds* ("The Blue Book"), incorporating IUPAC recommendations 1979 and 1993
> *Biochemical Nomenclature*
> *Chemical Terminology* ("The Gold Book"), with definitions of 7000 terms

See also the following printed publications:

> *A Guide to IUPAC Nomenclature of Organic Compounds*, Blackwell Scientific, London, 1993.
> *Biochemical Nomenclature and Related Documents,* Portland Press, London, 1992. Contains about forty reprints of articles taken from journals, on nomenclature of amino acids, peptides, and carbohydrates. This information is now mostly available on websites.

Updates to IUPAC recommendations are published on the website, usually with a summary in the IUPAC journal *Chemistry International*.

Algorithms are available that generate acceptable IUPAC names from structures, such as MARVIN from ChemAxon (www.chemaxon.com/marvin).

3.1.1   NUMBERING OF CHAINS

The first four members of the alkane series (methane, ethane, propane, butane) are irregular; subsequent members are named systematically by attaching -*ne* to the list of numerical prefixes given in Table 3.1.

TABLE 3.1
Common Numerical Prefixes

1	mono	27	heptacosa
2	di	28	octacosa
3	tri	29	nonacosa
4	tetra	30	triaconta
5	penta	31	hentriaconta
6	hexa	32	dotriaconta
7	hepta	33	tritriaconta
8	octa	40	tetraconta
9	nona	50	pentaconta
10	deca	60	hexaconta
11	undeca	70	heptaconta
12	dodeca	80	octaconta
13	trideca	90	nonaconta
14	tetradeca	100	hecta
15	pentadeca	101	henhecta
16	hexadeca	102	dohecta
17	heptadeca	110	decahecta
18	octadeca	120	eicosahecta or icosahecta
19	nonadeca	130	triacontahecta
20	eicosa or icosa	200	dicta
21	heneicosa or henicosa	300	tricta
22	docosa	400	tetracta
23	tricosa	1,000	kilia
24	tetracosa	2,000	dilia
25	pentacosa	3,000	trilia
26	hexacosa	4,000	tetrilia

3.1.1.1   Multiplicative Prefixes from Greek and Latin

In CAS Index Names, Greek prefixes are preferred, except for *sesqui*- (for one and one-half), *nona*- (for nine), and *undeca*- (for eleven). The terms *hemi*- (Greek) and *sesqui*- (Latin) are employed by CAS only in hydrate and ammoniate names. A full list is given in Table 3.2.

The terms *bis*, *tris*, *tetrakis*, etc. (meaning essentially "twice," "three times," etc.) are used to avoid ambiguity in nomenclature. This is best illustrated by the following example:

1, 2-cyclohexanedione
diphenylhydrazone
(strictly, mono(diphenylhydrazone))

1, 2-cyclohexanedione
bis(phenylhydrazone)

In naming ring assemblies the alternative prefixes *bi*-, *ter*-, *quater*-, *quinque*-, and *sexi*- are used.

TABLE 3.2
Greek and Latin Multiplicative Prefixes

	Greek	Latin		Greek
1/2	hemi	semi	25	pentacosa, pentacos
1	mono, mon	uni	26	hexacosa, hexacos
3/2		sesqui	27	heptacosa, heptacos
2	di	bi	28	octacosa, octacos
3	tri	tri, ter	29	nonacosa, nonacos
4	tetra, tert	quadric, quadr, quater	30	triconta, triacont
5	penta, pent	quinque, quinqu	31	hentriconta, hentriacont
6	hexa, hex	sexi, sex	32	dotriaconta, dotriacont
7	hepta, hept	septi, sept	33	tritriaconta, tritriacont
8	octa, oct, octo, octi		40	tetraconta, tetracont
9	ennea, enne	nona, non, novi	50	pentaconta, pentacont
10	deca, dec, deci		60	hexaconta, hexacont
11	hendeca, hendec	undeca, undec	70	heptaconta, heptacont
12	dodeca, dodec		80	octaconta, octacont
13	trideca, tridec		90	nonaconta, nonacont
14	tetradeca, tetradec		100	hecta, hect
15	pentadeca, pentadec		101	henhecta, henhect
16	hexadeca, hexadec		102	dohecta, dohect
17	heptadeca, heptadec		110	decahecta, decahect
18	octadeca, octadec		120	eicosahecta, eicosahect (or ic …)
19	nonadeca, nonadec		132	dotriacontahecta, dotriacontahect
20	eicosa, eicos (or ic …)		200	dicta, dict
21	henicosa, henicos		300	tricta
22	docosa, docos		400	tetracta
23	tricosa, tricos		1,000	kilia
24	tetracosa, tetracos			

3.1.2 NUMBERING OF SUBSTITUENTS: IUPAC PRINCIPLES

If a molecular skeleton can be numbered in more than one way, then it should be numbered so as to give the substituents the lowest set of locants. The locants for all the substituents (regardless of what the substituents are) are arranged in numerical order; the possible sets of locants are then compared *number by number* until a difference is found.

Decane, 6,7,8,9-tetrachloro-1-fluoro-, *not* decane, 2,3,4,5-tetrachloro-10-fluoro-

3.1.3 ALPHABETISATION

Substituent prefixes are placed in alphabetical order according to their name; only then are numerical prefixes (*di-*, *tri-*, etc.) placed in front of each as required and the locants inserted.

The substituents are 1-chloro, 2-nitro, 4-bromo-, 6-(dibromomethyl)-, and 7-bromo-. The substituents are cited in alphabetical order, i.e., bromo, chloro, (dibromomethyl), nitro. The Index Name is "Naphthalene, 4,7-dibromo-1-chloro-6-(dibromomethyl)-2-nitro-."

(Dibromomethyl) is an example of a complex substituent, one that is made up of two or more simple substituents. A complex substituent requires enclosing parentheses, and is alphabetised at its first letter, regardless of the origin of this letter, e.g., *b* from (bromomethyl), *d* from (dibromomethyl), and *t* from (tribromomethyl).

3.1.4 OTHER NOMENCLATURE CONVENTIONS

See Chapter 2 of Fox and Powell for the detailed application of the following IUPAC conventions in organic names: spelling, italics, punctuation, enclosing marks, locants, and detachable and non-detachable prefixes.

3.2 CAS NOMENCLATURE

CAS nomenclature in general accords with IUPAC principles and can be considered a special case of it, but because CAS needs to arrive at a unique name for each substance, its rules are more definitive. In addition, CAS (in consultation with the American Chemical Society nomenclature committees) has to operate on a short time frame, and often has to introduce names in areas where IUPAC has not yet formulated policy. Occasionally the IUPAC rules, when published, may differ from what CAS has already done, and CAS may not adopt IUPAC recommendations when they are eventually published. (For a fuller account, see Fox and Powell, pp. 6–7.)

Major changes in CAS nomenclature were made at the beginning of the ninth Collective Index period (1972), giving what became widely known as 9CI nomenclature. This is described in the publication *Naming and Indexing of Chemical Substances for Chemical Abstracts* (Appendix IV to the CAS 1992 Index Guide, but also available separately).

Nomenclature was then largely stable for organic compounds until 2006; further changes introduced are described in Section 3.2.2 and at appropriate places in the next chapter. Current CAS policy is described in the updated *Naming and Indexing of Chemical Substances for Chemical Abstract,* 2007 edition, available at cas.org.

The use of CI suffixes in CAS to indicate the Collective Index period during which the name was applied has now been discontinued, although labels 9CI, 8CI, etc., attached to existing names remain in place.

3.2.1 OLDER NAMES ENCOUNTERED IN CAS PRE-1972

At the changeover from the eighth to the ninth Collective Index periods (1972), the use of many older stem names was discontinued. These are all found in the older literature, and some can still be found in the literature today. The list in Table 3.3 equates many 9CI name fragments with those used in the 8CI and earlier. An asterisk indicates that the name was used in 8CI for the unsubstituted substance only; substituted derivatives were indexed elsewhere.

TABLE 3.3

8CI Name	9CI Name	8CI Name	9CI Name
Acetamidine	Ethanimidamine	Acetonaphthone	Ethanone, 1-(naphthalenyl)-
Acetanilide	Acetamide, *N*-phenyl-	Acetone*	2-Propanone
Acetanisidide	Acetamide, *N*-(methoxyphenyl)-	Acetophenetidide	Acetamide, *N*-(ethoxyphenyl)-
Acetoacetic acid	Butanoic acid, 3-oxo-	Acetophenone	Ethanone, 1-phenyl-

* Name used in 8CI for unsubstituted substance only.

TABLE 3.3 (continued)

8CI Name	9CI Name	8CI Name	9CI Name
Acetotoluidide	Acetamide, N-(methylphenyl)-	Chromone	4H-1-Benzopyran-4-one
Acetoxylidide	Acetamide, N-(dimethylphenyl)-	Cinchoninic acid	4-Quinolinecarboxylic acid
Acetylene	Ethyne	Cinnamic acid	2-Propenoic acid, 3-phenyl-
Acrolein	2-Propenal	Cinnamyl alcohol*	2-Propen-1-ol, 3-phenyl-
Acrylic acid	2-Propenoic acid	Citraconic acid*	2-Butenedioic acid, 2-methyl, (Z)-
Adamantane	Tricyclo[3.3.1.1³,⁷]decane	Citric acid	1,2,3-Propanetricarboxylic acid, 2-hydroxy-
Adipic acid*	Hexanedioic acid	Coumarin	2H-1-Benzopyran-2-one
Allene*	1,2-Propadiene	Cresol	Phenol, methyl-
Alloxan	2,4,5,6(1H,3H)-Pyrimidinetetrone	Cresotic acid	Benzoic acid, hydroxymethyl-
Alloxazine	Benzo[g]pteridine-2,4(1H,3H)-dione	Crotonic acid	2-Butenoic acid
Allyl alcohol*	2-Propen-1-ol	Cumene	Benzene, (1-methylethyl)-
Allylamine	2-Propen-1-amine	Cumidine	Benzenamine, 4-(1-methylethyl)-
Aniline	Benzenamine	Cymene	Benzene, methyl(1-methylethyl)-
Anisic acid	Benzoic acid, methoxy-	Cytosine	2(1H)-Pyrimidinone, 4-amino-
Anisidine	Benzenamine, ar-methoxy-		
Anisole	Benzene, methoxy-	Diacetamide	Acetamide, N-acetyl-
Anthranilic acid	Benzoic acid, 2-amino-	Dibenzamide	Benzamide, N-benzoyl-
Anthraquinone	9,10-Anthracenedione	Diethylamine	Ethanamine, N-ethyl-
Anthroic acid	Anthracenecarboxylic acid	Diethylene glycol*	Ethanol, 2,2'-oxybis-
Anthrol	Anthracenol	Diimide	Diazene
Anthrone	9(10H)-Anthracenone	Dimethylamine	Methanamine, N-methyl-
Atropic acid	Benzeneacetic acid, α-methylene-	Divicine	4,5-Pyrimidinedione, 2,6-diamino-1,6-dihydro-
Azelaic acid*	Nonanedioic acid		
Azobenzene	Diazene, diphenyl-	Elaidic acid	9-Octadecenoic acid, (E)-
Azoxybenzene	Diazene, diphenyl-, 1-oxide	Elaidolinolenic acid	9,12,15-Octadecatrienoic acid, (E,E,E)-
		Ethyl alcohol*	Ethanol
Barbituric acid	2,4,6(1H,3H,5H)-Pyrimidinetrione	Ethyl ether	Ethane, 1,1'-oxybis-
Benzanilide	Benzamide, N-phenyl-	Ethyl sulfide*	Ethane, 1,1'-thiobis-
Benzhydrol	Benzenemethanol, α-phenyl-	Ethylamine	Ethanamine
Benzidine	[1,1'-Biphenyl]-4,4'-diamine	Ethylene	Ethene
Benzil	Ethanedione, diphenyl-	Ethylene glycol*	1,2-Ethanediol
Benzilic acid	Benzeneacetic acid, α-hydroxy-α-phenyl	Ethylene oxide*	Oxirane
Benzoin	Ethanone, 2-hydroxy-1,2-diphenyl-	Ethylenimine	Aziridine
Benzophenone	Methanone, diphenyl-		
o-Benzoquinone	3,5-Cyclohexadiene-1,2-dione	Flavan	2H-1-Benzopyran, 3,4-dihydro-2-phenyl-
p-Benzoquinone	2,5-Cyclohexadiene-1,4-dione	Flavanone	4H-1-Benzopyran-4-one, 2,3-dihydro-2-phenyl
Benzyl alcohol	Benzenemethanol	Flavone	4H-1-Benzopyran-4-one, 2-phenyl-
Benzylamine	Benzenemethanamine	Flavylium	1-Benzopyrylium, 2-phenyl-
Bibenzyl	Benzene, 1,1'-(1,2-ethanediyl)bis-	Fulvene*	1,3-Cyclopentadiene, 5-methylene-
Bornane	Bicyclo[2.2.1]heptane, 1,7,7-trimethyl-	Fumaric acid	2-Butenedioic acid, (E)-
Butyl alcohol*	1-Butanol	2-Furaldehyde	2-Furancarboxaldehyde
sec-Butyl alcohol*	2-Butanol	Furfuryl alcohol	2-Furanmethanol
tert-Butyl alcohol*	2-Propanol, 2-methyl-	Furfurylamine	2-Furanmethanamine
Butylamine	1-Butanamine	Furoic acid	Furancarboxylic acid
Butyraldehyde	Butanal		
Butyric acid	Butanoic acid	Gallic acid	Benzoic acid, 3,4,5-trihydroxy-
Butyrophenone	1-Butanone, 1-phenyl-	Gentisic acid	Benzoic acid, 2,5-dihydroxy-
		Glutaconic acid	2-Pentenedioic acid
Caffeine	1H-Purine-2,6-dione,3,7-dihydro-1,3,7-trimethyl-	Glutaric acid	Pentanedioic acid
Camphene*	Bicyclo[2.2.1]heptane,2,2-dimethyl-3-methylene-	Glyceraldehyde	Propanal, 2,3-dihydroxy-
Camphor*	Bicyclo[2.2.1]heptan-2-one, 1,7,7-trimethyl-	Glyceric acid	Propanoic acid, 2,3-dihydroxy-
Carane	Bicyclo[4.1.0]heptane, 3,7,7-trimethyl-	Glycerol*	1,2,3-Propanetriol
Carbodiimide	Methanediimine	Glycidic acid	Oxiranecarboxylic acid
Carbostyril	2(1H)-Quinolinone	Glycolic acid	Acetic acid, hydroxyl-
Carvacrol	Phenol, 2-methyl-5-(1-methylethyl)-	Glyoxal	Ethanedial
Chalcone	2-Propen-1-one, 1,3-diphenyl-	Glyoxylic acid	Acetic acid, oxo-
Chroman	2H-1-Benzopyran, 3,4-dihydro-	Guanine	6H-Purin-6-one, 2-amino-1,7-dihydro-

* Name used in 8CI for unsubstituted substance only.

TABLE 3.3 (continued)

8CI Name	9CI Name	8CI Name	9CI Name
Heteroxanthine	1H-Purine-2,6-dione, 3,7-dihydro-7-methyl-	Maleic acid	2-Butenedioic acid, (Z)-
Hippuric acid	Glycine, N-benzoyl-	Maleic anhydride	2,5-Furandione
Hydantoin	2,4-Imidazolidinedione	Maleimide	1H-Pyrrole-2,5-dione
Hydracrylic acid	Propanoic acid, 3-hydroxy-	Malic acid	Butanedioic acid, hydroxy-
Hydratropic acid	Benzeneacetic acid, α-methyl-	Malonic acid	Propanedioic acid
Hydrazobenzene	Hydrazine, 1,2-diphenyl-	Mandelic acid	Benzeneacetic acid, α-hydroxy-
Hydrocinnamic acid	Benzenepropanoic acid	Melamine	1,3,5-Triazine-2,4,6-triamine
Hydrocoumarin	2H-1-Benzopyran-2-one, 3,4-dihydro-	Menthane	Cyclohexane, methyl(1-methylethyl)-
Hydroorotic acid	4-Pyrimidinecarboxylicacid,hexahydro-2,6-dioxo-	Mesaconic acid*	2-Butenedioic acid, 2-methyl-, (E)-
Hydroquinone	1,4-Benzenediol	Mesitol	Phenol, 2,4,6-trimethyl-
Hydrouracil	2,4(1H,3H)-Pyrimidinedione, dihydro-	Mesitylene	Benzene, 1,3,5-trimethyl
Hypoxanthine	6H-Purin-6-one, 1,7-dihydro-	Mesoxalic acid	Propanedioic acid, oxo-
		Metanilic acid	Benzenesulfonic acid, 3-amino-
Indan	1H-Indene, 2,3-dihydro-	Methacrylic acid*	2-Propenoic acid, 2-methyl
Indoline	1H-Indole, 2,3-dihydro-	Methyl sulfoxide*	Methane, sulfinylbis-
Indone	1H-Inden-1-one	Methylamine	Methanamine
Isobarbituric acid	2,4,5(3H)-Pyrimidinetrione, dihydro-	Methylenimine	Methanimine
Isobutyl alcohol*	1-Propanol, 2-methyl-	Myristic acid*	Tetradecanoic acid
Isobutyric acid*	Propanoic acid, 2-methyl-		
Isocaffeine	1H-Purine-2,6-dione,3,9-dihydro-1,3,9-trimethyl-	Naphthalic acid	1,8-Naphthalenedicarboxylic acid
Isocarbostyril	1(2H)-Isoquinolinone	Naphthoic acid	Naphthalenecarboxylic acid
Isochroman	1H-2-Benzopyran, 3,4-dihydro-	Naphthol	Naphthalenol
Isocoumarin	1H-2-Benzopyran-1-one	Naphthoquinone	Naphthalenedione
Isocytosine*	4(1H)-Pyrimidinone, 2-amino-	Naphthylamine	Naphthalenamine
Isoflavan	2H-1-Benzopyran, 3,4-dihydro-3-phenyl	Nicotinic acid	3-Pyridinecarboxylic acid
Isoflavanone	4H-1-Benzopyran-4-one, 2,3-dihydro-3-phenyl	Nipecotic acid	3-Piperidinecarboxylic acid
		Norbornane	Bicyclo[2.2.1]heptane
Isoflavone	4H-1-Benzopyran-4-one, 3-phenyl-	Norcarane	Bicyclo[4.1.0]heptane
Isoflavylium	1-Benzopyrylium, 3-phenyl-	Norpinane	Bicyclo[3.1.1]heptane
Isoguanine	2H-Purin-2-one, 6-amino-1,3-dihydro-		
Isohexyl alcohol*	1-Pentanol, 4-methyl-	Oleic acid	9-Octadecenoic acid, (Z)-
Isoindoline	1H-Isoindole, 2,3-dihydro-	Orotic acid	4-Pyrimidinecarboxylicacid,1,2,3,6-tetrahydro-2,6-dioxo-
Isonicotinic acid	4-Pyridinecarboxylic acid		
Isonipecotic acid	4-Piperidinecarboxylic acid	Oxalacetic acid	Butanedioic acid, oxo-
Isopentyl alcohol*	1-Butanol, 3-methyl-	Oxalic acid	Ethanedioic acid
Isophthalic acid	1,3-Benzenedicarboxylic acid		
Isoprene*	1,3-Butadiene, 2-methyl-	Palmitic acid*	Hexadecanoic acid
Isopropyl alcohol*	2-Propanol	Paraxanthine	1H-Purine-2,6-dione, 3,7-dihydro-1,7-dimethyl-
Isopropylamine	2-Propanamine	Pentaerythritol*	1,3-Propanediol, 2,2-bis-(hydroxymethyl)
Isoquinaldic acid	1-Isoquinolinecarboxylic acid	Pentyl alcohol*	1-Pentanol
Isovaleric acid*	Butanoic acid, 3-methyl-	tert-Pentyl alcohol*	2-Butanol, 2-methyl-
		Peroxyacetic acid	Ethaneperoxoic acid
Ketene	Ethenone	Peroxybenzoic acid	Benzenecarboperoxoic acid
		Phenethyl alcohol	Benzeneethanol
Lactic acid	Propanoic acid, 2-hydroxy	Phenethylamine	Benzeneethanamine
Lauric acid*	Dodecanoic acid	Phenetidine	Benzenamine, ar-ethoxy-
Lepidine	Quinoline, 4-methyl-	Phenetole	Benzene, ethoxy-
Levulinic acid	Pentanoic acid, 4-oxo-	Phenylenediamine	Benzenediamine
Linoleic acid	9,12-Octadecadienoic acid, (Z,Z)-	Phloroglucinol	1,3,5-Benzenetriol
Linolelaidic acid	9,12-Octadecadienoic acid, (E,E)-	Phthalan	Isobenzofuran, 1,3-dihydro
Linolenic acid	9,12,15-Octadecatrienoic acid, (Z,Z,Z)-	Phthalic acid	1,2-Benzenedicarboxylic acid
γ-Linolenic acid	6,9,12-Octadecatrienoic acid, (Z,Z,Z)-	Phthalic anhydride	1,3-Isobenzofurandione
Lumazine	2,4(1H,3H)-Pteridinedione	Phthalide	1(3H)-Isobenzofuranone
Lupetidine*	Piperidine, C,C′-dimethyl-	Phthalimide	1H-Isoindole-1,3(2H)-dione
Lutidine	Pyridine, dimethyl-	Phthalonic acid	Benzeneacetic acid, 2-carboxy-α-oxo-

* Name used in 8CI for unsubstituted substance only.

TABLE 3.3 (continued)

8CI Name	9CI Name	8CI Name	9CI Name
Phytol	2-Hexadecen-1-ol, 3,7,11,15-tetramethyl-	Stilbene	Benzene, 1,1'-(1,2-ethenediyl)bis-
Picoline	Pyridine, methyl-	Styrene	Benzene, ethenyl-
Picolinic acid	2-Pyridinecarboxylic acid	Suberic acid*	Octanedioic acid
Picric acid	Phenol, 2,4,6-trinitro-	Succinic acid	Butanedioic acid
Pimelic acid*	Heptanedioic acid	Succinic anhydride	2,5-Furandione, dihydro-
Pinane	Bicyclo[3.1.1]heptane, 2,7,7-trimethyl-	Succinimide	2,5-Pyrrolidinedione
Pipecolic acid	2-Piperidinecarboxylic acid	Sulfanilic acid	Benzenesulfonic acid, 4-amino-
Pipecoline	Piperidine, C-methyl-		
Piperonal	1,3-Benzodioxole-5-carboxaldehyde	Tartaric acid	Butanedioic acid, 2,3-dihydroxy-
Piperonylic acid	1,3-Benzodioxole-5-carboxylic acid	Tartronic acid	Propanedioic acid, hydroxy-
Pivalic acid*	Propanoic acid, 2,2-dimethyl-	Taurine	Ethanesulfonic acid, 2-amino-
Propiolic acid	2-Propynoic acid	Terephthalic acid	1,4-Benzenedicarboxylic acid
Propionaldehyde	Propanal	Tetrolic acid	2-Butynoic acid
Propionic acid	Propanoic acid	Theobromine	1H-Purine-2,6-dione, 3,7-dihydro-3,7-dimethyl-
Propionitrile	Propanenitrile	Theophylline	1H-Purine-2,6-dione, 3,7-dihydro-1,3-dimethyl
Propiophenone	1-Propanone, 1-phenyl-	Thujane	Bicyclo[3.1.0]hexane,4-methyl-1-(1-methylethyl)-
Propyl alcohol*	1-Propanol	Thymine	2,4(1H,3H)-Pyrimidinedione, 5-methyl-
Propylamine	1-Propanamine	Thymol	Phenol, 5-methyl-2-(1-methylethyl)-
Propylene oxide	Oxirane, methyl-	Toluene	Benzene, methyl-
Protocatechuic acid	Benzoic acid, 3,4-dihydroxy-	Toluic acid	Benzoic acid, methyl-
Pyridone	Pyridinone	Toluidine	Benzenamine, ar-methyl-
Pyrocatechol	1,2-Benzenediol	Triethylamine	Ethanamine, N,N-diethyl-
o-Pyrocatechuic acid	Benzoic acid, 2,3-dihydroxy	Trimethylamine	Methanamine, N,N-dimethyl-
Pyrogallol	1,2,3-Benzenetriol	Trimethylene oxide*	Oxetane
Pyruvic acid	Propanoic acid, 2-oxo-	Tropic acid*	Benzeneacetic acid, α-(hydroxymethyl)-
		Tropolone	2,4,6-Cycloheptatrien-1-one, 2-hydroxy-
Quinaldic acid	2-Quinolinecarboxylic acid		
Quinaldine	Quinoline, 2-methyl-	Uracil	2,4(1H,3H)-Pyrimidinedione
Quinolone	Quinolinone	Urete	1,3-Diazete
Quinuclidine	1-Azabicyclo[2.2.2]octane	Uretidine	1,3-Diazetidine
		Uric acid	1H-Purine-2,6,8(3H)-trione, 7,9-dihydro-
Resorcinol	1,3-Benzenediol		
α-Resorcylic acid	Benzoic acid, 3,5-dihydroxy-	Valeric acid	Pentanoic acid
β-Resorcylic acid	Benzoic acid, 2,4-dihydroxy-	Vanillic acid	Benzoic acid, 4-hydroxy-3-methoxy-
γ-Resorcylic acid	Benzoic acid, 2,6-dihydroxy-	Vanillin	Benzaldehyde, 4-hydroxy-3-methoxy-
Ricinelaidic acid	9-Octadecenoic acid, 12-hydroxy-, [R-(E)]-	Veratric acid	Benzoic acid, 3,4-dimethoxy-
Ricinoleic acid	9-Octadecenoic acid, 12-hydroxy-, [R-(Z)]-	o-Veratric acid	Benzoic acid, 2,3-dimethoxy-
		Vinyl alcohol	Ethenol
Salicylic acid	Benzoic acid, 2-hydroxy-		
Sarcosine	Glycine, N-methyl-	Xanthine	1H-Purine-2,6-dione, 3,7-dihydro
Sebacic acid*	Decanedioic acid	Xylene	Benzene, dimethyl-
Sorbic acid	2,4-Hexadienoic acid	Xylenol	Phenol, dimethyl-
Stearic acid*	Octadecanoic acid	Xylidine	Benzenamine, ar, ar'-dimethyl-

* Name used in 8CI for unsubstituted substance only.

3.2.2 Changes in CAS Nomenclature 1977–2006

CAS nomenclature was stable for most organics between 1977 and 2006 and the system was known as 9CI nomenclature.

The following specialised classes of organic substances or types of names were subject to changes during the twelfth (1987–1991) or thirteenth (1992–1996) Collective Index periods:

- Carbohydrate lactams
- Formazans
- Multiplicative names

- Nitrilimines
- Onium compounds (free radicals)
- Phosphonium ylides
- Phosphorylhaloids and halogenoids
- Zwitterions and sydnones
- List of common ring systems

Further major changes to CAS nomenclature affecting organics were made in 2006 and are described at www.cas.org.

Some examples of the 2006 changes affecting simple mainstream organics are shown here. Other changes affecting more specialised areas of nomenclature are referred to in the following chapter.

	9CI	New (2006) CAS Name
Ketones		
$Me_3Si–COCH_2CH_3$	Trimethyl(1-oxopropyl)silane	1-(Trimethylsilyl)-1-propanone
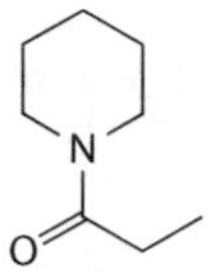	1-(1-Oxopropyl)piperidine	1(1-Piperidinyl)-1-propanone
Aldehydes substituted at the aldehydo hydrogen		
$H_3CCO–NO$	1-Nitrosoacetaldehyde	1-Nitrosoethanone
Silanes		
PhSiMe=O	Methyloxophenylsilane	(Methyloxosilyl)benzene
Acylheteroatom substances		
$Ph_2P–COCH_2CH_3$	(1-Oxopropyl)diphenylphosphine	1-(Diphenylphosphino)-1-propanone
Locants		
In various types of compounds where locants were previously omitted because the name was unambiguous without them, they are now inserted	Oxiranecarboxylic acid	2-Oxiranecarboxylic acid
	Bicyclo[2.2.2]octanone	Bicyclo[2.2.2]octan-2-one
	Propynoic acid	2-Propynoic acid
	Butanedioic acid, monoethyl ester	Butanedioic acid, 1-ethyl ester

3.3 TYPES OF NAME

Names may be of the following types:

- *Substitutive.* Substitution of hydrogen, usually, by another group, e.g., chloromethane. These names are the commonest.
- *Additive.* Addition of an atom or group of atoms, e.g., pyridine *N*-oxide, and decahydronaphthalene
- *Subtractive.* Loss of certain atoms or groups from a parent structure, e.g., *N*-demethylnitidine. Relatively common in natural product nomenclature, rare in mainstream organic chemistry.
- *Conjunctive*, e.g., cyclohexanemethanol. A conjunctive name may be applied when the principal functional group is attached to a *saturated* carbon chain that is directly attached to a cyclic component by a carbon-carbon *single* bond. A conjunctive name consists of the name of the parent ring system followed by the name of the alicyclic chain plus a suffix indicating the principal group. The ring retains its normal numbering; carbon atoms in the side chain are indicated by Greek letters. The terminal carbon atom of acids, acid halides, amides, aldehydes, and nitriles is *not* lettered. Extensively used in CAS.

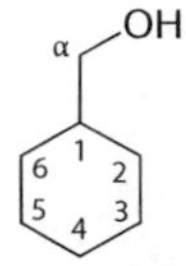

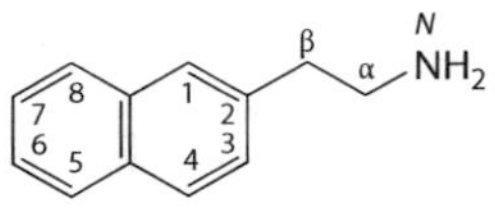

cyclohexanemethanol

2-naphthaleneethanamine

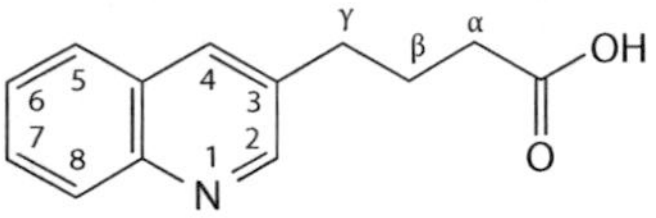

3-quinolinebutanoic acid
(substitutive equivalent is 4-(3-quinolinyl)butanoic acid)

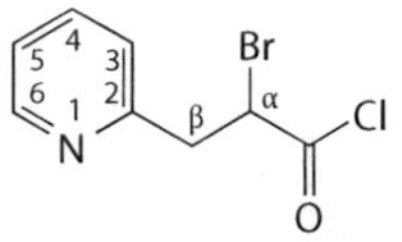

α-bromo-2-pyridinepropanoyl chloride

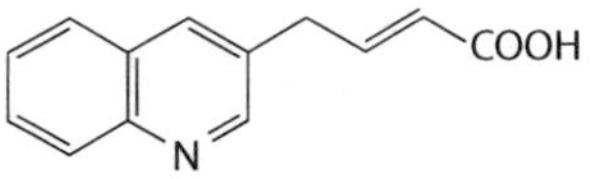

4-(3-quinolinyl)-2-butenoic acid

But note that in 4-(3-quinolinyl)-2-butenoic acid, the unsaturated chain means that substitutive nomenclature has to be used. Forms such as $\Delta^{\alpha,\beta}$-3-quinolinebutanoic acid are obsolete and should not be used.

- *Multiplicative,* e.g., 2,2′-thiobisacetic acid, $HOOCCH_2$-S-CH_2COOH. A multiplying radical, in this case *thio*, is used to join two or more identical fragments. These names are fairly extensively used in CAS, but only where the two joined fragments are completely identical, e.g., 2,2′-oxybispyridine but not 2,3′-oxybispyridine (CAS name 2-(3-pyridinyloxy)pyridine).
- *Radicofunctional,* e.g., methyl alcohol, ethyl methyl ketone, dimethyl peroxide. A name in which the principal function is expressed as a single-name term while the remainder of the structure attached to this function is described by one or more radicals. Largely obsolescent in organic chemistry, but still extensively used in the real world. Used by CAS only for disulfides, peroxides, and hydroperoxides.
- *Replacement,* e.g., azacyclotridecane. Organic replacement names are formed by denoting heteroatoms that replace skeletal atoms of a hydrocarbon molecular skeleton by organic replacement prefixes (Table 3.4). In nomenclature, the prefixes are cited in the order they are given in the table.

TABLE 3.4
Organic Replacement Prefixes

fluorine	fluora	phosphorus	phospha
chlorine	chlora	arsenic	arsa
bromine	broma	antimony	stiba
iodine	ioda	bismuth	bisma
oxygen	oxa	silicon	sila
sulfur	thia	germanium	germa
selenium	selena	tin	stanna
tellurium	tellura	lead	plumba
nitrogen	aza	boron	bora

Elision of vowels is not used in replacement nomenclature, thus *pentaoxa-* not *pentoxa-*. Prefixes *azonia*, *oxonia*, *thionia*, etc., denote replacement of a carbon atom by a positively charged atom.

Replacement names can be used for chains of atoms, usually when there are four or more heteroatoms. They are useful for naming polyethers:

$$H_3{}^1C-{}^2O-CH_2CH_2-O-CH_2CH_2-O-CH_2CH_2-O-CH_2CH_2-{}^{14}O-{}^{15}CH_3$$

2,5,8,11,14-pentaoxapentadecane

Replacement nomenclature is also used for some heterocyclic systems, including von Baeyer systems (see Chapter 4), large rings (>10 members) and some spiro compounds.

azacyclotridecane

silabenzene

3.4   CONSTRUCTING A SYSTEMATIC NAME

A systematic (e.g., CAS) name may have up to four components; the *heading parent*, the *substituents*, the *modifications*, and the *stereodescriptors*. Of these, only the first is always present; the others may or may not be.

3.4.1   THE HEADING PARENT

The heading parent, e.g., 2-butenoic acid, consists of a molecular skeleton (2-butene) and a suffix (-oic acid) detailing the *principal functional group*. There can only be one functional group in any one name.* (Note elision of the terminal -*e* in butene.) Where there is no functional group, the heading parent consists only of a molecular skeleton name, e.g., methane, pyridine.

The main types of molecular skeleton are the following:

- Unbranched chains of carbon atoms with or without multiple bonds, e.g., methane, propane, pentane, 1-butene, 1,3-pentadiyne.
- Rings or ring systems, e.g., cyclopentane, benzene, benzo[*b*]thiophene. The naming of the different types of ring systems is covered in Chapter 4.
- Conjunctive parents.

3.4.1.1   Choosing the Heading Parent

The first step in choosing the index heading parent is to identify the principal functional group (the term *characteristic group* is now preferred by IUPAC):

- If there is no functional group (alkanes, parent heterocyclic systems, etc.), just name the skeleton.
- If there is only one functional group, this takes precedence in nomenclature and numbering.

---

* Very occasional deviations from this IUPAC principle may sometimes be made for ease of nomenclature, e.g., in the *Dictionary of Natural Products* for compounds containing both lactone and carboxylic acid functions, e.g., 3,14-dihydroxycard-20(22)-enolid-19-oic acid. CAS does not do this.

TABLE 3.5
Functional Groups in Order of Priority

Functional Group		Suffix[a]	Prefix[a]
cations (e.g., ammonium)	E.g., $>N^+<$	-ium	
carboxylic acid	–COOH	-oic acid or -carboxylic acid[b]	carboxy
sulfonic acid	–SO$_3$H	-sulfonic acid	sulfo
carboxylic acid halide	–COX	-oyl halide or -carbonyl halide[b]	(haloformyl)
sulfonyl halide	–SO$_2$X	-sulfonyl halide	(halosulfonyl)
carboxamide	–CONH$_2$	-amide or -carboxamide[b]	(aminocarbonyl)
sulfonamide	–SO$_2$NH$_2$	-sulfonamide	(aminosulfonyl)
nitrile	–CN	-nitrile or -carbonitrile[b]	cyano
aldehyde	–CHO	-al or -carboxaldehyde[b]	formyl
ketone	=O	-one	oxo
thione	=S	-thione	thioxo
alcohol and phenol	–OH	-ol	hydroxy
thiol	–SH	-thiol	mercapto
amine	–NH$_2$	-amine	amino
imine	=NH	-imine	imino

[a] Only one type of function may be expressed as a suffix in a name. If more than one type of functional group is present, those of lower priority are expressed using substituent prefixes.

[b] The suffixes -oic acid, -oyl halide, -amide, -nitrile, and -al are used when the functional group is at the end of a carbon chain, as in pentanoic acid. The endings -carboxylic acid, etc., are used when the group is attached to a ring, as in 2-pyridinecarboxylic acid.

- If there are two or more different functional groups, consult Table 3.5, and the functional group highest in the list takes precedence. The other groups become substituents.
- If there are two or more identical functional groups, a choice of molecular skeletons is possible. The rules summarised below should give a choice, but in case of uncertainty, it is best to locate related compounds and name by analogy.

For example, consider the compound below:

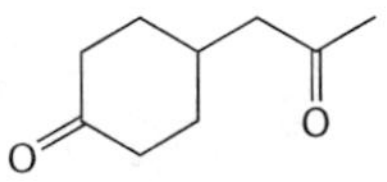

This contains two ketone groups which cannot be expressed as a single parent. The heading parent could either be cyclohexanone or 2-propanone but the correct name is 4-(2-oxopropyl)cyclohexanone. In order to arrive at this kind of conclusion, the following rules are applied in sequence until a decision is reached.

1. The preferred parent is that which expresses the maximum number of the principal function groups.

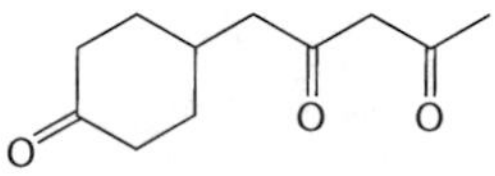

2,4-Pentanedione (expresses two ketone groups) > cyclohexanone (expresses only one ketone group) → **2,4-Pentanedione, 1-(4-oxocyclohexyl)-**.

2. A cyclic molecular skeleton is preferred to an acyclic carbon chain.

Cyclohexanone (cyclic skeleton) > 3-heptanone (acyclic skeleton) → **Cyclohexanone, 4-(3-oxoheptyl)-**.

3. The preferred parent is that which contains the maximum possible number of skeletal atoms.

1-Hexene (six atoms) > 1,4-pentadiene (five atoms) → **1-Hexene, 3-ethenyl-**.

4. For acyclic parents, the parent that expresses the maximum number of multiple bonds (double or triple) is preferred.

1,4-Pentadiene (two multiple bonds) > 1-pentene (one multiple bond) → **1,4-Pentadiene, 3-ethyl-**.

5. For acyclic parents with the same number of multiple bonds, double bonds are preferred to triple bonds.

1,4-Pentadiene (two double bonds) > 1-penten-4-yne (one double bond) → **1,4-Pentadiene, 3-ethynyl-**.

6. The preferred parent is that which contains the lowest locants for functional groups.

1,2-Benzenediol (locants 1,2) > 1,3-benzenediol (locants 1,3) → **1,2-Benzenediol, 3-[(2,4-dihydroxyphenyl)methyl]-**.

7. The preferred parent is that which contains the lowest locants for multiple bonds (double or triple).

2-Butyn-1-ol (multiple-bond locant 2) > 3-buten-1-ol (multiple-bond locant 3) → **2-Butyn-1-ol, 4-[(4-hydroxy-1-butenyl)oxy]-**.

8. The preferred parent is that which contains the lowest locants for double bonds.

2-Penten-4-yn-1-ol (double-bond locant 2) > 4-penten-2-yn-1-ol (double-bond locant 4)
→ **2-Penten-4-yn-1-ol, 5-[(5-hydroxy-1-penten-3-ynyl)oxy]-**.

9. The Index Name is based on that heading to which is attached the greatest number of substituents.

Propanoic acid, 3,3,3-trichloro-2-methyl-2-(nitromethyl)- (five substituents on the propanoic acid parent) > propanoic acid, 2-methyl-3-nitro-2-(trichloromethyl)- (three substituents attached to the parent propanoic acid) or propanoic acid, 2-(nitromethyl)-2-(trichloromethyl)- (two substituents on the propanoic acid parent).

10. The Index Name is based on that parent which gives the lowest locants for substituents.

Benzoic acid, 3-(4-carboxyphenoxy)- (substituent at the 3 position on the parent benzoic acid) > benzoic acid, 4-(3-carboxyphenoxy)- (substituents at the 4 position).

11. If no decision has been made at this point, a multiplicative name may be possible (see Section 3.3).

Ethanol, 2,2′-iminobis-.

12. If no decision can be made at this point, the CA Index Name will appear first in the CA Substance Index.

Propanoic acid, 2,3,3,3-tetrafluoro-2-(trichloromethyl)- > propanoic acid, 3,3,3-tri-chloro-2-fluoro-2-(trifluoromethyl)- because it would appear first alphabetically in the CA Substance Index (tetrafluoro comes before trichloro).

3.4.2 Functional Groups

If more than one type of functional group is present, the one highest in the list is treated as the principal functional group (Table 3.5). Some groups can never be functional groups, only substituents, e.g., *chloro-, nitro-* (distinct from the very early literature where nitro, for example, was treated as a functional group).

Fully substitutive names for certain types of compounds, especially heterocyclic, also occur. Examples are 2-aminopyridine for 2-pyridinamine, 2-formylpyridine for 2-pyridinecarboxaldehyde, and 2-cyanopyridine for 2-pyridinecarbonitrile. Such forms are technically incorrect, but frequently occur. Others, such as 2-carboxypyridine for 2-pyridinecarboxylic acid, are sometimes encountered but should not be used.

3.4.3 FUNCTIONAL REPLACEMENT NOMENCLATURE

This occurs when one or more oxygen atoms in a functional group are notionally replaced by other heteroatoms. Depending on the hierarchy, this may lead to the use of functional replacement prefixes (e.g., seleno in selenoacetic acid, $H_3C-C(=Se)OH$), infixes, or suffixes (e.g., in benzenecarbodithioic acid, $Ph-C(=S)-SH$).

Because of the large number of possible functional groups thus generated, IUPAC guidance is incomplete, and there is also considerable duplication of possible names, e.g., $-CH=Se$ is selenoformyl or selenoxomethyl. Table 3.6 gives a list of common replacement suffixes.

TABLE 3.6
Common Functional Replacement Suffixes

-aldehydic acid	Denotes that one COOH group of a trivially named dicarboxylic acid has been replaced by a CHO group; thus, malonaldehydic acid is $OHCCH_2COOH$
-azonic acid	$R_2N(O)OH$
-carbodithioic acid	$-C(S)SH$
-carbohydrazonic acid	$-C(OH)=NNH_2$
-carbohydroxamic acid	$-C(=NOH)OH$
-carbohydroximic acid	$-C(O)NHOH$
-carbonitrile	$-C\equiv N$
-carbonitrolic acid	$-C(=NOH)NO_2$
-carbonitrosolic acid	$-C(=NOH)NO$
-carboperoxoic acid	$-C(O)OOH$
-carboselenaldehyde	$-C(=Se)H$
-carboselenoic acid	$-C(=Se)OH$ or $-C(=O)SeH$
-carboselenothioic acid	$-C(=Se)SH$ or $-C(=S)SeH$
-carbothioaldehyde	$-C(=S)H$
-carbothioamide	$-C(=S)NH_2$
-carbothioic acid	$-C(=S)OH$ (-carbothioic O-acid) or $-C(O)SH$ (-carbothioic S-acid)
-carboxamide	$-CONH_2$
-carboxamidine	$-C(=NH)NH_2$
-carboxamidoxime	$-C(=NOH)NH_2$
-carboxamidrazone	$-C(=NHNH_2) NH_2$
-carboxanilide	$-CONHPh$
-carboximidamide	$-C(=NH)NH_2$
-carboximidic acid	$-C(=NH)OH$
-hydrazonic acid	$-C(=NNH_2)OH$
-hydroxamic acid	$-C(O)NHOH$
-hydroximic acid	$-C(=NOH)OH$
-imidic acid	$-C(=NH)OH$
-nitrolic acid	$-C(=NOH)NO_2$
-nitrosolic acid	$-C(=NOH)NO$

TABLE 3.6 (continued)
Common Functional Replacement Suffixes

-peroxoic acid	Suffix denoting –C(O)OOH as part of an aliphatic chain; thus, propaneperoxoic acid is $H_3CCH_2C(O)OOH$
-selenal	–C(Se)H
-selenamide	–$SeNH_2$
-selenenic acid	–SeOH; selenium analogues of sulfenic acids
-seleninamide	–$Se(O)NH_2$
-seleninic acid	–Se(O)OH; selenium analogues of sulfinic acids
-selenonamide	–$Se(O)_2NH_2$
-selenonic acid	–$Se(O)_2OH$; selenium analogues of sulfonic acids
-sulfenamide	–SNH_2; thus, ethanesulfenamide is $EtSNH_2$
-sulfenic acid	–S–OH
-sulfinamide	–$S(O)NH_2$
-sulfinamidine	–$S(=NH)NH_2$
-sulfinic acid	–S(O)OH
-sulfinimidic acid	–S(=NH)OH
-sulfinohydrazonic acid	–$S(OH)=NNH_2$
-sulfinohydroximic acid	–S(OH)=NOH
-sulfonamide	–SO_2NH_2
-sulfonic acid	–$S(O)_2OH$
-sulfonimidic acid	–S(O)(OH)=NH
-sulfonohydrazide	–SO_2NHNH_2
-sulfonohydrazonic acid	–$S(O)(OH)=NNH_2$
-sulfonohydroximic acid	–S(O)(OH)=NOH
-tellurenamide	–$TeNH_2$
-tellurenic acid	–TeOH
-tellurinamide	–$Te(O)NH_2$
-tellurinic acid	–Te(O)OH
-telluronamide	–$Te(O)_2NH_2$
-telluronic acid	–$Te(O)_2OH$
-thioamide	–$C(S)NH_2$ at the end of an aliphatic chain
-thioic acid	–C(S)OH (-thioic *O*-acid) or –C(O)SH (-thioic *S*-acid) at the end of an aliphatic chain; *-dithioic acid* denotes –C(S)SH

3.4.4 SUBSTITUENTS

Groups that are not the functional group become substituents (Table 3.7). In 3-amino-2-chloro-2-butenoic acid, the –COOH group is the principal functional group and the –Cl and –NH_2 groups are substituents. If the carboxylic group were not present, the amino group would become the principal functional group and the compound would be a chlorobutenamine. (The –Cl group can never be a functional group.)

Substituents marked with an asterisk should not be used in constructing formal names, either because they are definitely obsolete or because they are informal descriptors often used in free text but not approved for constructing actual names (e.g., aryl, brosyl). Apart from these, the list does not give a definite preference for one alternative over another, except in a few cases (e.g., caproyl), which should definitely be avoided because of inaccuracy or ambiguity. Different publications, including CAS, have different editorial preferences.

In the CAS indexes, substituents follow a dash and a comma of inversion.

TABLE 3.7
Substituents

Acetamido	(Acetylamino) $H_3CCONH-$
Acetimido	This radical name has been used both for (acetylimino) $AcN=$ and for (1-iminoethyl) $H_3CC(=NH)-$
Acetimidoyl	(1-Iminoethyl) $H_3CC(=NH)-$
Acetoacetyl	(1,3-Dioxobutyl) H_3CCOCH_2CO-
Acetohydrazonoyl	$H_3CC(NHNH_2)-$
Acetohydroximoyl	$H_3CC(NHOH)-$
Acetonyl*	(2-Oxopropyl) H_3CCOCH_2-
Acetoxy	(Acetyloxy) H_3CCOO-
Acetyl	H_3CCO-; often abbreviated to Ac in structural and line formulae
aci-Nitr(o)amino	$HON(O)=N-$
aci-Nitro	$HON(O)=$ (methyl-*aci*-nitro) is $MeON(O)=$; *aci*-nitro compounds are also known as nitronic acids
Acryl(o)yl*	(1-Oxo-2-propenyl) $H_2C=CHCO-$
Acyl*	General term for a radical formed from an acid by removal of a hydroxy group, e.g., H_3CCO-, $PhSO_2-$; names for acyl radicals are derived by changing the endings: *-ic acid* to *-yl*, *-oic acid* to *-oyl*, and *-carboxylic acid* to *-carbonyl*
Adipoyl*	Hexanedioyl, $-CO-(CH_2)_4-CO-$
Allophanyl*	$H_2NCONHCO-$
Allyl	2-Propenyl $H_2C=CCH_2$
β-Allyl*	(1-Methylethenyl) $H_2C=C(CH_3)-$
Allylidene*	2-Propenylidene $H_2C=CHCH=$
Amidino/guanyl/carbamimidoyl	$HN=C(NH_2)-$
Amido	Denotes a radical formed by loss of a hydrogen from an amide group; thus, acetamido is $H_3CCONH-$
Aminosulfinyl	H_2NSO- (*not* sulfinamoyl)
Aminosulfonyl/sulfamoyl/ sulfurimidoyl	H_2NSO_2-
Aminothio/aminosulfanyl	H_2NS-
Amin(o)oxy	H_2N-O-
Amyl*	Pentyl $H_3C(CH_2)_4-$
tert-Amyl*	(1,1-Dimethylpropyl) $H_3CCH_2C(CH_3)_2-$
Angeloyl	(Z)-(2-Methyl-1-oxo-2-butenyl), (Z)-$H_3CCH=C(CH_3)CO-$; the (E)-form is tigloyl
Anilino	(Phenylamino) $PhNH-$
Anisoyl*	(Methoxybenzoyl) thus, *o*-anisoyl is 2-$MeOC_6H_4CO-$
Anthran(il)oyl*	(2-Aminobenzoyl)-2-$H_2NC_6H_4CO-$
Anthroyl*	(Anthracenylcarbonyl) $(C_{14}H_9)CO-$
Anthryl	Anthracenyl $(C_{14}H_9)-$
Anthrylene	Anthracenediyl $-(C_{14}H_8)-$
Aralkyl*	A general name for a radical comprising an aryl group attached to an alkyl radical, e.g., $PhCH_2CH_2-$
Aryl*	General term for a monovalent radical derived by loss of hydrogen from an aromatic hydrocarbon
Arylene*	General term for a divalent radical derived by loss of hydrogens from two different atoms of an aromatic hydrocarbon
Azido	N_3-
Azimino	$-N=NNH-$; used as a bridge name in naming bridged fused ring systems

* Substituents not to be used in constructing formal names.

TABLE 3.7 (continued)
Substituents

Azinico/hydroxyazonoyl/ hydroxyazinylidene/ hydroxynitroroyl	$HO-N(O)(S)-$
Azino/hydrazinediylidene	$=N-N=$
Azinoyl/azinyl/dihydronitroryl	$H_2N(O)-$
Azinylidene/azonoyl/hydronitroroyl	$HN(O)<$ or $HN(O)=$
Azo/diazenediyl	$-N=N-$
Azono	$(HO)_2N(O)-$
Azonoyl/azinylidene/hydronitroryl	$HN(O)<$ or $-N=N(O)=$
Azoxy	$-N=N(O)-$
Benzal	(Phenylmethylene) $PhCH=$
Benzamido/benzoylamino/ benzenecarbonylamino	$PhCONH-$
Benzenesulfenamido/(phenylthio) amino	$Ph-S-NH-$
Benzenesulfinyl/phenylsulfinyl	$PhSO-$
Benzenesulfonamido/ benzenesulfonylamino/ (phenylsulfonyl)amino	$PhSO_2NH-$
Benzenesulfony/phenylsulfonyl	$PhSO_2-$
Benzhydryl*	(Diphenylmethyl) Ph_2CH-
Benzhydrylidene/ diphenylmethylidene/ diphenylmethylene*	$Ph_2C=$
Benzimidoyl/benzenecarboximidoyl	$PhC(=NH)-$
Benzohydroximoyl/ benzenecarbohydroximoyl	$PhC(=NOH)-$
Benzoyl/phenylcarbonyl/ benzenecarbonyl	$Ph-CO-$
Benzyl	(Phenylmethyl) $PhCH_2-$
Benzylidene	(Phenylmethylene) $PhCH=$
Benzylidyne	(Phenylmethylidyne) $PhC\equiv$
Benzyloxy/phenylmethoxy	$PhCH_2O-$
Boranediyl	$BH<$
Boranetriyl	$-B<$
Boryl	H_2B-
Borylene/boranylidene	$HB=$
Borylidyne	$B\equiv$, $-B<$ or, $-B=$; the three possibilities are more accurately described as boranylidyne, boranetriyl, and boranylylidene, respectively
Bromonio	H^+Br-
Bromonium	H_2Br^+-
Brosyl*	p-Bromobenzenesulfonyl
Butyryl*	(1-Oxobutyl) $H_3CCH_2CH_2CO-$
sec-Butyl*	(1-Methylpropyl) $H_3CCH_2CH(CH_3)-$; often abbreviated to Bu^s or s-Bu in structural formula
tert-Butyl	(1,1-Dimethylethyl) $(H_3C)_3C-$; often abbreviated to Bu^t or t-Bu in structural formula

(continued on next page)

* Substituents not to be used in constructing formal names.

TABLE 3.7 (continued)
Substituents

Caprinoyl*	Decanoyl; *definitely avoid*; strong possibilities for confusion with hexanoyl or octanoyl; see below
Caproyl*	Hexanoyl; *definitely avoid*; see below
Capryl*	Decanoyl; *definitely avoid*; the derived acyl group becomes caproyl, which is identical with the obsolete name for hexanoyl above (caprinoyl was used instead); in addition, capryl was sometimes used in the old literature for octyl
Capryl(o)yl*	Octanoyl; *definitely avoid*; see above
Carbamido	[(Aminocarbonyl)amino] $H_2NCONH–$
Carbam(o)yl	(Aminocarbonyl) $H_2NCO–$
Carbaniloyl	[(Phenylamino)carbonyl] PhNHCO–
Carbazimidoyl/ hydrazinecarboximidoyl	$H_2NNHC(=NH)–$
Carbazono/2-diazenecarbonylhydrazinyl	HN=NCONHNH–
Carbazoyl/hydrazinecarbonyl/ hydrazinylcarbonyl	$H_2NNHCO–$
Carb(o)ethoxy/ethoxycarbonyl	EtOOC–
Carbobenzoxy/ phenylmethoxycarbonyl	$PhCH_2OOC–$
Carbomethoxy/methoxycarbonyl	MeOOC–
Carbonimidoyl/iminomethylene	=C=NH or >C(=NH); the two possibilities can be systematically distinguished as iminomethylidene and iminomethanediyl, respectively
Carbonothioyl/thiocarbonyl	>C(=S)
Carbonyl	>C=O
Cathyl*	(Ethoxycarbonyl) EtOC(O)–
Cetyl*	Hexadecyl $H_3C(CH_2)_{15}–$
Chlorocarbonyl/carbonochloridoyl/ chloroformyl	ClCO–
Chlorosyl	OCl–
Chloryl	$O_2Cl–$
Cinnamoyl	(1-Oxo-3-phenyl-2-propenyl) PhCH=CHCO–; usually refers to the *E*-form
Cinnamyl*	(3-Phenyl-2-propenyl) $PhCH=CHCH_2–$
Cinnamylidene*	(3-Phenyl-2-propenylidene) PhCH=CHCH=
Cresoxy*	(Methylphenoxy) $H_3CC_6H_4O–$
Cresyl*	(Methylphenyl) $H_3CC_6H_4–$ or (hydroxymethylphenyl) $HO(H_3C)C_6H_3–$
Croton(o)yl*	(1-Oxo-2-butenyl) $H_3CCH=CHCO–$
Crotyl*	2-Butenyl $H_3CCH=CHCH_2–$
Cumenyl*	Isopropylphenyl $(H_3C)_2CHC_6H_4–$
Cumoyl*	4-Isopropylbenzoyl $4-(H_3C)_2CHC_6H_4CO–$
Cumyl*	Isopropylphenyl $(H_3C)_2CHC_6H_4$
α-Cumyl*	(1-Methyl-1-phenylethyl) $PhC(CH_3)_2–$
Cyanato	NCO–
Cyano	NC–
Dansyl*	[[5-(Dimethylamino)-1-naphthalenyl]sulfonyl]
Desyl*	(2-Oxo-1,2-diphenylethyl) PhCOCHPh–
Diazeno	Diazenyl HN=N–

* Substituents not to be used in constructing formal names.

TABLE 3.7 (continued)
Substituents

Diazo	N_2=; thus, diazomethane is H_2CN_2; diazo compounds are compounds containing the diazo group, R_2CN_2; the term *diazo* has also been used in naming compounds RN=NX; for example, benzenediazohydroxide is PhN=NOH, benzenediazocyanide is PhN=NCN, and benzenediazosulfonic acid is PhN=NSO$_3$H
Diazoamino	–N=NNH–
Diazonio	N_2^+–
Diphosphino/diphosphanyl	H_2PPH–
Disilanyl	H_3Si–SiH$_2$–
Dithio/disulfanediyl	–S–S–
Dithiocarboxy	HSC(S)–
Dithioperoxy/thiosulfeno/disulfanyl	HS–S–
Dithiosulfonyl/sulfonodithioyl	–S(=S)$_2$–
Duryl*	(2,3,5,6-Tetramethylphenyl)
Durylene*	(2,3,5,6-Tetramethyl-1,4-benzenediyl)
Enanth(o)yl*	(1-Oxoheptyl) H_3C(CH$_2$)$_5$CO–
Epidioxy	–O–O– (connecting two atoms in the same ring or chain)
Epidithio	–S–S– (bridge)
Epimino	–NH– (bridge)
Epithio	–S– (bridge)
Epox(y)imino	–O–NH– (bridge)
Epoxymethano	–O–CH$_2$– (bridge)
Epoxythio	–O–S– (bridge)
1,2-Ethanediyl	–CH$_2$CH$_2$–; also called ethano when a bridge
Ethano	–CH$_2$CH$_2$– (bridge)
Ethenyl/vinyl	H_2C=CH–
Ethenylidene	H_2C=C=
Ethoxy	EtO–
Ethoxycarbonyl	EtO$_2$C–
Ethyl	H_3CCH$_2$–; often abbreviated as Et in structural and line formulae
Ethylenebis(oxy)	–OCH$_2$CH$_2$O–
Ethylenedioxy	–CH$_2$CH$_2$–O–O–
Ethylidene	H_3CCH=
Ethylidyne	H_3CCH=
Ethylthio	EtS–
Ethynyl	HC≡C–
Fluoryl	O_2F–
Formamido/formylamino	HCONH–
1-Formazanyl (hydrazonomethyl)azo or (diazanylidenemethyl)diazenyl	H_2NN=CHN=N–
3-Formazanyl	(Diazenehydrazono)methyl H_2NN=C(N=NH)–
5-Formazanyl (diazanylmethylene) hydrazinyl	HN=NCH=NNH–
Formazyl	[(Phenylazo)(phenylhydrazonyl)methyl] PhN=NC(=NNHPh)–
Formimidoyl	(Iminomethyl) HN=CH–

(continued on next page)

* Substituents not to be used in constructing formal names.

TABLE 3.7 (continued)
Substituents

Forminato*	–CNO
Formyl/methanoyl	–CH=O; sometimes used as a substituent in fully substitutive names for aldehydes, e.g., 2-formylpyridine (technically incorrect) = 2-pyridinecarboxaldehyde
Formyloxy	–O–CHO
Fumar(o)yl*	(E)-(1,4-Dioxo-2-butene-1,4-diyl) –COCH=CHCO–; the (Z)-form is maleoyl
Furfuryl*	(2-Furanylmethyl)
Furfurylidene*	(2-Furanylmethylene)
Furoyl*	(Furanylcarbonyl)
Furyl*	A contracted form of furanyl
Galloyl*	(3,4,5-Trihydroxybenzoyl) 3,4,5-$(HO)_3C_6H_2CO$–
Gentisoyl*	(2,5-Dihydroxybenzoyl) 2,5-$(HO)_2C_6H_3CO$–
Germyl	H_3Ge
Germylene	$H_2Ge<$ or $H_2Ge=$. These can be distinguished by the more formal names germanediyl and germanylidene, respectively
Glutar(o)yl	(1,5-Dioxo-1,5-pentanediyl) –$CO(CH_2)_3CO$–
Glyceroyl*	(2,3-Dihydroxy-1-oxopropyl) $HOCH_2CH(OH)CO$–
Glyceryl*	1,2,3-Propanetriyl –$CH(CH_2–)_2$
Glycidyl*	Oxiranylmethyl
Glyco(l)loyl/glyco(l)lyl*	(Hydroxyacetoxy) $HOCH_2CO$–
Glycyl*	(Aminoacetyl) H_2NCH_2CO–
Glyoxal(in)yl*	Imidazolyl
Glyoxyl(o)yl*	(Oxoacetyl) OHCCO–
Guanidino/amidinoamino/ carbamidoylamino/ aminoiminomethyl (CAS)	$HN=C(NH_2)$–NH–
Guanyl	(Aminoiminomethyl) $H_2NC(=NH)$–
Hal(gen)o*	A general term for a monovalent substituent derived from a halogen atom F–, Cl–, Br–, I–
Hippur(o)yl*	N-Benzoylglycyl $PhCONHHCH_2CO$–
Homoallyl*	3-Butenyl $H_2C=CHCH_2CH_2$–
Hydantoyl*	(Carbamoylamino) acetyl or [(aminocarbonyl)amino}acetyl, $H_2NCONHCH_2CO$–
Hydrazino/hydrazinyl/diazanyl	H_2NNH–
Hydrazono/hydrazinylidene	$H_2NN=$
Hydrocinnamoyl*	(1-Oxo-3-phenylpropyl) $PhCH_2CH_2CO$–
Hydrocinnamyl*	(3-Phenylpropyl) $Ph(CH_2)_3$–
Hydrohydroxynitroroyl/ hydroxyazin(o)yl	HONH(O)–
Hydroperoxy	HO–O–
Hydroperoxycarbonyl/peroxycarboxy	HO–O–CO–
Hydroseleno	HSe–
Hydrox(y)amino	HONH–
Hydrox(y)imino	HONH=
Hydrox(y) iminomethyl/C-hydroxycarbonimidoyl	HN=C(OH)–
Hydroxyphosphinidine	>POH or =POH

* Substituents not to be used in constructing formal names.

TABLE 3.7 (continued)
Substituents

Hydroxyphosphinyl/ hydrohydroxyphosphoryl	$-PH(=O)OH$
Hydroxysulfonothioyl/ hydroxy(thiosulfonyl)	$HO–S(=O)(=S)–$
Imidiocarbonyl/carbonimidoyl	$-C(=NH)–$
Imidodicarbonyl/iminodicarbonyl	$-CONHCO–$
Iminio	$H_2N^+=$
Imino	$HN=$ or $HN<$; the two types can more accurately be described as azanylidene and azanediyl, respectively
Iminomethylene	$HN=C(NH)<$ or $HN=C=$; the two types can more accurately be described as iminomethanediyl and iminomethylidene, respectively
Indyl	A contracted form of indolyl
Iodonio	$HI^+–$
Iodonium	$H_2I^+–$
Iodoso/iodosyl	$OI–$
Iodoxy/iodyl	$O_2I–$
Isoallyl*	1-Propenyl $H_3CCH=CH–$
Isoamyl*	(3-Methylbutyl) $(H_3C)_2CHCH_2CH_2–$ (in the old literature, usually italicised as *iso*-amyl, so indexes under *a*)
Isobutenyl*	2-Methyl-1-propenyl, $(H_3C)_2C=CH–$
Isobutoxy*	(2-Methylpropoxy) $(H_3C)_2CHCH_2O–$
Isobutyl*	(2-Methylpropyl) $(H_3C)_2CHCH_2–$; often abbreviated to Bu^i or *i*-Bu in structural and line formulae; in the old literature, usually italicised as *iso*-butyl, so indexes under *b*
Isobutylidene*	(2-Methylpropylidene) $(H_3C)_2CHCH–$
Isobutyryl*	(2-Methyl-1-oxopropyl) $(H_3C)_2CHCO–$
Isocarbazido/isocarbonohydrazido	$H_2N=C(OH)NHNH–$
Isocrotyl*	(2-Methyl-1-propenyl) $(H_3C)_2C=CH–$
Isocyanato	$OCN–$
Isocyano	$CN–$
Isohexyl*	(4-Methylpentyl) $(H_3C)_2CH(CH_2)_3–$
Isoleucyl	$H_3CCH(CH_3)CH(NH_2)CO–$; the acyl radical from isoleucine used in naming peptides
Isonicotinoyl*	(4-Pyridinylcarbonyl)
Isonitro	*aci*-Nitro $HON(O)=$
Isonitroso(hydroxyimino)	$HON=$; *isonitroso compounds* is an obsolete term for oximes
Isopentenyl*	3-Methyl-2-butenyl; *definitely avoid*; use either the systematic form or, for brevity, the trivial prefix name *prenyl*
Isopentyl*	(3-Methylbutyl) $(H_3C)_2CHCH_2CH_2–$ (in the old literature, usually italicised as *iso*pentyl, so indexes under *p*)
Isopentylidene*	(3-Methylbutylidene) $(H_3C)_2CHCH_2CH=$
Isophthaloyl*	1,2-Phenylenedicarbonyl $1,3-C_6H_4(CO–)_2$
Isopropenyl*	(1-Methylethenyl) $H_2C=C(CH_3)–$
Isopropoxy	(1-Methylethoxy) $(H_3C)_2CHO–$
Isopropyl	(1-Methylethyl) $(H_3C)_2CH–$ (in the old literature, usually italicised as *iso*propyl, so indexes under *p*)

(continued on next page)

* Substituents not to be used in constructing formal names.

TABLE 3.7 (continued)
Substituents

Isopropylidene	(1-Methylethylidene) $(H_3C)_2C=$
Isoselenocyanato	SeCN–
Isosemicarbazido	HN=C(OH)NHNH–
Isothiocyanato	SCN–
1-Isoureido*	[(Iminohydroxymethyl)amino] HN=C(OH)NH–
3-Isoureido*	[(Aminohydroxymethylene)amino] $H_2NC(OH)=N–$
Isovaleryl*	(3-Methyl-1-oxobutyl) $(H_3C)_2CHCH_2CO–$
Isovalyl	$H_3CCH_2C(CH_3)(NH_2)CO–$; the acyl radical from isovaline used in naming peptides
Lactoyl*	(2-Hydroxy-1-oxopropyl) $H_3CCH(OH)CO–$
Lauroyl*	(1-Oxododecyl) $H_3C(CH_2)_{10}CO–$
Lauryl*	Dodecyl $H_3C(CH_2)_{11}$
L(a)evulinoyl*	(1,4-Dioxopentyl) $H_3CCOCH_2CH_2CO–$
Maleoyl*	(Z)-(1,4-Dioxo-2-butene-1,4-diyl) –COCH=CHCO–; the E-form is fumaroyl
Maleyl*	(Z)-(3-Carboxy-1-oxo-2-propenyl) HOOCCH=CHCO–
Malon(o)yl*	(1,3-Dioxo-1,3-propanediyl) $–COCH_2CO–$
Maloyl*	(2-Hydroxy-1,4-dioxo-1,4-butanediyl) $–COCH_2CH(OH)CO–$
Mandeloyl*	(Hydroxyphenylacetyl) PhCH(OH)CO–
Mercapto/sulfanyl	–SH
Mercaptocarbonyl/sulfanylcarbonyl	HS–CO–
Mercaptooxy/sulfanyloxy	HS(O)–
Mercaptophosphinyl/ hydromercaptophosphoryl/ mercaptooxophosphoranyl	HS–PH(=O)–
Mercaptosulfonyl	$HS–SO_2–$
Mesaconoyl*	E-[2-Methyl-1,4-dioxo-2-butene-1,4-diyl] $–COCH=C(CH_3)CO–$; the Z-form is citraconyl
Mesidino*	[(2,4,6-Trimethylphenyl)amino] $2,4,6-(H_3C)_3C_6H_2NH–$
Mesityl*	(2,4,6-Trimethylphenyl) $2,4,6-(H_3C)_3C_6H_2–$
α-Mesityl*	[(3,5-Dimethylphenyl)methyl] $3,5-(H_3C)_2C_6H_3CH_2–$
Mesoxalo*/carboxyoxoacetyl	HOOCCOCO–
Mesoxyalyl*	(1,2,3-Trioxo-1,3-propanediyl) –COCOCO–
Mesyl	Methanesulfonyl $MeSO_2–$
Metanilyl*	[(3-Aminophenyl)sulfonyl] $3-H_2NC_6H_4SO_2–$
Methacryloyl*	(2-Methyl-1-oxo-2-propenyl) $H_2C=C(CH_3)CO–$
Methallyl*	(2-Methyl-2-propenyl) $H_2C=C(CH_3)CH_2–$
Methanediylidene	=C=
Methanesulfinyl	Me–SO–
Methanesulfonamido	(Methylsulfonyl)amino $MeSO_2NH–$
Methanetetrayl	>C<
Methanetriyl	–CH<
Methano	$–CH_2–$ (bridge)
Methanylylidene	–CH=
Methenyl*	Methylidyne HC≡
Methoxalyl*	Methoxyoxoacetyl or (methoxycarbonyl)acetyl MeOCO–CO–
Methoxycarbonyl	$MeO_2C–$
Methoxythio	MeO–S–

* Substituents not to be used in constructing formal names.

TABLE 3.7 (continued)
Substituents

Methyl	H_3C-; often denoted by Me in structural and line formulae
Methyldioxy/methylperoxy	Me–O–O–
Methyldithio/methyldisulfanyl	Me–S–S–
Methylene	–CH$_2$– or CH$_2$=; the former is more correctly called methanediyl and the latter methylidene, although *methylene* remains in widespread use for both; compounds containing two CH$_2$= groups should be called bis(methylene) not dimethylene
Methylenedioxy/methylenebis(oxy)	–O–CH$_2$–O–
Methylidene	Methylene H$_2$C= or –CH$_2$–
Methylidyne	HC≡
Methylol*	(Hydroxymethyl) HOCH$_2$–
Methylthio/methylsulfanyl	Me–S–
Methyltrithio/methyltrisulfanyl	Me–S–S–S–
Morpholino	4-Morpholinyl
Myristoyl*	(1-Oxotetradecyl) H$_3$C(CH$_2$)$_{12}$CO–
Myristyl*	Tetradecyl H$_3$C(CH$_2$)$_{13}$–
Naphthenyl*	(Naphthalenylmethylidyne) (C$_{10}$H$_7$)C≡
Naphthionyl*	[(4-Amino-1-naphthalenyl)sulfonyl] 4,1-H$_2$NC$_{10}$H$_7$SO$_2$–
Naphthobenzyl*	(Naphthalenylmethyl) (C$_{10}$H$_7$)CH$_2$–
Naphthoxy	(Naphthalenyloxy) (C$_{10}$H$_7$)O–
Naphthoyl	(Naphthalenylcarbonyl) (C$_{10}$H$_7$)CO–
Naphthyl	Contracted form of naphthalenyl
Naphthylene	Naphthalenediyl
Nazyl*	(Naphthalenylmethyl) (C$_{10}$H$_7$)CH$_2$–
Neopentyl*	(2,2-Dimethylpropyl) (H$_3$C)$_3$CCH$_2$–
Neophyl*	2-Methyl-2-phenylpropyl PhC(CH$_3$)$_2$CH$_2$–
Nicotinoyl*	(3-Pyridinylcarbonyl)
Nitramino	(Nitroamino) O$_2$NNH–
Nitrilio	HN$^+$≡
Nitrilo	≡N or –N= or –N<; the three types can be distinguished using the more precise prefixes *azanylidyne*, *azanylylidene*, and *azanetriyl*, respectively, but these are not yet widely used
aci-Nitro	HON(O)=
Nitroryl	≡NO
Nitros(o)amino	ON–NH–
Nitros(o)imino	ON–N=
Nitroso	ON–; nitroso compounds are compounds RNO
Norbornyl*	A contracted form of norbornanyl, the radical derived from norbornane
Norcaryl*	A contracted form of norcaranyl, the radical derived from norcarane
Norleucyl*	H$_3$C(CH$_2$)$_3$CH(NH$_2$)CO–; the acyl radical from norleucine used in naming peptides; in this case the prefix *nor* means normal, i.e., the straight-chain isomer of leucine
Norpinyl*	A contracted form of norpinanyl, the radical derived from norpinane
Nosyl*	[(4-Nitrophenyl)sulfonyl] 4-O$_2$NC$_6$H$_4$SO$_2$–
tert-Octyl*	(1,1,3,3-Tetramethylbutyl) (H$_3$C)$_3$CCH$_2$C(CH$_3$)$_2$–
Oenanthyl*	See *enanthoyl*
Oleoyl*	(1-Oxo-9-octadecenoyl) H$_3$C(CH$_2$)$_7$CH=CH(CH$_2$)$_7$CO–

(continued on next page)

* Substituents not to be used in constructing formal names.

TABLE 3.7 (continued)
Substituents

Oleyl*	(Z)-9-Octadecenyl $H_3C(CH_2)_7CH=CH(CH_2)_8-$
Oxalaceto*	(3-Carboxy-1,3-dioxopropyl) $HOOCCOCH_2CO-$
Oxal(o)acetyl*	(1,2,4-Trioxo-1,4-butanediyl) $-COCH_2COCO-$
Oxalo*	(Carboxycarbonyl) $HOOCCO-$
Oxal(o)yl*	(1,2-Dioxo-1,2-ethanediyl) $-COCO-$
Oxam(o)yl*	(Aminooxoacetyl) $H_2NCOCO-$
Oximido	(Hydroxyimino) $HON=$
Oxonio	H_2O^+-
Oxy	$-O-$
Palmitoyl*	(1-Oxohexadecyl) $H_3C(CH_2)_{14}CO-$
Pelargon(o)y*	(1-Oxononyl) $H_3C(CH_2)_7CO-$
tert-Pentyl*	(1,1-Dimethylpropyl) $H_3CCH_2C(CH_3)_2-$
Perchloryl	O_3Cl-
Peroxy/dioxy	$-O-O-$
Phenacyl*	(2-Oxo-2-phenylethyl) $PhCOCH_2-$
Phenacylidene*	(2-Oxo-2-phenylethylidene) $PhCOCH=$
Phenenyl*	Benzenetriyl; *as*-phenenyl is 1,2,4-benzenetriyl, *s*-phenenyl is 1,3,5-benzenetriyl, and *vic*-phenenyl is 1,2,3-benzenetriyl
Phenethyl*	(2-Phenylethyl) $PhCH_2CH_2-$
Phenethylidene*	(2-Phenylethylidene) $PhCH_2CH=$
Phenoxy	$PhO-$
Phenylazo/phenyldiazenyl/ benzeneazo	$Ph-N=N-$
Phenylene	$-(C_6H_4)-$; aso called benzenediyl; thus, *o*-phenylene or 1,2-phenylene is 1,2-benzenediyl
Phosphanediyl/phosphinediyl	$HP<$
Phosphazo	$-P=N-$
Phosphinico/hydroxyphosphoryl/ hydroxyphosphinylidene	$HOP(O)<$
Phosphinidene/phosphanylidene	$HP=$
Phosphinidyne	$P\equiv$
Phosphinim(ido)yl	$H_2P(=NH)-$
Phosphino/phosphanyl	H_2P-; the name *phosphinyl* would logically be used for this radical, but phosphinyl is well-established for $H_2P(O)-$
Phosphinothioyl/ dihydrophosphorothioyl/ thiophosphinoyl	$H_2P(=S)-$
Phosphinoyl/phosphinyl/ dihydrophosphoryl	$H_2P(O)-$
Phosphinylidene/phosphonoyl/ hydrophosphoryl	$HP(=O)=$ or $HP(O)<$
Phospho	O_2P-; *phospho* is occasionally used in place of *phosphono* to denote the group $-P(O)(OH)_2$ when attached to atoms other than C, e.g., as in phosphocholine, $Me_3N^+CH_2CH_2OP(O)(OH)_2$
Phosphonio	H_3P^+-
Phosphonitridyl	$H_2P(\equiv N)-$
Phosphono	$(HO)_2P(O)-$

* Substituents not to be used in constructing formal names.

TABLE 3.7 (continued)
Substituents

Phosphonoyl/phosphinylidene/ hydrophosphoryl	$=PH(=O)$ or $>PH(=O)$
Phosphoranyl/λ^5-phosphanyl	H_4P-
Phosphoranylidene	$H_3P=$
Phosphoranylidyne	$H_2P\equiv$
Phosphoro	1,2-Diphosphophenediyl $-P=P-$
Phosphorodiamidothioyl/ diaminophosphinothioyl	$-P(=S)(NH_2)_2$
Phosphoroso	$OP-$
Phosphoryl/phosphinylidyne	$\equiv P(=O)$ or $>P(=O)-$ or $=P(=O)-$
Phthalimido	(1,3-Dihydro-1,3-dioxo-2H-isoindol-2-yl)
Phthaloyl	(1,2-Phenylenedicarbonyl) 1,2-$C_6H_4(CO-)_2$
Phthalyl	(2-Carboxybenzoyl) 2-$HOOCC_6H_4CO-$
Picolinoyl*	(2-Pyridinylcarbonyl)
Picryl*	(2,4,6-Trinitrophenyl) 2,4,6-$(O_2N)_3C_6H_2-$
Pimeloyl*	(1,7-Dioxo-1,7-heptanediyl) $-CO(CH_2)_5CO-$
Pipecol(o)yl*	(2-Piperidinylcarbonyl)
Piperidino*	1-Piperidinyl
Piperidyl	A contracted form of piperidinyl
Piperonyl*	1,3-Benzodioxol-5-ylmethyl or 3,4-methylenedioxybenzyl
Pipsyl*	[(4-Iodophenyl)sulfonyl] 4-$IC_6H_4SO_2-$
Pivaloyl(pivalyl)*	(2,2-Dimethyl-1-oxopropyl) $(H_3C)_3CCO-$
Prenyl*	(3-Methyl-2-butenyl) $(H_3C)_2C=CHCH_2-$; also called isoprenyl or γ,γ-dimethylallyl (avoid these)
Prolyl	(2-Pyrrolidinylcarbonyl); the acyl radical from proline used in naming peptides
Propanamido/propionamido	H_3CCH_2CONH-
Propano	$-CH_2CH_2CH_2-$ (bridge)
Propargyl*	2-Propynyl $HC\equiv CCH_2-$
Propiol(o)yl*	(1-Oxo-2-propynyl) $HC\equiv CCO-$
Propionyl	(1-Oxopropyl) H_3CCH_2CO-
Propoxy	$H_3CCH_2CH_2O-$
Propyl or n-propyl	$H_3CCH_2CH_2-$; often abbreviated to Pr (or Pr^n or n-Pr) in structural and line formulae
sec-Propyl*	(1-Methylethyl) or isopropyl, $(H_3C)_2CH-$
Propylene	(Radical) (1-methyl-1,2-ethanediyl) $-CH(CH_3)CH_2-$
Propylidene	$H_3CCH_2CH=$
Prop(an)ylidyne	$H_3CCH_2C\equiv$
Pyrocatechuoyl*	(3,4-Dihydroxybenzoyl) 3,4-$(HO)_2C_6H_3CO-$
Pseudo(o)allyl*	(1-Methylethenyl) or isopropenyl $H_2C=C(CH_3)-$
Pseudocumyl*	(Trimethylphenyl); as-pseudocumyl is 2,3,5-trimethylphenyl, s-pseudocumyl is 2,4,5-trimethylphenyl. and v-pseudocumyl is 2,3,6-trimethylphenyl
Pyroglutamyl*	(5-Oxoprolyl)
Pyromucyl*	(2-Furanylcarbonyl)
Pyrr(o)yl*	(Pyrrolylcarbonyl)
Pyruvoyl*	(1,2-Dioxopropyl) $H_3CCOCO-$
Quinaldoyl*	(2-Quinolinylcarbonyl)

(continued on next page)

* Substituents not to be used in constructing formal names.

TABLE 3.7 (continued)
Substituents

Salicyl*	[(2-Hydroxyphenylmethyl] 2-HOC$_6$H$_4$CH$_2$–
Salicylidene*	[(2-Hydroxyphenyl)methylene] 2-HOC$_6$H$_4$CH=
Salicyloyl*	(2-Hydroxybenzoyl) 2-HOC$_6$H$_4$CO–
Sarcosyl*	(N-Methylglycyl) MeNHCH$_2$CO–
Sebacoyl*	(1,10-Dioxo-1,10-decanediyl) –CO(CH$_2$)$_8$CO–
Seleneno	HOSe–
Selenienyl	The radical formed from selenophene by loss of a hydrogen
Selenino	HOSe(O)–
Seleninyl	OSe=
Selenocyanato	NCSe–
Selenonio	H$_2$Se$^+$–
Selenonium	HSe$^+$
Selenono	(HO)Se(O)$_2$–
Selenonyl	O$_2$Se–
Selenoxo	Se=; usually used when both free valencies are attached to the same atom
Selenyl/hydroseleno	HSe–
Semicarbazido*	[2-(Aminocarbonyl)hydrazino] H$_2$NCONHNH–
Semicarbazono*	2-Carbamoylhydrazono or (2-aminocarbonyl)hydrazinylidene, H$_2$NCONHN=
Senecioyl*	(3-Methyl-1-oxo-2-butenyl) (H$_3$C)$_2$C=CHCO–
Siamyl*	(1,2-Dimethylpropyl) (H$_3$C)$_2$CHCH(CH$_3$)–
Silanediyl	H$_2$Si<
Silanediylidene	=Si=
Silanetetrayl	>Si<
Silanylylidene	=SiH–
Sil(yl)oxy	H$_3$SiO–
Silyl	H$_3$Si–
Silylene	H$_2$Si=
Silylidyne	HSi≡
Sinapoyl*	[3-(4-Hydroxy-3,5-dimethoxyphenyl)-1-oxo-2-propenyl]
Sorboyl*	(1-Oxo-2,4-hexadienyl) H$_3$CCH=CHCH=CHCO–
Stannyl	H$_3$Sn–
Stannylene	H$_2$Sn< or H$_2$Sn=; the two situations can be distinguished by the more accurate names stannanediyl and stannylidene, respectively
Stearoyl*	(1-Oxooctadecyl) H$_3$C(CH$_2$)$_{16}$CO–
Stearyl*	Octadecyl H$_3$C(CH$_2$)$_{17}$
Stibyl	H$_2$Sb–
Stibylene	HSb< or HSb=; the two situations can be distinguished by the more accurate names stibenediyl/stibanediyl and stibanylidene, respectively
Styryl*	(2-Phenylethenyl) PhCH=CH–
Suberoyl*	(1,8-Dioxo-1,8-octanediyl) –CO(CH$_2$)$_6$CO–
Succinimido*	(2,5-Dioxo-1-pyrrolidinyl)
Succin(o)yl*	(1,4-Dioxo-1,4-butanediyl) –COCH$_2$CH$_2$CO–
Sulfamino(sulfoamino)	HOSO$_2$NH–
Sulfamoyl/sulfamyl/aminosulfonyl	–SO$_2$NH$_2$
Sulfanilyl*	[(4-Aminophenyl)sulfonyl] 4-H$_2$NC$_6$H$_4$SO$_2$–
Sulfenamoyl	H$_2$N–S–

* Substituents not to be used in constructing formal names.

TABLE 3.7 (continued)
Substituents

Sulfeno/hydroxythio/hydroxysulfanyl	HO–S–
Sulfhydryl*	Mercapto HS–
Sulfido	–S–
Sulfinamoyl	$H_2NS(O)$–
Sulfino	$HOS(O)$–
Sulfinyl	OS=
Sulfo	HO_3S–
Sulfonio	H_2S^+–
Sulfonium	H_3S^+–
Sulfonyl	$–SO_2$–
Sulfonylbis(oxy)	$–O–SO_2–O$–
Sulfonyldioxy	$–SO_2–O–O$–
Sulfoxonium	$H_3S^+=O$
Sulfuryl*	Sulfonyl $–SO_2$–
Supermesityl*	[2,4,6-Tris (1,1-dimethylethyl)phenyl]
Tartronoyl*	(2-Hydroxy-1,3-dioxo-1,3-propanediyl) –COCH(OH)CO–
Tauryl*	[(2-Aminoethyl)sulfonyl] $H_2NCH_2CH_2SO_2$–
Tellureno	HOTe–
Tellurino	HOTe(O)–
Tellurono	$HOTe(O)_2$–
Telluroxo	Te=; used when both free valencies are attached to the same atom
Telluryl	HTe–
Terephthaloyl*	(1,4-Phenylenedicarbonyl) $1,4-C_6H_4(CO–)_2$
Tetramethylene*	1,4-Butanediyl $–(CH_2)_4$–
Thenoyl*	(Thienylcarbonyl)
Thenyl*	(Thienylmethyl)
Thenylidene*	(Thienylmethylene)
Thenylidyne*	(Thienylmethylidyne)
Thexyl*	(1,1,2-Trimethylpropyl) $(H_3C)_2CHC(CH_3)_2$–
Thienyl	The radical derived from thiophene
Thio/sulfanediyl	–S–
Thioacetyl/ethanethioyl	Me–C(=S)–
Thiocarbamoyl/carbamothioyl	–C(=S)NH_2
Thiocarbonyl*	Carbonothioyl –C(S)–
Thiocyano	NCS–
Thiocyano*	Thiocyanato NCS–
Thioformyl	–CH(=S)
Thionyl*	Sulfinyl –S(O)–
Thiosulfeno/disulfanyl/ dithiohydroperoxy	HS–S–
Thiosulfinyl/thiosulfino/sulfinothioyl	–S(=S)–
Thiosulfonyl/sulfonothioyl	–S(=O)(=S)–
Thioxo/sulfanylidene	=S
Threonyl*	$H_3CCH(OH)CH(NH_2)CO$–; the acyl radical from threonine used in naming peptides

(continued on next page)

* Substituents not to be used in constructing formal names.

TABLE 3.7 (continued)
Substituents

Tigloyl*	E-(2-Methyl-1-oxo-2-butenyl) (E)-H₃CCH=C(CH₃)CO–; the Z-form is angeloyl
Toloxy*	(Methylphenoxy) $H_3CC_6H_4O-$
Toluidino*	[(Methylphenyl)amino] $H_3CC_6H_4NH-$
Tolu(o)yl*	(Methylbenzoyl) $H_3CC_6H_4CO-$
Tolyl*	(Methylphenyl) $H_3CC_6H_4-$
α-Tolyl*	(Phenylmethyl) or benzyl $PhCH_2-$
Tolylene*	(Methylphenylene) $-(H_3CC_6H_3)-$
Tosyl*	[(4-Methylphenyl)sulfonyl] $4-H_3CC_6H_4SO_2-$
Triazano	–NHNHNH– (bridge)
Triazeno/azimino	–N=N–NH– (bridge)
Triazenyl	$-N=N-NH_2$
Triflyl*	[(Trifluoromethyl)sulfonyl] F_3CSO_2-
Trimethylene/1,3-propanediyl	$-CH_2CH_2CH_2-$
Trithio/trisulfanyl	–S–S–S–
Trithiosulfo/mercaptosulfonyldithio/ mercapto(dithiosulfonyl)	HS–S(=S)–
Trityl*	(Triphenylmethyl) Ph_3C-
Tropoyl*	(3-Hydroxy-1-oxo-2-phenylpropyl) $PhCH(CH_2OH)CO-$
Ureido*	[(Aminocarbonyl)amino] $H_2NCONH-$
Urylene*	Carbonyldiimino, –NHCONH–
Valer(o)yl*	(1-Oxopentyl) $H_3C(CH_2)_3CO-$
Valyl	$(H_3C)_2CHCH(NH_2)CO$; the acyl radical from valine used in naming peptides
Vanilloyl*	(4-Hydroxy-3-methoxybenzoyl)
Vanillyl*	[(4-Hydroxy-3-methoxyphenyl)methyl]
Veratroyl*	(3,4-Dimethoxybenzoyl) $3,4-(MeO)_2C_6H_4CO-$
o-Veratroyl*	(2,3-Dimethoxybenzoyl) $2,3-(MeO)_2C_6H_4CO-$
Veratryl*	[(3,4-Dimethoxyphenyl)methyl] $3,4-(MeO)_2C_6H_4CH_2-$
Vinyl	Ethenyl $H_2C=CH-$
Vinylene*	1,2-Ethenediyl –CH=CH–
Vinylidene/ethenylidene	$H_2C=C=$ or $H_2C=C<$; the latter better named as ethene-1,2-diyl
Xanthyl*	Contracted form of xanthenyl
Xenyl*	-Biphenylyl PhC_6H_4-
Xylidino*	[(Dimethylphenyl)amino] $(H_3C)_2C_6H_3NH-$
Xyloyl*	(Dimethylbenzoyl) $(H_3C)_2C_6H_3CO-$
Xylyl*	(Dimethylphenyl) $(H_3C)_2C_6H_3-$
Xylylene*	[Phenylenebis(methylene)] $-CH_2C_6H_4CH_2-$

* Substituents not to be used in constructing formal names.

3.4.5 Modifications

If present, these modify the functional group(s), e.g., in 3-amino-2-chloro-2-butenoic acid, ethyl ester, hydrochloride. Modifications are used for anhydrides, esters, and salts of acids, oxides, sulfides, and selenides of ring systems containing P and As, hydrazones, and oximes of carbonyl compounds, salts of amines, etc.

Note that in the case of esters, reinversion is allowed, so that, for example, the correct name for *acetic acid, ethyl ester* is *ethyl acetate*. In CAS, esters are usually indexed at the name of the component acid. However, esters of some very common acids (class I acids) are indexed at the names of the component alcohol/phenol or thiol unless the alcohol/phenol or thiol component is also very common (a class I alcohol).

Table 3.8 lists the class I acids. All other acids are class II acids.

TABLE 3.8
Class I Acids

Acetic acid	Methylcarbamic acid
Aminobenzoic acid	Nitric acid
(all isomers)	Nitrobenzoic acid (all isomers)
Benzenesulfonic acid	Phenylcarbamic acid
Benzoic acid	Phosphinic acid
Boric acid (H_3BO_3)	Phosphonic acid
Carbamic acid	Phosphoric acid
Carbonic acid	Phosphorodithioic acid
Dinitrobenzoic acid	Phosphorothioic acid
(all isomers)	Phosphorous acid
Formic acid	Propanoic acid
Methanesulfonic acid	Sulfuric acid
4-Methylbenzenesulfonic acid	Sulfurous acid

Table 3.9 lists the class I alcohols and phenols. The list of class I thiols is completely analogous.

TABLE 3.9
Class I Alcohols/Phenols

Benzeneethanol	1-Hexanol
Benzenemethanol	Methanol
1-Butanol	Methylphenol
2-Butanol	(all isomers)
Chlorophenol (all isomers)	2-Methyl-1-propanol
Cyclohexanol	2-Methyl-2-propanol
1-Decanol	Nitrophenol
2-(Diethylamino)ethanol	(all isomers)
2-(Dimethylamino)ethanol	1-Nonanol
1-Dodecanol	1-Octanol
Ethanol	1-Pentanol
Ethenol	Phenol
2-Ethyl-1-butanol	1-Propanol
2-Ethyl-1-hexanol	2-Propanol
1-Heptanol	2-Propen-1-ol

The combinations shown in Table 3.10 occur.

TABLE 3.10

	Acid	Alcohol	Indexed at
1.	Class I	Class I	Acid
2.	Class I	Class II	Alcohol
3.	Class II	Class I	Acid
4.	Class II	Class II	Acid

Examples of each of these combinations follow:

1. Methyl acetate is indexed at *acetic acid, methyl ester.*
2. Chloromethyl acetate is indexed at *methanol, chloro-, acetate.*
3. Methyl chloroacetate is indexed at *acetic acid, chloro-, methyl ester.*
4. Chloromethyl chloroacetate is indexed at *acetic acid, chloro-, chloromethyl ester.*

There is one exception. Where a polybasic class I acid, e.g., phosphoric acid, is esterified by two or more different alcohols, the acid heading is always used. Thus, chloromethyl dimethyl phosphate is indexed at *phosphoric acid, chloromethyl dimethyl ester* because the alcoholic components are not alike.

3.4.6 STEREODESCRIPTOR(S)

These are dealt with in Chapter 7.

3.5 NOMENCLATURE ALGORITHMS

A number of programs are available for generating names from chemical structures, and vice-versa. The best-known of these are:

ACD/Name (ACD Labs). Available in Windows and Linux versions. Continually upated, latest version is 12.0. There is a free basic version ACD/ChemSketch capable of naming compounds with not more than 50 common atoms and not more than 3 rings.

AutoNOM (Beilstein Institute) incorporated in *ISISDraw* (believed no longer being developed)

StructName included in *ChemDraw*

Other programs include *NameIt*, *LexiChem* and *Nomenclator*.

In most relatively straightforward cases these programs will produce an acceptable name which accords with IUPAC principles. However; (1) The different algorithms will not in general produce the same name, (2) In general, these will not correspond with the CAS name.

For a review giving examples of the results obtained by the three main algorithms (versions available *ca.* 2005) on a random selection of structures see Eller, G.A., *Molecules*, 2006, **11**, 915–925.

4 Nomenclature of Ring Systems

4.1 RING SYSTEMS (GENERAL)

Various publications from the Chemical Abstracts Service can be used to find the name of a known ring system. The most comprehensive source of ring system names is the *Ring Systems Handbook* (RSH). Entries are in ring analysis order, i.e., according to the following hierarchy of ring data:

1. Number of component rings
2. Sizes of component rings
3. Elemental analysis of component rings

For example, the ring system

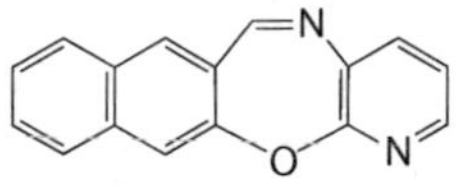

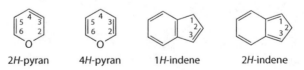

contains four rings, with sizes 6,6,6,7, and with elemental compositions $C_5N–C_6–C_6–C_5NO$. *The preferred parent contains the senior ring system.* For ring systems, nitrogen heterocycles > other heterocycles > carbocycles. Thus, pyridine > furan > naphthalene. If two ring systems are of a type, then that with the greater number of individual rings is preferred, e.g., quinoline > pyridine, and naphthalene > benzene. A further twelve criteria are needed to allow a decision to be made in all cases. These can be found in the *Chemical Abstracts* Index Guide, Appendix IV, paragraph 138.

A list of common hydrocarbon and heterocyclic parent skeletons and their numbering appears in Table 4.1.

4.1.1 INDICATED HYDROGEN

An italic *H* appearing with the name of a ring or ring system usually denotes an indicated or added hydrogen atom. For some fused polycyclic ring systems and certain monocyclic heterocycles that contain the maximum number of cumulative double bonds, it is possible to have more than one isomer differing in the positions of the double bonds. They are distinguished by using *H* with the appropriate locant to indicate that atom which is not connected to either neighbouring ring atom by a double bond. The *H* is known as *indicated hydrogen.*

2H-pyran   4H-pyran   1H-indene   2H-indene

Indicated hydrogen has the highest priority in naming compounds.

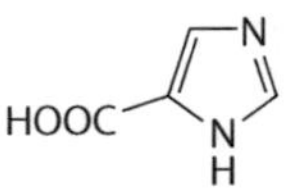

1*H*-imidazole-5-carboxylic acid > 3*H*-imidazole-4-carboxylic acid.

71

4.1.2 Added Hydrogen

Sometimes a hydrogen atom needs to be added to a ring system in order to accommodate structural features such as principal groups. For example, introduction of an oxo group into a naphthalene will mean the removal of one double bond, and there will then be a CH_2 unit in the ring. The position of this CH_2 unit is indicated by using *H* with the appropriate locant.

1(2*H*)-naphthalenone   1(4*H*)-naphthalenone

TABLE 4.1
Hydrocarbon and Heterocyclic Parent Skeletons

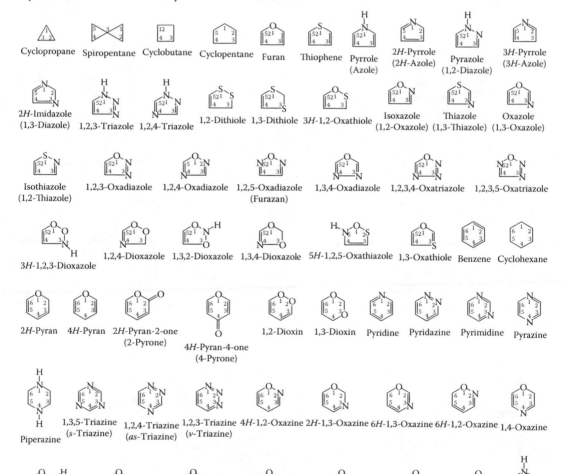

TABLE 4.1 (continued)
Hydrocarbon and Heterocyclic Parent Skeletons

     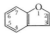 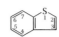

Oxepin   Thiepin   4H-1,2-Diazepine   Indene   2H-Indene (Isoindene)   Benzofuran   Isobenzofuran   Benzo[b]thiophene

 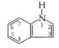 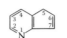 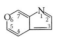 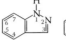

Benzo[c]thiophene   Indole   3H-Indole   1H-Indole   Cyclopenta[b]pyridine   Pyrano[3,4-b]-pyrrole   Indazole   Benzisoxazole (Indoxazene)

 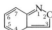   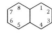 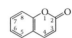

Benzoxazole   2,1-Benzisoxazole   Naphthalene   1,2,3,4-Tetra-hydronaphthalene (Tetralin)   Octahydronaphthalene (Decalin)   2H-1-Benzopyran (2H-Chromene)   2H-1-Benzopyran-2-one (Coumarin)

 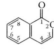 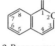 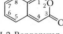 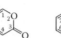   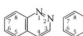

4H-1-Benzopyran-4-one (Chromen-4-one)   1H-2-Benzopyran-1-one (Isocoumarin)   3H-2-Benzopyran-1-one (Isochromen-3-one)   Quinoline   Isoquinoline   Cinnoline   Quinazoline

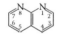 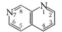 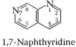 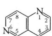 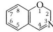 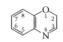

1,8-Naphthyridine   1,7-Naphthyridine   1,5-Naphthyridine   1,6-Naphthyridine   2H-1,3-Benzoxazine   2H-1,4-Benzoxazine

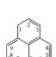 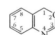 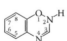 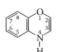 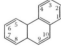 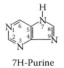

1H-2,3-Benzoxazine   4H-3,1-Benzoxazine   2H-1,2-Benzoxazine   4H-1,4-Benzoxazine   Anthracene   Phenanthrene

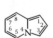 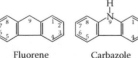 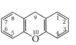 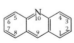

Phenalene   Fluorene   Carbazole   Xanthene   Acridine   Norpinane (Bicyclo[3.1.1]heptane)   7H-Purine

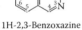 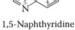

Indolizine   2H-form Quinolizine

Note: When a nitrogen or other heteroatom is at a ring junction position, that position is included in the main numbering, e.g., indolizine.

Note the irregular numbering of anthracene and purine.

4.2   BRIDGED RING SYSTEMS

Many bridged ring systems are named by the von Baeyer system. Von Baeyer names are used mostly for bridged ring systems and occasionally for nonbridged ring systems. Examples of von Baeyer names are bicyclo[3.2.1]octane and tricyclo[7.4.1.0³,⁶]tetradecane.

Bicyclo[3.2.1]octane

Bicyclo denotes two rings and *octane* denotes a total of eight skeletal atoms in the ring system. [3.2.1] gives the sizes of the three bridges connecting two bridgehead atoms.

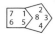

bicyclo[3.2.1]octane

The system is numbered starting from one of the bridgeheads and numbering by the longest possible path to the second bridgehead; numbering is then continued via the longer unnumbered path back to the first bridgehead and is completed via the third bridge.

Tricyclo[7.4.1.0³,⁶]tetradecane

Tricyclo denotes three rings and *tetradecane* denotes a total of fourteen skeletal atoms in the ring system. [7.4.1] gives the sizes of three bridges connecting two bridgehead atoms as in the previous example; these three bridges are numbered as in the previous example. 0³,⁶ denotes that there is a bridge of zero atoms (i.e., a bond) between the atoms numbered 3 and 6.

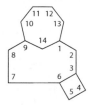

Fused ring systems that have other bridges are usually named by prefixing the name of the bridge to the name of the fused ring system. The names of hydrocarbon bridges are derived from the names of the parent hydrocarbons by replacing the final -*ane*, -*ene*, etc., by -*ano*, -*eno*, etc. Thus, –CH₂– is methano and –CH=CH– is etheno.

Names for bridges containing heteroatoms include:

–O–	Epoxy
–S–	Epithio
–NH–	Imino
–N=N–	Azo
–O–O–	Epidioxy
–S–S–	Epidithio
–N=	Nitrilo
–OCH₂–	(Epoxymethano)

Some examples are the following:

1,4-dihydro-1,4-ethanonaphthalene

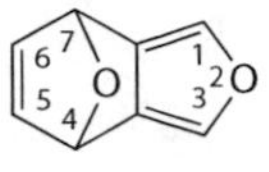

4,7-dihydro-4,7-epoxyisobenzofuran

Heterocyclic systems are named by replacement nomenclature. Unsaturation is denoted by *-ene* and *-yne* suffixes. For more information, see Eckroth, D. R., *J. Org. Chem.*, 32, 3312, 1967.

Some common cage structures are usually named trivially as parents. CAS names all of these systematically.

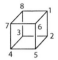

cubane

Pentacyclo[4.2.0.0^{2,5}.0^{3,8}.0^{4,7}]octane (CAS,9CI name)

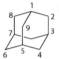

adamantane

Tricyclo[3.3.1.1^{3,7}]decane (CAS,9CI name)

4.3   SPIRO COMPOUNDS

Spiro[3.4]octane

This name denotes that there is one spiro atom and a total of eight atoms (from octane) in the structure. The numbers in square brackets, [3,4], show that there are three atoms linked to the spiro atom in one ring and four atoms linked to the spiro atom in the other ring.

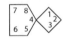

spiro[3.4]octane

Numbering starts with a ring atom next to the spiro atom and proceeds first around the smaller ring, then through the spiro atom, and then around the second ring. Heteroatoms are denoted by replacement nomenclature.

Dispiro[5.1.7.2]heptadecane

This name indicates that there are two spiro atoms and a total of seventeen atoms in the structure. The numbers in square brackets, [5.1.7.2], are the numbers of skeletal atoms linked to the spiro atoms in the same order that the numbering proceeds about the ring. Thus, 5, 1, 7, and 2 correspond to atoms 1–5, 7, 9–15, and 16–17, respectively.

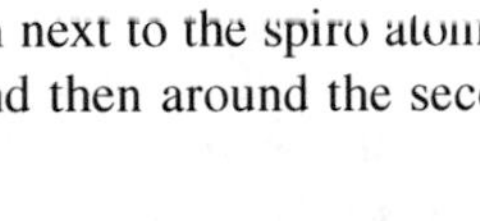

dispiro[5.1.7.2]heptadecane

Numbering starts with a ring atom next to a terminal spiro atom and proceeds around this terminal ring so as to give the spiro atoms as low numbers as possible. Trispiro names, etc., are formed similarly.

1,1′-Spirobiindene or 1,1′-spirobi[1*H*-indene]

Spirobi indicates that two similar components are joined through a spiro atom. The numbers of one component are distinguished by primes.

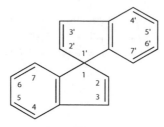

1.1'-spirobi[1*H*-indene]

Spiro[cyclopentane-1,2′-[2H]indene]

This name shows that a cyclopentane ring is joined to a 2*H*-indene ring through a spiro atom at the 1 position of the cycopentane and the 2 position of the indene. The numbers of the second component (indene) are distinguished by primes.

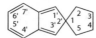

spiro[cyclopentane-1,2'-[2*H*]indene]

Alternatively, the term *spiro* may be placed between the components. Thus, cyclopentanespiro-2′-indene and indene-2-spiro-1′-cyclopentane are alternative names for the above compounds.

4.4   HETEROCYCLIC RING SYSTEMS

Some common monocyclic hetero systems have trivial names, for example, pyridine, furan (see Table 4.1).

Hantzsch-Widman names are used for one-ring heterocyclic systems that do not have trivial names. The names are applied to monocyclic compounds containing one or more heteroatoms in three- to ten-membered rings. The names are derived by combining the appropriate prefix or prefixes for the heteroatoms with a stem denoting the size of the ring (see below). The state of hydrogenation is indicated either in the stem or by the prefixes *dihydro-*, *tetrahydro-*, etc.

The prefixes are the normal replacement prefixes (see "Replacement Nomenclature," page 50), although elision of the final *a* often occurs. The prefixes are cited in the following order: *fluora-*, *chlora-*, *broma-*, *ioda-*, *oxa-*, *thia-*, *selena-*, *tellura-*, *aza-*, *phospha-*, *bora-*, and *mercura-*. *Chemical Abstracts* does not use Hantzsch-Widman names for rings containing silicon.

The stems used originally are as shown in Table 4.2.

The stems for unsaturated rings imply the maximum possible number of noncumulative double bonds. Rings with more than ten members are named by replacement nomenclature, e.g., azacycloundecane.

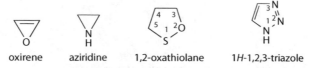

oxirene   aziridine   1,2-oxathiolane   1*H*-1,2,3-triazole

Several modifications were later made in order to avoid confusion with other compounds; for example, phosphorine was used instead of phosphine. The modified (extended) Hantzsch-Widman system (*Pure Appl. Chem.*, 55, 409, 1983) uses the stems shown in Table 4.3.

TABLE 4.2
Original Hantzsch-Widman Stems

No. of Members in Ring	Rings Containing Nitrogen		Rings Containing No Nitrogen	
	Unsaturation	Saturation	Unsaturation	Saturation
3	-irine	-iridine	-irene	-irane
4	-ete	-etidine	-ete	-etane
5	-ole	-olidine	-ole	-olane
6	-ine	—	-in	-ane
7	-epine	—	-epin	-epane
8	-ocine	—	-ocin	-ocane
9	-onine	—	-onin	-onane
10	-ecine	—	-ecin	-ecane

TABLE 4.3
Extended Hantzsch-Widman Stems[a]

No. of Members in Ring	Unsaturation	Saturation
3	-irene	-irane
4	-ete	-etane
5	-ole	-olane
6A[b]	-ine	-ane
6B[b]	-ine	-inane
6C[b]	-inine	-inane
7	-epine	-epane
8	-ocine	-ocane
9	-onine	-onane
10	-ecine	-ecane

[a] The stem for the least preferred heteroatom is selected.

[b] 6A applies to rings containing O, S, Se, Te, Bi, Hg;
6B applies to rings containing N, Si, Ge, Sn, Pb;
6C applies to rings containing B, F, Cl, Br, I, P, As, Sb.

Special stems were previously used for four- and five-membered rings containing one double bond. These stems are *-etine* for four-membered rings containing nitrogen, *-etene* for four-membered rings containing no nitrogen, *-oline* for five-membered rings containing nitrogen, and *-olene* for five-membered rings containing no nitrogen. These stems are no longer recommended.

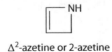

Δ^2-azetine or 2-azetine

4.5   RING ASSEMBLIES

Ring assemblies are polycyclic systems consisting of two or more identical rings or ring systems directly joined to each other by single or double bonds. Linear assemblies joined by single bonds are named by citing a numerical prefix (Table 4.4) with the name of the ring or ring system (except for benzene and the cycloalkanes, when the appropriate radical name is used).

TABLE 4.4
Prefixes Used in Naming Ring Assemblies

No. of Components	Numerical Prefixes
2	bi
3	ter
4	quater
5	quinque
6	sexi
7	septi
8	octi
9	novi
10	deci
11	undeci
12	dodeci
13	trideci
	etc.

The numbering of the assembly is that of the component system. One terminal component is assigned unprimed numbers as locants, the locants of the other components being primed serially.

1,1'-bicyclohexyl   2,2'-bipiperidine   4,2':6',4"-terpyridine   1,1':2',1":2",1"'-quaterphenyl or *o*-quaterphenyl

Ring assembly names are sometimes applied to ring systems joined by a double bond.

1,1'-bicyclopentylidene $\Delta^{2,2'}$-bi-2*H*-indene

4.6   RING FUSION NAMES

Examples of ring fusion names are:

- Naphtho[2,3-*b*]furan
- Benzo[*a*]cyclopent[*j*]anthracene
- Dibenzo[*de,rst*]pentaphene
- Pyrido[1',2':1,2]imidazo[4,5-*b*]quinoxaline

They are derived by prefixing to the name of a component ring or ring system (the base component) designations of the other components. The prefixes are normally obtained by changing the ending *-e* of the name of the ring or ring system to *-o*; there are exceptions, such as *benzo-*, *pyrido-*, and *cyclopenta-*. Isomers are distinguished by lettering the peripheral sides of the base component *a, b, c*, etc., beginning with *a* for side 1 → 2. To the letter denoting where fusion occurs are prefixed, if necessary, the numbers of the positions of attachment of the other components. The resulting name denotes the ring system containing the maximum number of noncumulative double bonds. In cases where the parent ring system is unsystematically numbered, e.g., anthracene, the fusion lettering uses the 1 → 2 face as *a*, then proceeds around the ring sequentially, regardless of the unsystematic numbering.

Benzo- is used in the normal manner when naming fused systems such as benz[*a*]anthracene and benzo[*b*]thiophene. However, bicyclic hetero ring systems consisting of a benzene ring fused to a monocyclic hetero ring named by the Hantzsch-Widman system (q.v.) receive a slightly different treatment. *Benzo-* or *benz-* is placed directly in front of the Hantzsch-Widman name of the monocyclic hetero ring, and indicated hydrogen and locants describing the position of the heteroatoms are cited, when necessary, in front of the resulting name.

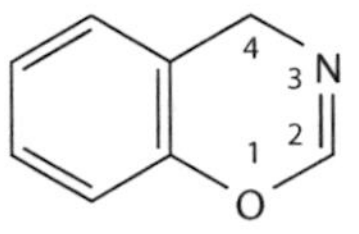

4*H*-1,3-benzoxazine 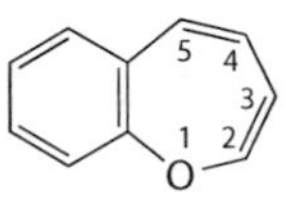   1-benzoxepin 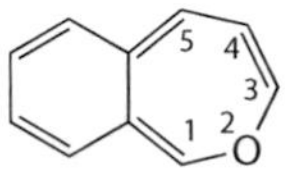   2-benzoxepin

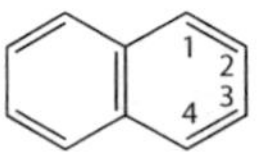

naphthalene
fusion prefix = naphtho

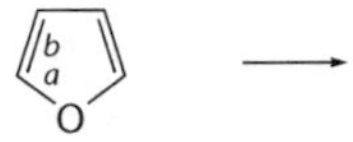

furan
(base component)

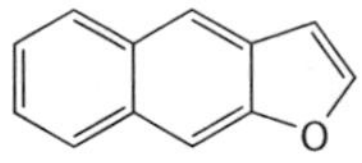

naphtho[2,3-*b*]furan

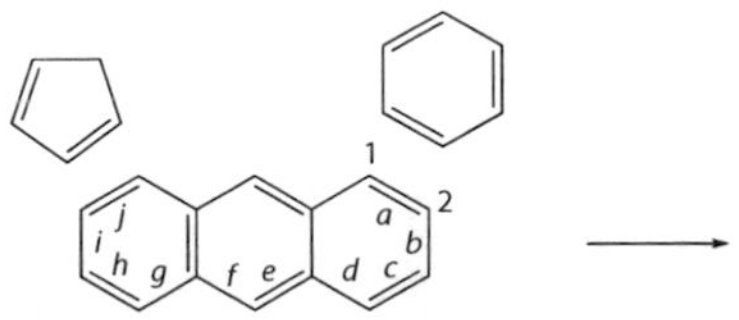

anthracene (base component) 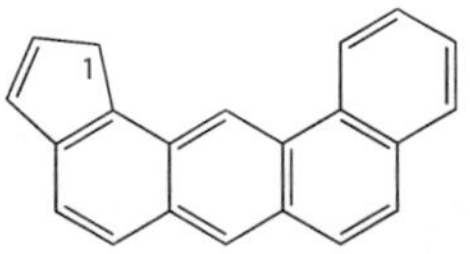   1*H*-benzo[*a*]cyclopent[*j*]anthracene

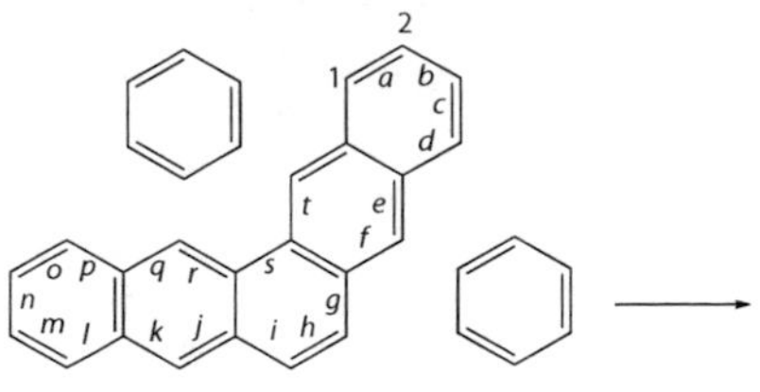

pentaphene (base component) 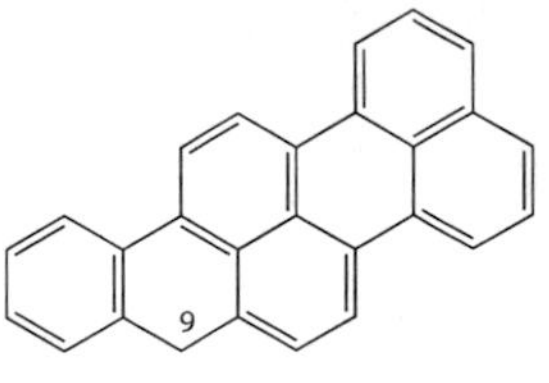   9*H*-dibenzo[*de,rst*]pentaphene

quinoxaline   imidazo   pyrido
(base component)

pyrido[1',2':1,2]imidazo[4,5-b]quinoxaline

   Ring systems produced by fusion are completely renumbered, and the numbering bears no rela-
tion to the numbering of the fusion components. The rules for deciding correct numbering of a fused
system involve orienting the skeleton so as to put the maximum number of rings in a horizontal
row and the largest possible number of rings in the upper-right-hand quadrant. Numbering then
goes clockwise starting in the upper-right quadrant. In case of uncertainty, always consult the *Ring
Systems Handbook*.

5 Nomenclature of Individual Classes of Compound

5.1 CARBOHYDRATES

Carbohydrate nomenclature impacts on stereochemistry, and on the nomenclature of compounds other than mainstream carbohydrates (e.g., hydroxylactones), often named as modified carbohydrates in Chemical Abstracts Service (CAS) and elsewhere. For further stereochemical information on carbohydrates, see Chapter 7.

For IUPAC guidelines on carbohydrate nomenclature see *Pure Appl. Chem.*, 68, 1919–2008, 1996.

5.1.1 FUNDAMENTAL ALDOSES

The fundamental carbohydrates are polyhydroxyaldehydes (aldoses) and -ketones (ketoses). Of these, the most important for nomenclature are the aldoses. An aldose, $HOCH_2(CHOH)_{n-2}CHO$, has (n–2) chiral centres. The stereochemical designation of a fundamental aldose is arrived at by assigning it to the D- or L-series depending on the absolute configuration of the *highest-numbered chiral centre (penultimate carbon atom)* of the chain, together with the aldose name, which defines the relative configuration of all the chiral centres, thus D-glucose. This system of stereodescription is used extensively in organic chemistry to specify the absolute configurations of compounds that can be related to carbohydrates. When applied in this general sense, the descriptors are italicised, e.g., L-*erythro-*, D-*gluco-*.

The *Dictionary of Carbohydrates*, ed. P. M. Collins (see Section 1.2.1), is recommended for an overview of all the fundamental types of carbohydrate. Each compound is classified under one or more types of compound code, and perusal of the printed or electronic version can often resolve uncertainties of nomenclature. The dictionary also forms part of the *Combined Chemical Dictionary*.

Carbohydrates may be represented as *Fischer, Haworth,* or *planar (Mills)* diagrams, as well as zigzag diagrams, as used for noncarbohydrates. Figure 5.1 shows how these representations are related, and how to go from one to another.

In a *Fischer projection* of an open-chain carbohydrate, the chain is written vertically with carbon number 1 at the top. The OH group on the highest-numbered chiral carbon atom is depicted on the right in monosaccharides of the D-series and on the left in the L-series. To go from a Fischer projection to the correct absolute configuration, the groups attached to the *horizontal* bonds are pulled *above* the plane of the paper. Rotation of a Fischer diagram by 180° in the plane of the paper is an allowed operation that leaves the configuration unchanged.

Caution: Rotating a Fischer projection by 90° inverts the stereochemistry. Occasionally Fischer diagrams are drawn horizontally to save space. This should never be done!

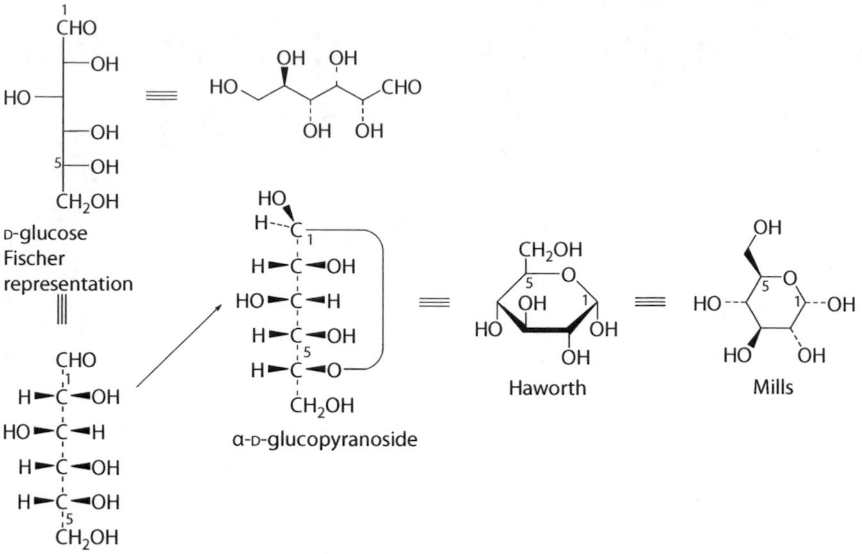

FIGURE 5.1

The configuration of a group of consecutive asymmetric carbon atoms (such as >CHOH) containing one to four centres of chirality is designated by one of the configurational prefixes shown in Table 5.1.

Each prefix is preceded by D- or L-, depending on the configuration of the highest-numbered chiral carbon atom in the Fischer projection of the prefix.

TABLE 5.1
Configurational Prefixes

No. of Carbon Atoms	Prefixes
1	*glycero-*
2	*erythro-, threo-*
3	*arabino-, lyxo-, ribo-, xylo-*
4	*allo-, altro-, galacto-, gluco-,*
	gulo-, ido-, manno-, talo-

The names of the aldoses and their formulae are:

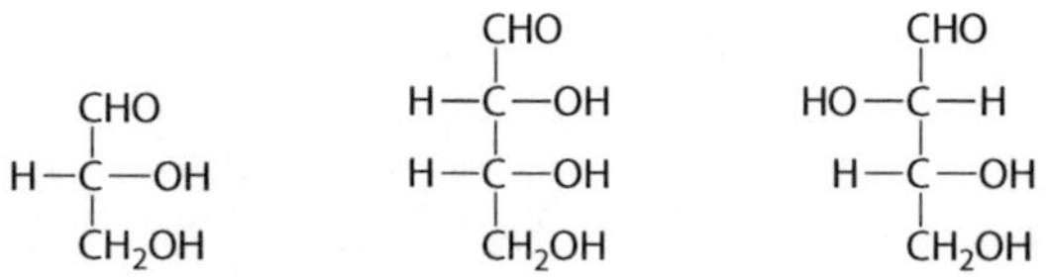

D-glycerose D-erythrose D-threose

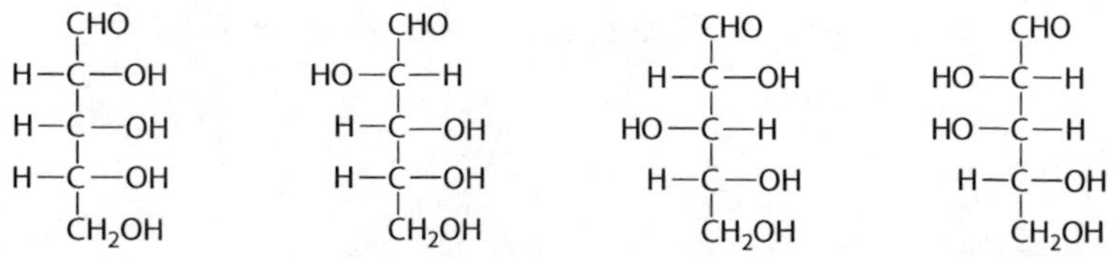

D-ribose D-arabinose D-xylose D-lyxose

```
    CHO              CHO              CHO              CHO
 H—C—OH          HO—C—H           H—C—OH          HO—C—H
 H—C—OH          H—C—OH           HO—C—H          HO—C—H
 H—C—OH          H—C—OH           H—C—OH          H—C—OH
 H—C—OH          H—C—OH           H—C—OH          H—C—OH
   CH₂OH            CH₂OH            CH₂OH            CH₂OH
  D-allose         D-altrose        D-glucose        D-mannose


    CHO              CHO              CHO              CHO
 H—C—OH          HO—C—H           H—C—OH          HO—C—H
 H—C—OH          H—C—OH           HO—C—H          HO—C—H
 HO—C—H          HO—C—H           HO—C—H          HO—C—H
 H—C—OH          H—C—OH           H—C—OH          H—C—OH
   CH₂OH            CH₂OH            CH₂OH            CH₂OH
  D-gulose         D-idose         D-galactose       D-talose
```

Strictly, carbohydrates containing one chiral centre should have their configuration specified as D- or L-*glycero*-. In practice this is often omitted, and such compounds can often be named equally well as aliphatics.

```
   1
CH₂CH₂CHO                          HO              CHO
  |—OH              ≡                  \    /
CH₂OH                                   OH
```

2,3-Dideoxy-D-*glycero*-copentose   (S)-4,5-Dihydroxypentanal
                                       (note different numbering)

```
              OH
           1 /
CH₂CH₂C —H                 HO                  H  OH
 5|—O                ≡          \    /             ≡    HO      5    2
CH₂OH                             O                            O       OH
```

2,3-Dideoxy-D-*glycero*-pentofuranose
= tetrahydro-5-(hydroxymethyl)-2-furanol
or Tetrahydro-5-hydroxy-2-furanmethanol
(note different numbering)

The consecutive asymmetric carbon atoms need not be contiguous. Thus, the following four arrangements are all L-*erythro*- (X is attached to the lowest-numbered carbon atoms).

```
                                             X
                              X           HO—C—H           X
              X            HO—C—H           CH₂          HO—C—H
           HO—C—H            CH₂            CH₂            C=O
           HO—C—H         HO—C—H         HO—C—H         HO—C—H
              Y              Y              Y              Y
```

L-*erythro*-

5.1.2　Fundamental Ketoses

The most important ketoses are the hexos-2-uloses $HOCH_2(CH2)_{n-3}COCH_2OH$, such as fructose. They have one less chiral centre than the aldoses of the same chain length; i.e., there are only four diastereomerically different hexos-2-uloses.

Trivial names for the 2-hexuloses and their formulae are:

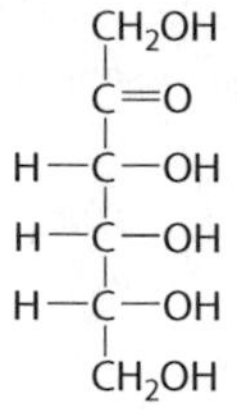

CH$_2$OH	CH$_2$OH	CH$_2$OH	CH$_2$OH
C=O	C=O	C=O	C=O
H—C—OH	HO—C—H	H—C—OH	HO—C—H
H—C—OH	H—C—OH	HO—C—H	HO—C—H
H—C—OH	H—C—OH	H—C—OH	H—C—OH
CH$_2$OH	CH$_2$OH	CH$_2$OH	CH$_2$OH
D-psicose	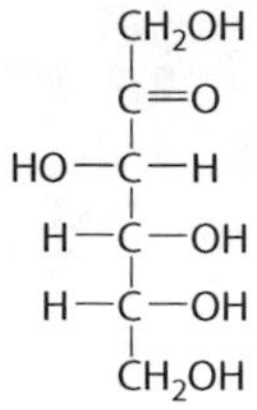 D-fructose	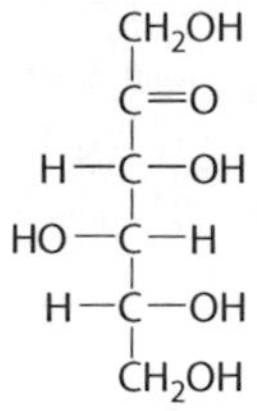 D-sorbose	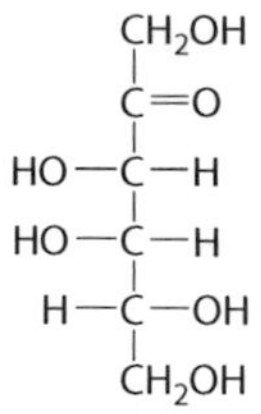 D-tagatose

5.1.3　Modified Aldoses and Ketoses

Suffixes are employed to denote modification of functional groups in an aldose or ketose, e.g., by oxidation of an OH group (Table 5.2).

5.1.4　Higher Sugars

Sugars having more than six carbon atoms are named using two prefixes, one defining the configuration at C(2)–C(5) as in a hexose, and the other, which appears first in the name, defining the configuration at the remaining chiral centres.

Examples of the use of configurational prefixes are:

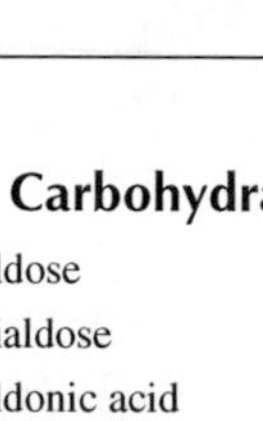

CH$_2$OH
HO—C—H
C=O
H—C—OH
H—C—OH
CH$_2$OH

D-*arabino*-3-hexulose

1 CHO
2 H—C—OH ⎤
3 HO—C—H ⎥
4 H—C—OH ⎥ D-gluco
5 H—C—OH ⎦
6 H—C—OH } D-glycero
7 CH$_2$OH

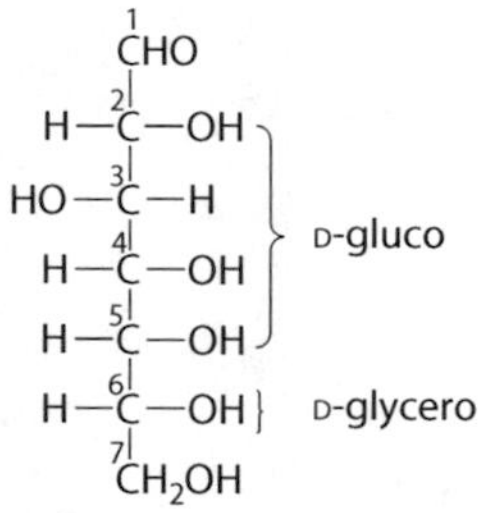

D-*glycero*-D-*gluco*-heptose

TABLE 5.2
Suffixes Used in Carbohydrate Nomenclature

-ose	Aldose	X = CHO, Y = CH$_2$OH	
-odialdose	Dialdose	X = Y = CHO	X
-onic acid	Aldonic acid	X = COOH, Y = CH$_2$OH	|
-uronic acid	Uronic acid	X = CHO, Y = COOH	(CHOH)$_x$
-aric acid	Aldaric acid	X = Y = COOH	|
-itol	Alditol	X = Y = CH$_2$OH	Y

-ulose	Ketose	X = Y = CH$_2$OH	X
-osulose	Ketoaldose	X = CHO, Y = CH$_2$OH	|
-ulosonic acid	Ulosonic acid	X = COOH, Y = CH$_2$OH	C=O
-ulosuronic acid	Ulosuronic acid	X = CHO, Y = COOH	(CHOH)$_2$ (2-hexulose series)
-ulosaric acid	Ulosaric acid	X = Y = COOH	|
-odiulose	Diketose		Y

5.1.5 CYCLIC FORMS: ANOMERS

When a monosaccharide exists in the heterocyclic intramolecular hemiacetal form, the size of the ring is indicated by the suffixes *-furanose*, *-pyranose*, and *-septanose* for five-, six-, and seven-membered rings, respectively.

Two configurations known as anomers may result from the formation of the ring. These are distinguished by the anomeric prefixes α- and β-, which relate the configuration of the anomeric carbon atom to the configuration at a reference chiral carbon atom (normally the highest-numbered chiral carbon atom). For example, consider the glucopyranoses:

- In the D-series, the CH$_2$OH is projected above the ring.
- In the L-series, the CH$_2$OH is projected below the ring.
- In the α-series, the anomeric OH (at position 1) is on the opposite side of the ring from the CH$_2$OH group.
- In the β-series, the anomeric OH (at position 1) is on the same side of the ring as the CH$_2$OH group.

Suffixes used in carbohydrate nomenclature to indicate cyclic forms are as follows:

-ose (acyclic form), *-ofuranose* (five-membered ring), *-opyranose* (six membered ring), *-heptanose* (seven-membered ring).

Similar suffixes can be constructed for dicarbonyl sugars and other modifications, for example:

-ulose   *-ulopyranose*
-osulose   *-opyranosulose* or *-osulopyranose*
-odialdose *-odialdopyranose*.

The suffixes for the acids can be modified to indicate the corresponding amide, nitriles, acid halides, etc., e.g., *-uronamide*, *-ononitrile*, and *-ulosonyl chloride*.

5.1.6 GLYCOSIDES

These are mixed acetals resulting from the replacement of the hydrogen atom on the anomeric (glycosidic) OH of the cyclic form of a sugar by a radical R derived from an alcohol or phenol (ROH). They are named by changing the terminal *-e* of the name of the corresponding cyclic form of the saccharide to *-ide*; the name of the R radical is put at the front of the name followed by a space.

Methyl β-D-glucopyranoside

5.1.7 DISACCHARIDES AND OLIGOSACCHARIDES

These are sugars produced where the alcohol forming the glycoside of a sugar is another sugar. Where the resulting sugar has a (potentially) free aldehyde function, it is called a reducing disaccharide, and where both aldehyde functions are involved in the linkage (1 → 1) glycoside, it is a non-reducing disaccharide.

maltose (4-O-α-D-glucopyranosyl-
D-glucose), a reducing disaccharide

α-D-galactopyranosyl α-D-galactopyranoside,
a non-reducing disaccharide

Abbreviations for use in representing oligosaccharides are shown in Table 5.3. See *Pure Appl. Chem.*, 54, 1517, 1982.

Examples are:

Ara*f*	Arabinofuranose
Glc*p*	Glucopyranose
Gal*p*A	Galactopyranuronic acid
D-Glc*p*N	2-Amino-2-deoxy-D-glucopyranose
3,6-AnGal	3,6-Anhydrogalactose

5.1.8 TRIVIALLY NAMED SUGARS

A number of names for modified sugars, which occur frequently in natural glycosides, are in common use.

Allomethylose	6-Deoxyallose
Cymarose	2,6-Dideoxy-3-*O*-methyl-*ribo*-hexose
Diginose	2,6-Dideoxy-3-*O*-methyl-*lyxo*-hexose
Digitoxose	2,6-Dideoxy-*ribo*-hexose

Fucose	6-Deoxygalactose
Quinovose	6-Deoxyglucose
Rhamnose	6-Deoxymannose
Olandrose	2,6-Dideoxy-3-*O*-methyl-*arabino*-hexose
Thevetose	6-Deoxy-3-O-methylglucose

TABLE 5.3
Abbreviations for Use in
Representing Oligosaccharides

Hexoses	All	allose
	Alt	altrose
	Gal	galactose
	Glc	glucose
	Gul	gulose
	Ido	idose
	Man	mannose
	Tal	talose
Pentoses	Ara	arabinose
	Lyx	lyxose
	Rib	ribose
	Xyl	xylose
Other	Rha	rhamnose
	Fuc	fucose
	Fru	fructose
Suffixes	*f*	furanose
	p	pyranose
	A	uronic acid
	N	2-deoxy-2-amino sugar
Prefixes	D-	configurational descriptor
	L-	configurational descriptor
	An	anhydro

Note that if the absolute configuration of a sugar is not clear from the literature, CAS makes certain assumptions, e.g., rhamnose is assumed to be L-.

5.2 ALDITOLS AND CYCLITOLS

5.2.1 ALDITOLS

Reduction of the carbonyl group of an aldose (or of the oxo group in a ketose) gives the series of alditols (called tetritols, pentitols, hexitols, etc., with 4, 5, 6, ..., carbon atoms).

Because of their higher symmetry compared to the aldoses, the number of possible isomers is lower, and some isomers are *meso*-forms or, in the C_7 series, some isomers show pseudoasymmetry (further described in Chapter 7).

```
CH₂OH              CH₂OH
 ├─OH         HO ─┤
 ├─OH              ├─OH
CH₂OH             CH₂OH
erythritol        D-threitol
(meso-)
```

```
CH₂OH              CH₂OH              CH₂OH
 ├─OH         HO ─┤                    ├─OH
 ├─OH              ├─OH          HO ─┤
 ├─OH              ├─OH                ├─OH
CH₂OH             CH₂OH             CH₂OH
ribitol           D-arabinitol       xylitol
(meso-)           ≡ D-lyxitol        (meso-)
```

```
CH₂OH        CH₂OH        CH₂OH        CH₂OH        CH₂OH        CH₂OH
 ├─OH    HO─┤             ├─OH     HO─┤        HO─┤              ├─OH
 ├─OH        ├─OH     HO─┤         HO─┤              ├─OH    HO─┤
 ├─OH        ├─OH         ├─OH         ├─OH     HO─┤        HO─┤
 ├─OH        ├─OH         ├─OH         ├─OH         ├─OH         ├─OH
CH₂OH       CH₂OH       CH₂OH       CH₂OH       CH₂OH       CH₂OH
allitol      D-altritol   D-glucitol   D-mannitol   D-iditol    galactitol
(meso-)      ≡ D-talitol  ≡ L-gulitol                           (meso-)
```

FIGURE 5.2 The alditols derived from the C4, C5, and C6 monosaccharides in the D-series. Degenerate symmetry means that there are only three pentitols and six hexitols.

Some isomers can therefore be named in more than one way. A choice is made according to a special carbohydrate rule that says that allocation to the D-series takes precedence over alphabetical assignment to the parent carbohydrate diastereoisomer.

5.2.2 CYCLITOLS

Posternak, L., *The Cyclitols* (San Francisco: Holden-Day, 1965).
For more information see: Hudlicky, T., and Cebulak, M., *Cyclitols and Their Derivatives* (New York: VCH, 1993).

The most important cyclitols are the inositols (1,2,3,4,5,6-cyclohexanehexols). The relative arrangement of the six hydroxyl groups below or above the plane of the cyclohexane ring is denoted by an italicised configurational prefix in the eight inositol stereoparents (the numerical locants indicate OH groups that are on the same side of the ring):

cis-Inositol   (1,2,3,4,5,6)
epi-Inositol   (1,2,3,4,5)
allo-Inositol   (1,2,3,4)
myo-Inositol   (1,2,3,5)
muco-Inositol   (1,2,4,5)
neo-Inositol   (1,2,3)
chiro-Inositol   (1,2,4)
scyllo-Inositol   (1,3,5)

Six of these isomers (*scyllo*-, *myo*-, *epi*-, *neo*-, *cis*-, and *muco*-) have one or more planes of symmetry and are *meso*-compounds; *chiro*-inositol lacks a plane of symmetry and exists as the D- and

L-forms. In *myo*-inositol, the plane of symmetry is C-2/C-5; unsymmetrically substituted derivatives on C-1, C-3, C-4, and C-6 are chiral. Substitution at C-2 and/or C-5 gives a *meso*-product. *allo*-Inositol appears to have a plane of symmetry, but at room temperature it is actually a racemate formed of two enantiomeric conformers in rapid equilibrium.

5.2.2.1 Assignment of Locants for Inositols

(From the IUPAC-IUB 1973 Recommendations for the Nomenclature of Cyclitols; *Biochem. J.*, 153, 23–31, 1976; based upon proposals first issued in 1967; *Biochem. J.*, 112, 17–28, 1969.)

- The lowest locants are assigned to the set (above or below the plane) that has the most OH groups.
- For *meso*-inositols only, the C-1 locant is assigned to the (prochiral) carbon atom, which has the L-configuration (see Chapter 7).

5.2.2.2 Absolute Configuration

Using a horizontal projection of the inositol ring, if the substituent on the lowest-numbered asymmetric carbon is above the plane of the ring and the numbering is counterclockwise, the configuration is assigned D, and if clockwise, the configuration is L (illustrated in Figure 5.3 for *myo*-inositol 1-phosphate enantiomers).

Note that 1D-*myo*-inositol 1-phosphate is the same as 1L-*myo*-inositol 3-phosphate (and 1L-*myo*-inositol 1-phosphate is the same as 1D-*myo*-inositol 3-phosphate), but the lower locant has precedence over the stereochemical prefix (D or L) in naming the derivative. A consequence of applying the 1973 IUPAC-IUB rules to *myo*-inositol is that the numbering of C-2 and C-5 remains invariant.

Before 1968, the nomenclature for inositols assigned the symbols D- and L- to the *highest*-numbered chiral centre, C-6. This convention was based on the rules for naming carbohydrates. For substituted *myo*-inositols, in particular where C-1 and C-6 hydroxyl groups are *trans*, compounds identified in the literature before 1968 as D- are now assigned 1L-.

Locants for unsubstituted inositols other than *myo*-inositol are shown in Figure 5.4.

In order to clarify the metabolic pathways for substituted *myo*-inositols (in practice *myo*-inositol phosphates), the lowest-locant rule, which gives priority to a 1L-locant has been relaxed, and numbering based on the 1D-series is now allowed (*Biochem. J.*, 258, 1–2, 1989). This is to allow substances related by simple chemical or biochemical transformations to carry the same labels. Thus, 1L-*myo*-inositol 1-phosphate may now be called 1D-*myo*-inositol-3-phosphate.

In a further simplification, the symbol Ins may be used to denote *myo*-inositol, with the numbering of the 1D-configuration implied (unless the prefix L is explicitly added).

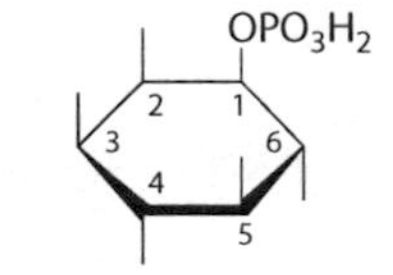

1D-*myo*-inositol 1-(dihydrogen phosphate)

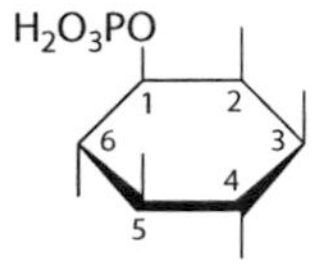

1L-*myo*-inositol 1-(dihydrogen phosphate)

FIGURE 5.3

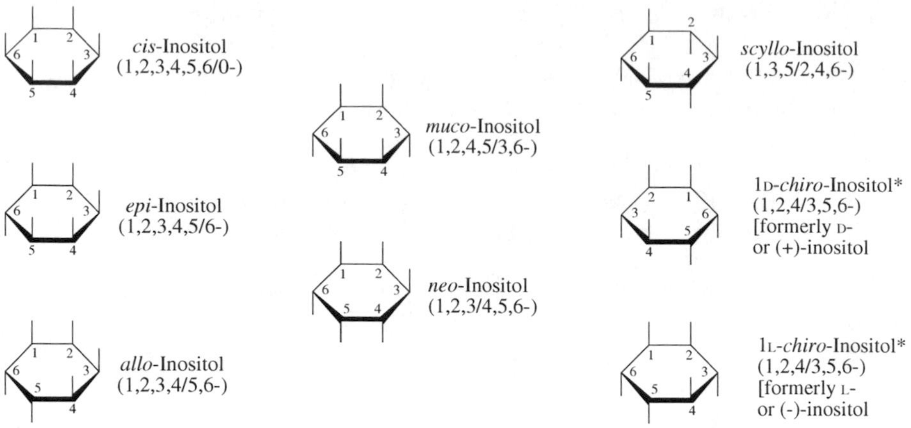

FIGURE 5.4

5.3   AMINO ACIDS AND PEPTIDES

See *Pure Appl. Chem.*, 56, 595, 1984.

5.3.1   AMINO ACIDS

In α-amino acids, the L-compounds are those in which the NH_2 group is on the left-hand side of the Fischer projection in which the COOH group appears at the top.

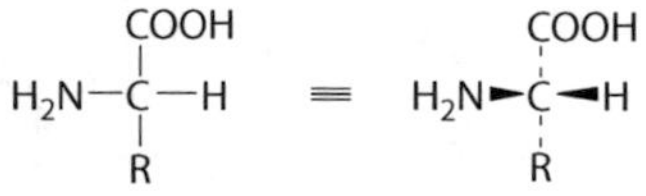

Table 5.4 lists the common α-amino acids. Most of these are found in proteins. Those marked * are nonproteinaceous but common in peptides and are also used as stem names in CAS. The list is in order of nomenclatural priority according to current CAS practice (2006), e.g., CAS name *alanyl-arginine* not *argininylalanine*. The order pre-2006 was different.

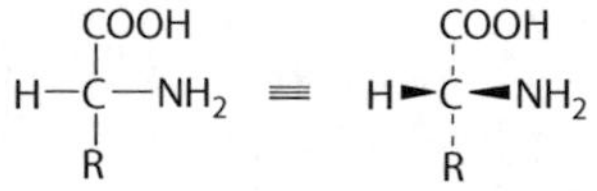

For all the amino acids in the table, except for cysteine, the L-form has the *S*-configuration. For cysteine, the L-form has the *R*-configuration, because the –CH_2SH group has higher priority than –COOH according to the sequence rule (see Chapter 7).

Other one-letter abbreviations are as follows:

B Asparagine or aspartic acid
X Unspecified amino acid
Z Glutamine or glutamic acid

Other abbreviations that may be encountered in the literature include those listed in Table 5.5.

TABLE 5.4
α-Amino Acids Listed in Order of Precedence in CAS Nomenclature (2006 Revision)

Name		Abbreviations	R Group (Side Chain)	Molecular Formula
Glutamic acid	Glu	E	$-CH_2CH_2COOH$	$C_5H_9NO_4$
Aspartic acid	Asp	D	$-CH_2COOH$	$C_4H_7NO_4$
Tryptophan	Trp	W	*(structure)*	$C_{11}H_{12}N_2O_2$
Histidine	His	H	*(structure)*	$C_6H_9N_3O_2$
Proline	Pro	P	*(structure)*	$C_5H_9NO_2$
Tyrosine	Tyr	Y	*(structure)* –OH	$C_9H_{11}NO_3$
Phenylalanine	Phe	F	$-CH_2Ph$	$C_9H_{11}NO_2$
Lysine	Lys	K	$-CH_2CH(CH_3)_2$	$C_6H_{14}N_2O_2$
Norleucine*	Nle		$-(CH_2)_3CH_3$	$C_6H_{13}NO_2$
Glutamine	Gln (or Glu(NH$_2$))	Q	$-CH_2CH_2CONH_2$	$C_5H_{10}N_2O_3$
Arginine	Arg	R	$-(CH_2)_3NHC(NH_2)=NH$	$C_6H_{14}N_4O_2$
Ornithine*	Orn		$-(CH_2)_3NH_2$	$C_5H_{12}N_2O_2$
Isoleucine	Ile	I	$-CH(CH_3)CH_2CH_3$ (R^*,R^*-)	$C_6H_{13}NO_2$
Alloisoleucine	aIle		$-CH(CH_3)CH_2CH_3$ (R^*,S^*-)	$C_6H_{13}NO_2$
Leucine	Leu	L	$-CH_2CH(CH_3)_2$	$C_6H_{13}NO_2$
Norvaline*	Nva (or Avl)		$-CH_2CH_2CH_3$	$C_5H_{11}NO_2$
Asparagine	Asn		$-CH_2CONH_2$	$C_4H_8N_2O_2$
Threonine	Thr	T (also stands for thymine)	$-CH(OH)CH_3$ (R^*,S^*-)	$C_4H_9NO_3$
Allothreonine	aThr		$CH(OH)CH_3$ (R^*,R^*-)	$C_4H_9NO_3$
Homoserine*	Hse		$-CH_2CH_2OH$	$C_4H_9NO_3$
Methionine	Met	M	$-CH_2CH_2SMe$	$C_5H_{11}NO_2S$
Homocysteine	Hcy		$-CH_2CH_2SH$	$C_4H_9NO_2S$
Valine	Val	V	$-CH(CH_3)_2$	$C_5H_{11}NO_2$
Isovaline	Iva		$-CH_2CH_3 + \alpha CH_3$	$C_5H_{11}NO_2$
Serine	Ser	S	$-CH_2OH$	$C_3H_7NO_3$
Cystine				$C_6H_{12}N_2O_4S_2$
Cysteine	Cys	C (also stands for cytosine)	$-CH_2SH$	$C_3H_7NO_2S$
Alanine	Ala	A (also stands for adenine)	$-CH_3$	$C_3H_7NO_2$
β-Alanine*	βAla		$-CH_2NH_2$ (replaces α-NH$_2$)	$C_3H_7NO_2$
Glycine	Gly	G (also stands for guanine)	$-H$	$C_2H_5NO_2$

Note: Nonprotein amino acids are marked *. Three-letter codes in brackets are not recommended.

TABLE 5.5
Other Amino Acid–Related Abbreviations Found in the Literature

βAad	3-Aminoadipic acid	Hsl	Homoserine lactone
Aad	2-Aminoadipic acid	Hyl	5-Hydroxylysine
A2bu	2,4-Diaminobutanoic acid	5Hyl	5-Hydroxylysine
Abu	2-Aminobutanoic acid	Hyp	4-Hydroxyproline
εAhx	6-Aminohexanoic acid	4Hyp	4-Hydroxyproline
Ahx	2-Aminohexanoic acid (norleucine)	J (one-letter code)	Indistinguishable leucine or isoleucine
2-MeAla	2-Methylalanine	MetO	Methionine S-oxide
Ape	2-Aminopentanoic acid (norvaline)	MetO$_2$	Methionine S,S-dioxide
Apm	2-Aminopimelic acid	Mur	Muramic acid
A2pr	2,3-Diaminopropionic acid	Neu	Neuraminic acid
Asp(NH$_2$)	Asparagine	Neu5Ac	N-Acetylneuraminic acid
Asx	Asparagine or aspartic acid	5-oxoPro	5-Oxoproline (pyroglutamic acid)
Dpm	2,6-Diaminopimelic acid	Sar	Sarcosine
Dpr	2,3-Diaminopropionic acid	Sec or U	Selenocysteine (one-letter code U;
Gla	4-Carboxyglutamic acid		also stands for uridine)
Glp or pGlu or <Glu	5-Oxoproline (pyroglutamic acid)	Ser(P)	Phosphoserine
		Thx	Thyroxine
Glx	Glutamine or glutamic acid	Tyr(I$_2$)	3,5-Diiodotyrosine
		Tyr(SO$_3$H)	O^4-Sulfotyrosine
		Xaa	Unspecified amino acid

5.3.2 PEPTIDES

Peptides are oligomers notionally derived from amino acids by condensation to produce amide linkages. They are named either systematically or trivially.

The *primary structure* of a peptide is the amino acid sequence. The *secondary structure* is that resulting from modifying bonds, especially hydrogen bonds and cysteine/cysteine dimerisation, and the *tertiary structure* is the three-dimensional organisation resulting from the folding of a peptide chain into helices, sheets, etc. The *quaternary structure* of a protein comprises the macrostructure formed by the coming together of two or more smaller subunits.

Trivial names of peptides can be modified in the following ways to denote a change in the amino acid sequence:

Replacement. When a peptide with a trivial name has an amino acid replaced by another amino acid, the modified peptide can be named as a derivative of the parent peptide by citing the new amino acid as a replacement. The new amino acid is designated by the appropriate amino acid residue number:

H-Arg-Pro-Pro-Gly-Phe-Ser-Pro-Phe-Arg-OH = bradykinin
H-Arg-Pro-Pro-Gly-Phe-Ser-Phe-Phe-Arg-OH = 7-L-phenylalaninebradykinin

Extension. Extension of a trivially named peptide at the N-terminal end is denoted by substitutive nomenclature. Extension at the C-terminal end is made by citing the new amino acid residues with locants derived by suffixing the highest locant with a, b, etc. Extension in the middle of the chain is denoted by use of the term *endo*-:

H-Lys-Arg-Pro-Pro-Gly-Phe-Ser-Pro-Phe-Arg-OH = N^2-L-lysylbradykinin
H-Arg-Pro-Pro-Gly-Phe-Ser-Pro-Phe-Arg-Arg-OH = 9*a*-L-argininebradykinin
H-Arg-Pro-Pro-Gly-Phe-Ser-Ala-Pro-Phe-Arg-OH = 6*a-endo*-L-alaninebradykinin

Removal. Removal of an amino acid residue is denoted using *de-*:

H-Pro-Pro-Gly-Phe-Ser-Pro-Phe-Arg-OH = 1-de-L-argininebradykinin

Various numbering methods have been used to indicate substitution or other modification in or of the residues of a peptide. The method now recommended by IUPAC and introduced into the *Dictionary of Natural Products* (see Section 1.2.1) uses numerical locants of the type 3^2, where 3 is the locant of the substituent in the amino acid residue and 2 is the amino acid position in the ring or chain, numbered from the N-terminal end, which is standard for all peptides). $N^{5.4}$-methyloxytocin would indicate a methyl substituent on N-5 of the glutamine residue at position 4 of oxytocin.

5.3.2.1 Recent CAS Peptide Nomenclature Revisions

For the 14th Collective Index period, several revisions in CAS peptide nomenclature have been made, and further changes were made as part of the 2006 revisions.

- No structure is assigned a peptide name unless it contains at least two standard amino acid residues. A standard amino acid residue is any amino acid that can stand alone as a stereoparent (e.g., glycine or tryptophan), plus asparagine and glutamine. 2-Aminobutanoic acid and 2,4-diaminobutanoic acid are now considered nonstandard amino acids.
- The 2006 changes to CAS nomenclature have reduced the number of peptide parent names from about three thousand to fewer than one hundred of the most studied examples, e.g., bradykinin. All others are now named systematically.
- The nomenclature of linear peptides has been simplified. The C-terminal residue is the index heading parent, and the other residues are cited in the substituent, beginning with the N-terminal residue and continuing from left to right in the sequence, e.g., L-lysine, D-alanylglycyl-L-leucyl-. This replaces the many locants and enclosing marks that have been used in the past, e.g., L-lysine, N^2-[N-(N-D-alanylglycyl)-L-leucyl]-.
- S-oxides of sulfur-containing amino acids are now named at the peptide, e.g.:

$$MeS(O)CH_2CH_2CH(NH_2)COOH$$

Butanoic acid, 2-amino-4-(methylsulfinyl), 9CI → methionine *S*-oxide

5.4 NATURAL PRODUCTS (GENERAL)

The best information source on the names of natural products is the *Dictionary of Natural Products* (DNP), which is part of the Chapman & Hall/CRC chemical database (see Section 1.2.1). DNP does not give CAS names where these are lengthy, but it does have extensive coverage of CAS numbers, from which the current CAS name can be readily obtained if needed.

Four different types of names can be applied to natural products:

1. *Trivial names.* Example: Corynoxine. These convey no structural information, and if the structure has not been determined, this will be the only name available. Often derived from the Latin binomial or other name for the originating species, e.g., strychnine from *Strychnos nux-vomica*. They have the advantage that they are unchanged if there is a structure revision. There are, however, numerous duplications of trivial names in the literature. IUPAC has promulgated proposals to systematise the endings of trivial names depending on the functional groups present, but this is not widely used. The ending *–in(e)* is well established for alkaloids, however.
2. *Systematic names.* Example: Methyl 6′-ethyl 1,2,2′3,6′,7′,8′,8′-octahydro-α-(methoxy-methylene)-2-oxospiro[3*H*-indole-3,1′(5′*H*-indolizine)]7′-acetate, (α*E*,1′*S*,6′*S*,7′*S*,8′a*S*)- is the

current CAS name for corynoxine. There are many cases in which CAS numbering does not correspond with the biogenetic schemes used by most natural products specialists. Biogenetic schemes may be discontinuous where, for example, one or more carbon atoms appear to have been lost during biosynthesis or new bonds formed.

3. *Semisystematic names.* Examples of semisystematic parents are corynoxan and labdane. DNP makes widespread use of semisystematic names for terpenoids and steroids (where skeletons such as labdane have not been used in CAS nomenclature since 8CI). IUPAC gives tables of recognised semisystematic parent skeletons and directions for introducing new ones, but in view of the discovery of ever more structurally complex types of natural products, most authors have avoided this route. Semisystematic parents can be modified by operators such as *nor-, abeo.*

    CAS still uses this type of name for some types of natural product, but the 2006 CAS nomenclature revisions have reduced the number in use by more than 3000.

4. *Semitrivial names.* These are names that are derived by appending a systematically derived operator to a trivial parent. Examples are 8-(1,1-dimethylallyl)confusameline and *N*-cyano-*sec*-pseudostrychnine. In general, such names should be avoided because of the possibilities for confusion, especially when there is a structure revision or where there is more than one numbering scheme in use for the parent skeleton. Trivial names should be preferred.

5.5   STEROIDS

These are naturally occurring compounds and synthetic analogues based on the cyclopenta[*a*]phenanthrene skeleton. For further details, see *Pure. Appl. Chem.*, 61, 1783, 1989.

Steroids are numbered, and rings are lettered as follows:

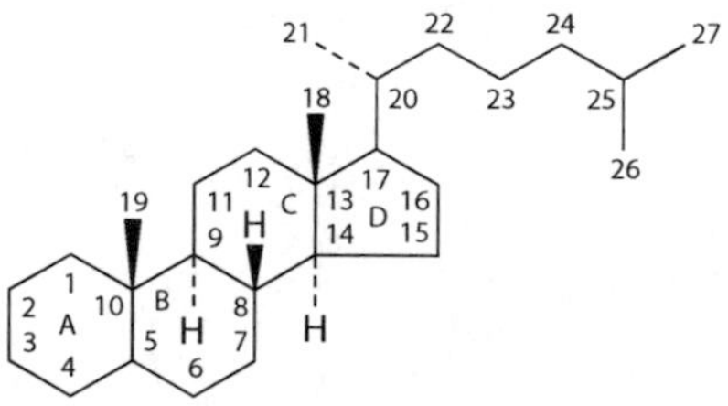

The following steroid names are the ones usually used as parent names:

androstane, bufanolide, campestane, cardanolide, cholane, cholestane, ergostane, estrane (oestrane), furostan, gonane, gorgostane, poriferastane, pregnane, spirostan, and stigmastane. CAS has restricted the number of semisystematic skeletons in use.

Stereochemistry is denoted by α and β; ξ (xi) is used for positions of unknown stereochemistry. For a steroid structure drawn in the normal manner, α- denotes that a substituent projects below the plane of the paper and β- indicates that a substituent projects above the plane of the paper. At a ring junction position, it is the H or Me group that determines whether the configuration is α- or β-. The configuration of steroids at the ring junctions is assumed to be $8\beta,9\alpha,10\beta,13\beta,14\alpha$ unless otherwise stated. The configuration at position 5 is not assumed and should be specified as 5α- or 5β-. The side chain at C(17) is normally 17β. In pregnane the stereochemistry at C(20) was formerly designated 20α or 20β based on a Fischer projection, as follows:

$$\beta X - \underset{\underset{\displaystyle \wedge}{|}}{\overset{\overset{\displaystyle CH_3}{|}}{C}} - Y^\alpha \quad \equiv \quad X \blacktriangleright \underset{\underset{\displaystyle \wedge}{|}}{\overset{\overset{\displaystyle CH_3}{|}}{C}} \blacktriangleleft Y$$

Terms used to describe modified steroid skeletons include *nor* (shortening of a side chain or contraction of a ring), *homo* (expansion of a ring), *cyclo* (formation of an additional ring), *seco* (fission of a ring), and *abeo* (migration of a bond).

5.6 LIPIDS

For a detailed discussion see:

> *The Lipid Handbook with CD-ROM,* 3rd ed., ed. F. D. Gunstone, J. L. Harwood, and A. J. Dijkstra (Boca Raton, FL: CRC Press, 2007).

Lipids are fatty acids and their derivatives, and substances related biosynthetically or functionally to them. Many fatty acids are still known by their trivial names (e.g., palmitic, linoleic).

The systematic names are often replaced by abbreviations of the form A:B(C). A indicates the number of carbon atoms in the molecule, B represents the number of unsaturated centres, which are usually *cis*-(Z-) alkenic, and C indicates the position and configuration of the unsaturation.

Palmitic = Hexadecanoic 16:0
Oleic = *cis*-9-Octadecenoic 18:1 (9Z)
Arachidonic = All-*cis*-5,8,11,14-eicosatetraenoic 20:4 ($n - 3$)

There are times when it is more appropriate to count from the methyl end and to use symbols such as $\omega - 3$ or $n - 3$ to indicate the position of the unsaturated centre closest to the methyl group. In this case it is assumed that all unsaturation is methylene interrupted and has *cis*-(Z-) configuration.

sn- (stereospecifically numbered) is used to indicate the configuration of glycerol derivatives. The carbon atom that appears at the top of that Fischer projection showing a vertical chain with the OH group of C(2) to the left is designated as C(1).

$$\overset{1}{C}H_2OH \qquad\qquad CH_2OPO_3H_2$$
$$HO \blacktriangleright \overset{2}{C} \blacktriangleleft H \qquad\qquad HO \blacktriangleright \overset{}{C} \blacktriangleleft H$$
$$\overset{3}{C}H_2OPO_3H_2 \qquad\qquad CH_2OH$$

sn-glycerol-3-phosphate   sn-glycerol-1-phosphate

Iso acids are isomers branched at the ($\omega - 1$) position, e.g., isopalmitic acid = $(H_3C)_2CH(CH_2)_{12}COOH$.

Anteiso acids are branched at the ($\omega - 2$) position, e.g., anteisopalmitic acid = $H_3CCH_2CH(CH_3)(CH_2)_{11}COOH$.

5.7 CAROTENOIDS

Carotenoids are a class of hydrocarbons consisting of eight isoprenoid units.

The name of a specific carotenoid hydrocarbon is constructed by adding two Greek letters as prefixes to the stem name *carotene*, these prefixes being characteristic of the two C_9 end groups. The prefixes are β- (beta), ε- (epsilon), κ- (kappa), φ- (phi), χ- (chi), and ψ- (psi).

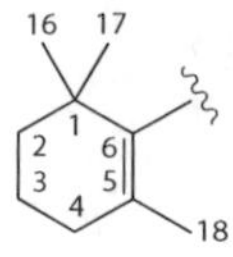

β-   ε-   κ-

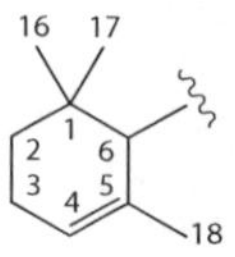

φ-   χ-   ψ-

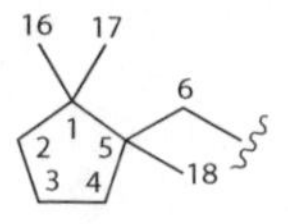

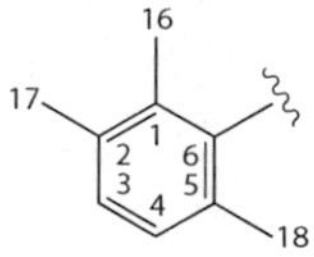

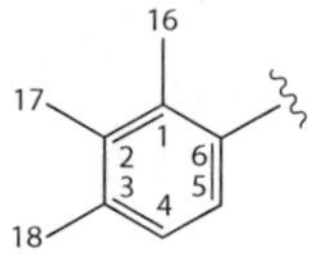

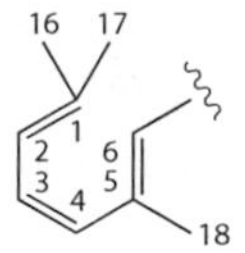

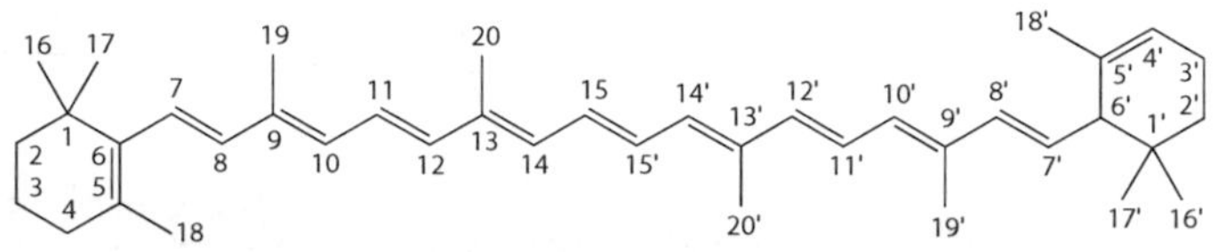

β,ε-carotene

For example, β,ε-carotene is as above.

5.8 LIGNANS

This is an extensive class of natural products typically formed by linkage of two (or more) C_9 (cinnamyl) residues. Linkage occurs in a multitude of ways in addition to the β,β-bonding of the originally discovered lignan types. (Compounds with unusual linkages are often called neolignans.) They can be named systematically, but this gives a large variety of different indexing parents. A more attractive method is the Freudenberg/Weinges/Moss (now IUPAC-approved) scheme based on linkage of the two "lign" fragments. Application of this scheme is not completely straightforward. See *Pure Appl. Chem.*, 72, 1493–1523, 2000 and http://www.chem.qmul.ac.uk/iupac/lignan.

5.9 NUCLEOTIDES AND NUCLEOSIDES

Nucleic acids, e.g., DNA, are ladder polymers of *nucleotides*, the heterocyclic bases of which (purines and pyrimidines) encode the genetic information. The nucleosides are linked together through the carbohydrate residues of the nucleotides to form the polymer. Nucleotides consist of *nucleosides O*-phosphorylated in the sugar residues. The nucleosides, e.g., thymidine (below), consist of a heterocyclic base (in this case thymine) attached to a carbohydrate residue as an *N*-glycoside. The most common bases found in nucleosides are shown in Table 5.6, and the most common nucleosides in Table 5.7.

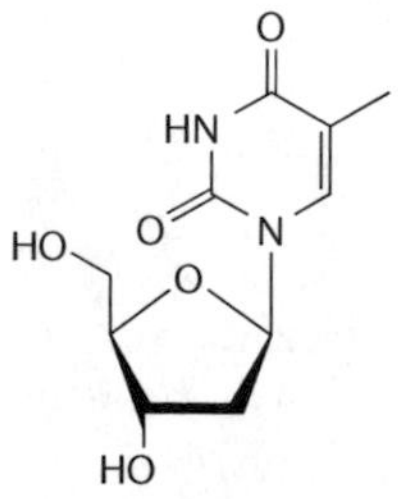

Thymidine

TABLE 5.6
Common Nucleoside Bases
and Their Abbreviated Forms

Ade	adenine
Cyt	cytosine
Gua	guanine
Hyp	hypoxanthine
Oro	orotate
Pur	unknown purine
Pyr	unknown pyrimidine
Shy	thiohypoxanthine
Sur	thiouracil
Thy	thymine
Ura	uracil
Xan	xanthine

TABLE 5.7
Abbreviations for Nucleosides

Ado	A	adenosine
BrUrd	B	5-bromouridine
Cyd	C	cytidine
	D or hU	5,6-dihydrouridine
Guo	G	guanosine
Ino	I	inosine
Nuc	N	unspecified nucleoside
Oro	O	orotidine
Puo	R	unspecified purine nucleoside
Pyd	Y	unspecified pyrimidine nucleoside
Ψrd	ψ or Q	pseudouridine
Sno	M or sI	thiouridine
Srd	S or sU	6-thioinosine
Thd	T	ribosylthymine (not thymidine)
Urd	U	uridine
Xao	X	xanthosine
D		2-deoxy
dThd	dT	thymidine
Nir		ribosylnicotinamide
–P		phosphoric residue

5.10   TETRAPYRROLES

This is a general term for porphyrins and bilane derivatives (cyclic and open-chain tetrapyrroles, respectively), centered around a numerically limited number of natural products. Other IUPAC parent skeletons are phorbine, corrin, chlorin, and phthalocyanine (synthetic). See *Pure Appl. Chem.*, 59, 779–782, 1987, for the numbering of these skeletons.

The parent porphyrin system is called porphyrin (IUPAC) or porphine (CAS). In the old literature, the so-called Fischer numbering may be encountered.

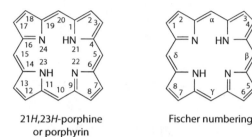

21*H*,23*H*-porphine   Fischer numbering
or porphyrin

5.11   ORGANOBORON COMPOUNDS

This is an extremely complex field, requiring major modifications to organic nomenclature and the use of terms and techniques from inorganic nomenclature. "Even so, there are a significant number of boron compounds whose names are not satisfactory to members of either the organic or inorganic community" (see Fox and Powell, loc. cit., Chapter 27, for details). Because the number of hydrogen atoms in neutral and anionic boron hydrides often bears no simple relationship to the number of boron atoms, borane names must express the number of both.

Special prefixes *closo-, nido- arachno-, catena-, hypho-, clado-, isocloso-, isonido-, isoarachno-, canasto-, anello-, precloso-, hypercloso-, pileo-*, and *conjuncto-* are found in the literature to describe borane structures.

CAS uses the names *boronic* [BH(OH)$_2$] and *borinic* [H$_2$BOH] *acid* as parents. Inorganic chemists prefer the names *dihydroxyborane* and *hydroxyborane*, since they are not really acids. However, the CAS system allows their derivatives to be named by analogy with other acids, such as the phosphorus acids.

5.12   ORGANOPHOSPHORUS (AND ORGANOARSENIC) COMPOUNDS

Organophosphorus chemistry is complicated by the stability of P(*V*) species in addition to trivalent species such as phosphines, and the possibility of tautomerism between them. In addition, many phosphorus compounds have been named as inorganics or biochemicals, as well as by the methods of organic nomenclature, leading to a proliferation of names.

An extensive *Dictionary of Organophosphorus Compounds* (compiled by R. E. Edmundson) was published in 1988, and has been updated as part of the CRC database (see Section 1.2.1). It gives an extensive selection of alternative names. Substructure searching to locate compounds of analogous structure can often resolve nomenclature difficulties for the commoner types.

Organoarsenic nomenclature is analogous.

Many phosphorus (and arsenic) compounds are named using functional replacement nomenclature in which replacement affixes are inserted into the names of the appropriate phosphorus (arsenic) acids (Table 5.8).

TABLE 5.8
Parent Acid Names Used in Functional Replacement
Nomenclature of Phosphorus and Arsenic Compounds

Trivalent Acids

$(HO)_3P$	Phosphorous acid	$(HO)_3As$	Arsenous acid
$(HO)_2HP$	Phosphonous acid	$(HO)_2HAs$	Arsonous acid
$(HO)H_2P$	Phosphinous acid	$(HO)H_2As$	Arsinous acid
$(HO)PO$	Phosphenous acid	$(HO)AsO$	Arsenenous acid

Pentavalent Acids

$(HO)_3PO$	Phosphoric acid	$(HO)_3AsO$	Arsenic acid
$(HO)_2HPO$	Phosphonic acid	$(HO)_3HAsO$	Arsonic acid
$(HO)H_2PO$	Phosphinic acid	$(HO)H_2AsO$	Arsinic acid
$(HO)PO_2$	Phosphenic acid	$(HO)AsO_2$	Arsenenic acid

TABLE 5.9
Functional Replacement Affixes for
Phosphorus and Arsenic Compounds

Affix	Replacement Operation
Amido	–OH by –NH_2
Azido	–OH by –N_3
Bromide	–OH by –Br
Chloride	–OH by –Cl
Cyanatido	–OH by –OCN
Cyanide	–OH by –CN
(Dithioperoxo)	–OH by –SSH
Fluoride	–OH by –F
Hydrazido	–OH by –$NHNH_2$
Imido	=O by =NH
Iodide	–OH by –I
Isocyanitido	–OH by –NCO
(Isothiocyanitido)	–OH by NCS
Nitride	=O and –OH by ≡N
Peroxo	–OH by –OOH
Seleno	=O by =Se or –OH by –SeH
Telluro	=O by =Te or –OH by –ThE
Thio	=O by =S or –OH by –SH
(Thiocyanitido)	–OH by –SCN

Acidic functional replacement analogues of mononuclear phosphorus and arsenic acids are named by citing the functional replacement affixes in alphabetical order just preceding the *-ic acid* or *-ous acid*. The affixes used are listed in Table 5.9.

The examples below are derived from phosphoric acid.

$(H_2N)(HO)_2PO$	Phosphoramidic acid
$Br(HO)_2PO$	Phosphorobromidic acid
$Cl_2(HO)PO$	Phosphorodichloridic acid
$(HS)_3P=NH$	Phosphorimidotrithioic acid

Non-acidic functional replacement analogues are named by replacing the word *acid* with the appropriate class name occurring earliest in the following list: hydrazide, halide, azide, amide, cyanide, nitride, imide. Other replacing groups are denoted by infixes, as described earlier for acidic functional replacement analogues. The examples below are derived from phosphoric acid.

$(H_2N)3PO$	Phosphoric triamide
$Cl_3P{=}NH$	Phosphorimidic trichloride
$(H_2N)_2(N_3)PO$	Phosphorodiamidic azide

See also Fox and Powell, Chapter 25. On pages 243–245 there is a tabulation of substituting group prefixes for phosphorus-containing groups, showing alternatives. For example, the group HP= is called phosphinidene in CAS, phosphinediyl by IUPAC (1979), and phosphanylidene by IUPAC (1993).

5.13   AZO AND AZOXY COMPOUNDS

Traditional nomenclature for azo compounds uses the multiplicative prefix *azo* –N=N–, e.g., Ph–N=N–Ph = azobenzene, Ph–N=N–$C_{10}H_7$ = 2-benzeneazonaphthalene or 2-phenylazonaphthalene. This is difficult to apply for more complex unsymmetrical compounds, but remains in use. Another form found in the older literature, especially for azo dyes, is naphthalene-2-azobenzene.

More recently, the parent name diazene –N=N– (has also been called diimide; not recommended) was introduced, e.g., Ph–N=N–Ph = diphenyldiazene. The 2006 CAS nomenclature changes have included the following:

Azo, 9CI → diazenyl or 1,2-diazenediyl
Hydrazo, 9CI → 1,2-hydrazinediyl

In naming unsymmetrical azoxy compounds, the prefixes *NNO-* or *ONN-* are used to indicate the position of the oxygen atom, e.g., Ph–N(O)=N–$C_{10}H_7$ = phenyl-*ONN*-azoxynaphthalene. However, post-2006, such azoxy compounds are named in CAS as (1-oxidodiazenyl) or (2-oxidodiazenyl).

5.14   LABELLED COMPOUNDS

There are two main methods used for naming isotopically labelled compounds. For specifically labelled compounds, IUPAC recommends forming the name by placing the nuclide symbols (plus locants if necessary) in square brackets before the name of the unlabelled compounds or that part of the name which is isotopically modified.

Chemical Abstracts uses the Boughton system, in which italicized nuclide symbols follow the name or part of the name of the unlabelled compound as shown below. The symbols -*d* and -*t* are used to denote deuterium and tritium, respectively.

	CA	**IUPAC**
CH_2D_2	Methane-*d$_2$*	[^{2}H$_2$]Methane
$H_3C^{14}CH_2OH$	Ethanol-*1-^{14}C*	[1-^{14}C]Ethanol

The prefix *deutero-* (*deuterio-*) is used to denote replacement of H by D, and *tritio-* for replacement by T.

5.15　TAUTOMERIC COMPOUNDS

The indexing and organisation of information relating to tautomeric or potentially tautomeric substances present severe difficulties to all information products. The issue is not how to name or document each individual tautomer, but in what assumptions to make about which structures are tautomeric, and how to organise information that may be imprecisely given in the literature under various structures, often without clear experimental data.

CAS has fairly precise rules for denoting which structural systems are deemed to be tautomeric, and to which tautomer indexing is directed. In CAS nomenclature 1972–2006, tautomeric substances were often indexed under theoretical tautomers, e.g., the 1*H*- form of purines, which had no practical existence. CAS numbers for tautomeric substances therefore often referred to unknown tautomers.

This nomenclature-based CAS policy has now been replaced by a structure-based policy for selecting the preferred tautomer, giving a closer relationship with physical reality.

6(5*H*)-Pteridinone, 1,7-dihydro, 9CI → 6(5*H*)-pteridinone, 7,8-dihydro

6 Acronyms and Miscellaneous Terms Used in Describing Organic Molecules

6.1 ABBREVIATIONS AND ACRONYMS FOR REAGENTS AND PROTECTING GROUPS IN ORGANIC CHEMISTRY

This list is based, in part, on the compilation of abbreviations and acronyms by Daub, G. H., et al., *Aldrichimica Acta*, 17(1), 13–23, 1984 (reproduced with permission), augmented by some acronyms used in *Science of Synthesis: Houben-Weyl Methods of Molecular Transformations*, Vols. 1–48 (Stuttgart: Thieme, 2000–2009) and in Kocieński, P. J., *Protecting Groups*, 3rd ed. (Stuttgart: Thieme, 2004), respectively, which are reproduced by permission of the publisher. More acronyms, particularly those currently in use for protecting groups, may be found in P. G. M. Wuts and T. W. Greene, *Greene's Protective Groups in Organic Synthesis*, 4th ed. (New York: Wiley, 2006). At the time of publication of this book, there is a useful website hosted by the Freie Universität Berlin, which lists abbreviations and acronyms, with an emphasis on those from the organic chemistry literature: http://www.chemie.fu-berlin.de/cgi-bin/ acronym. The German company FIZ CHEMIE Berlin also identifies acronyms used in organic chemistry together with their chemical structures at http://www.fiz-chemie.de/akronyme/akronyme.pl.

In the list printed below, the same abbreviation is sometimes used for different reagents or protecting groups, and a few acronyms are based on obsolete or misleading nomenclature (e.g., DMPU for *N*,*N*′-dimethylpropyleneurea, which is usually named 1,3 dimethyl-3,4,5,6-tetrahydro-2(1*H*)-pyridmidinone). The use of *o*- (ortho), *m*- (meta), and *p*- (para) is retained in the name of the reagent or protecting group to emphasise the derivation of the abbreviation or acronym. Abbreviations for amino acids, nucleotides, nucleosides, and carbohydrates are omitted in this section but may be found in Chapter 5.

AA	Anisylacetone
AAA	Acetoacetanilide
AAAF	2-(*N*-Acetoxyacetylamino)fluorene
AAMX	Acetoacet-*m*-xylidide (*m*-acetoacetoxylidide)
AAO	Acetaldehyde oxime
AAOA	Acetoacet-*o*-anisidide (*o*-acetoacetanisidide)
AAOC	Acetoacet-*o*-chloroanilide (*o*-acetochloranilide)
AAOT	Acetoacet-*o*-toluidide (*o*-acetoacetotoluidide)
ABA	Abscisic acid
ABL	α-Acetyl-γ-butyrolactone
ABO	2,7,8-Trioxabicyclo[3.2.1]octyl
ABTS	2,2′-Azinobis(3-ethylbenzothiazoline-6-sulfonic acid)
Ac	Acetyl
7-ACA	7-Aminocephalosporanic acid
acac	Acetylacetonato
ACAC (or acac)	Acetylacetonate

ACES	*N*-(2-Acetamido)-2-aminoethanesulfonic acid
Acm	Acetamidomethyl
AcOH	Acetic acid
AcOZ	*p*-Acetoxybenzyloxycarbonyl
Ad	Adamantyl
ADA	*N*-(2-Acetamido)iminodiacetic acid [*N*-(carbamoylmethyl)iminodiacetic acid]
7-ADCA	7-Aminodesacetoxycephalosporanic acid
ADDC	Ammonium diethyldithiocarbamate
ADMA	Alkyldimethylamine
Adoc	1-Adamantyloxycarbonyl
Adpoc	1-(1-Adamantyl)-1-methylethoxycarbonyl
AEP (or AEPZ)	1-(2-Aminoethyl)piperazine
AET	*S*-2-Aminoethylisothiouronium bromide hydrobromide
AIBN	2,2′-Azobis(isobutyronitrile)
AICA	5(4)-Aminoimidazole-4(5)-carboxamide
AIP	Aluminium isopropoxide
All	Allyl
Alloc (or aloc)	Allyloxycarbonyl
Alocam	Allyloxycarboxylaminomethyl
Am	Amyl
AMBA	3-Amino-4-methoxybenzanilide
AMEO	3-Aminopropyltriethoxysilane
AM-ex-OL	4-Chloro-2-phenylquinazoline
AMMO	2-Aminopropyltrimethoxysilane
bis-AMP	*N*-Bis(hydroxyethyl)-2-amino-2-methyl-1-propanol
AMPD	2-Amino-2-methyl-1,3-propanediol
AMPS	2-Acrylamido-2-methylpropanesulfonic acid
AMTCS	Amyltrichlorosilane
ANM	*N*-(4-Anilino-1-naphthyl)maleimide
ANPP	4-Azido-2-nitrophenyl phosphate
ANS-NH$_4$	8-Anilinonaphthalene-1-sulfonic acid, ammonium salt
AOC	Allyloxycarbonyl
AOM	*p*-Anisyloxymethyl [(4-methoxyphenoxy)methyl]
6-APA	6-Aminopenicillanic acid
APAP	*N*-Acetyl-*p*-aminophenol
APDC	Ammonium 1-pyrrolidinecarbodithioate
APDTC	Ammonium 1-pyrrolidinedithiocarbamate
APG	*p*-Azidophenylglyoxal hydrate
APTP	*N*-(4-Azidophenylthio)phthalimide
Ar	Aryl
ASC	*p*-Acetylaminobenzenesulfonyl chloride
ATA	Anthranilamide
ATC	Ethyltrichlorosilane
ATEE	*N*-Acetyl-ʟ-tyrosine ethyl ester monohydrate
1,3-BAC	1,3-Bis(aminomethylmethyl)cyclohexane)
BAL	2,3-Dimercapto-1-propanol (British anti-Lewisite)
BAO	Bis(4-aminophenyl)-1,3,4-oxadiazole
BaP (BAP)	Benzo[*a*]pyrene
BBA	Barbituric acid
9-BBN	9-Borabicyclo[3.3.1]nonane

9-BBN-H	9-Borabicyclo[3.3.1]nonane
BBO	2,5-Bis(4-biphenylyl)oxazole
BBOD	2,5-Bis(4-biphenylyl)-1,3,4-oxadiazole
BBOT	2,5-Bis(5-*tert*-butyl-2-benzoxazolyl)thiophene
BBP	Benzyl butyl phthalate
BCA	*N*-Benzylcyclopropylamine
BCNU	1,3-Bis(2-chloroethyl)-1-nitrosourea
BCP	Butyl carbitol piperonylate
BCPC	*sec*-Butyl *N*-(3-chlorophenyl)carbamate
bda	Benzylidene acetone
BDA	Butane-2,3-diacetal
BDMA	Benzyldimethylamine
BDPA	α,γ-Bisdiphenylene-β-phenylallyl, free radical
BDT	1,3-Benzodithiolan-2-yl
Benzostabase	1,1,3,3-Tetramethyl-1,3-disilaisoindoline
BES	*N*,*N*-Bis(2-hydroxyethyl)-2-aminoethanesulfonic acid
BGE	Butyl glycidyl ether
BHA	3-*tert*-Butyl-4-hydroxyanisole
BHC	Benzene hexachloride
BHMF	2,5-Bis(hydroxymethyl)furan
BHMT	Bis(hexamethylene)triamine
BHT	2,6-Di-*tert*-butyl-4-methylphenol (butylated hydroxytoluene)
BIC	5-Benzisoxazolylmethoxycarbonyl
BICINE	*N*,*N*-Bis(2-hydroxyethyl)glycine
BINAL-H	2,2′-Dihydroxy-1,1′-binaphthyllithium aluminium hydride
BINAP	2,2′-Bis(diphenylphosphino)-1,1′binaphthyl
bipy	2,2′-Bipyridyl
bis-DHP	6,6′-Bis(3,4-dihydo-2*H*-pyran)
BLO	γ-Butyrolactone
Bmpc	2,4-Dimethylthiophenoxycarbonyl
Bmpm	1,1-Bis(4-methoxyphenyl)-1-pyrenylmethyl
BMS	Borane-methyl sulfide complex
Bn	Benzyl (also Bzl or Bnz)
BN	Benzonitrile
BNAH	1-Benzyl-1,4-dihydronicotinamide
BNB	2,4,6-Tri-*tert*-butylnitrosobenzene
Bnz	(See Bn)
BOC (or Boc or t-BOC)	*tert*-Butoxycarbonyl
BOC-ON	2-(*tert*-Butoxycarbonyloxyimino)-2-phenylacetonitrile
BOC-OSU	*N*-(*tert*-Butoxycarbonyloxy)succinimide
BOC-OTCP	*tert*-Butyl 2,4,5-trichlorophenyl carbonate
BOM	Benzyloxymethyl
BOMBr	Benzyl bromomethyl ether
BOMCl	benzyl chloromethyl ether
BON	β-Hydroxynaphthoic acid
BOP	Benzotriazol-1-yloxytris(dimethylamino)phosphonium hexafluorophosphate
BOPCl	Bis(2-oxo-3-oxazolidinyl)phosphinic chloride
BPBG	Butyl phthalyl butyl glycolate
BPC	Butylpyridinium chloride
BPCC	2,2′-Bipyridinium chlorochromate

BPO	2-(4-Biphenylyl)-5-phenyloxazole
Bpoc	1-Methyl-1-(4-biphenylyl)ethoxycarbonyl
BPPM	(2*S*,4*S*)-*N*-*tert*-Butoxycarbonyl-4-diphenylphosphino-2-diphenylphosphinomethylpyrrolidine
Bromo-PADAP	2-(5-Bromo-2-pyridylazo)-5-diethylaminophenol
Bs	4-Bromobenzenesulfonyl (brosyl)
BSA	*N,O*-Bis(trimethylsilyl)acetamide
BSC	*N,O*-Bis(trimethylsilyl)carbamate
BSH	Benzenesulfonyl hydrazide
BSOCOES	Bis[2-(succinimidooxycarbonyloxy)ethyl] sulfone
BST chloride	2-(2-Benzothiazolyl)-5-styryl-3-(4-phthalhydrazidyl)tetrazolium chloride
BSTFA	*N,O*-Bis(trimethylsilyl)trifluoroacetamide
Bt	Benzotriazol-1-yl (1-benzotriazolyl)
BTA	Benzotrifluoroacetone
BTAF	Benzyltrimethylammonium fluoride
BTDA	3,3′,4,4′-Benzophenonetetracarboxylic dianhydride
BTEAC	Benzyltriethylammonium chloride
BTFA	Bis(trifluoroacetamide)
BTMSA	Bis(trimethylsilyl)acetylene
Bts	Benzothiazole-2-sulfonyl
Bu	Butyl
t-Bumeoc	1-(3,5-Di-*tert*-butylphenyl)-1-methylethoxycarbonyl
iBu	*iso*-Butyl
sBu	*sec*-Butyl
tBu	*tert*-Butyl
BuOH	Butanol
t-BuOK	Potassium *tert*-butoxide
Bus	*tert*-Butylsulfonyl
Bz	Benzoyl
Bzh	Diphenylmethyl (benzhydryl)
Bzl	Benzyl (also Bn)
CAM	Carboxamidomethyl
CAN	Cerium(*IV*) ammonium nitrate
CAP	Cellulose acetate phthalate
CAP-Li$_2$	Carbamoyl phosphate, dilithium salt
CAPS	3-Cyclohexylamino-1-propanesulfonic acid
CAT	2-Chloro-4,6-bis(ethylamino)-*s*-triazine
CBC	Carbomethoxybenzenesulfonyl chloride
Cbm	Carbamoyl
CBn (or Cb or Cbo)	Benzyloxycarbonyl (or carbobenzoxy)
Cbz (or CBZ or Z)	Benzyloxycarbonyl
CBZ-HONB	*N*-Benzyloxycarbonyloxy-5-norbornene 2,3-dicarboximide
Cbz-OSu	*N*-[(Benzyloxycarbonyl)oxy]succinimide
CCH	Cyclohexylidenecyclohexane
CCNU	1-(2-Chloroethyl)-3-cyclohexyl-1-nitrosourea
CD	Cyclodextrin
CDA	Cyclohexane-1,2-diacetal
CDAA	Chlorodiallylacetamide
CDC	Cycloheptaarylose-dansyl chloride complex
CDEC	2-Chloroallyl *N,N*-diethyldithiocarbamate
CDTA	*trans*-1,2-Diaminocyclohexane-*N,N,N′,N′*-tetraacetic acid

CE	Cyanoethyl
Cee	1-(2-Chloroethoxy)ethyl
CEEA	*N*-(2-Cyanoethyl)-*N*-ethylamine
CEEMT	*N*-(2-Cyanoethyl)-*N*-ethyl-*m*-toluidine
CEMA	*N*-(2-Cyanoethyl)-*N*-methylaniline
CEPEA	*N*-(2-Hydroxyethyl)-*N*-(2-cyanoethyl)aniline
CHAPS	3-[(3-Cholamidopropyl)dimethylammonio]propanesulfonate
CHES	2-(Cyclohexylamino)ethanesulfonic acid
Chiraphos	2,3-Bis(diphenylphosphino)butane
CHP	*N*-Cyclohexyl-2-pyrrolidone
CHT	Cycloheptatriene
5-CIA	5-Chloroisatoic anhydride
CMA	Carbomethoxymaleic anhydride
CMC	Carboxymethyl cellulose
CMC	1-Cyclohexyl-3-(2-morpholinoethyl)carbodiimide
CMDMCS	(Chloromethyl)dimethylchlorosilane
CMPI	2-Chloro-1-methylpyridinium chloride
CNAP	2-Naphthylmethyl carbamate
CNT	Cyanotoluene
Coc	Cinnamyloxycarbonyl
cod (or COD)	1,5-Cyclooctadiene
cot (or COT)	Cyclooctatetraene
Cp (or cp)	η^5-Cyclopentadienyl
Cp* (or cp*)	η^5-Pentamethylcyclopentadienyl
4-CPA	4-Chlorophenoxyacetic acid
m-CPBA	*m*-Chloroperbenzoic acid
CPTEO	3-Chloropropyltriethoxysilane
CPTMO	3-Chloropropyltrimethoxysilane
CPTr	4,4′,4″-Tris(4,5-dichlorophthalimido)triphenylmethyl
CSA	10-Camphorsulfonic acid
CSI	Chlorosulfonyl isocyanate
CTA	Citraconic anhydride
CTAB (or CTABr)	Cetyltrimethylammonium bromide
CTACl	Cetyltrimethylammonium chloride
CTACN	Cetyltrimethylammonium cyanide
CTAOH	Cetyltrimethylammonium hydroxide
CTFB	4-Trifluoromethylbenzyl carbamate
CTMP	1-[(2-Chloro-4-methylphenyl)-4-methoxy-4-piperidinyl]
Cy	Cyclohexyl
CYAP	*O,O*-Dimethyl *O*-(*p*-cyanophenyl) phosphorothioate
cyclam	1,4,8,11-Tetraazacyclotetradecane
CYP	*p*-Cyanophenyl ethyl phenylphosphonothioate
2,4-D	2,4-Dichlorophenoxyacetic acid
D	2,2′-Dithiodibenzoic acid
DAA	Diacetone acrylamide
DAA	Diacetone alcohol
DAB	*p*-Dimethylaminoazobenzene
DAB	Diaminobenzidine (usually 3,3′)
DABCO (or TED)	1,4-Diazabicyclo[2.2.2]octane
DABITC	4-(*N,N*-Dimethylamino)azobenzene-4′-isothiocyanate

DABS-Cl	4-(*N*,*N*-Dimethylamino)azobenzene-4′-sulfonyl chloride
3,5-DACB	3,5-Diaminochlorobenzene
DACH	*trans*-1,2-Diaminocyclohexane
DACM-3	*N*-(7-Dimethylamino-4-methyl-3-coumarinyl)maleimide
DAD	(See DEAD)
DAM	Di(4-methoxyphenyl)methyl
DAMN	Diaminomaleonitrile
DANSYL	5-Dimethylaminonaphthalene-1-sulfonyl
DAP	Diallyl phthalate
DAP	Diammonium phosphate
DAPI	4′,6-Diamidino-2-phenylindole dihydrochloride
DAS	4,4′-Diaminostilbene-2,2′-disulfonic acid
DAST	*N*,*N*-Diethylaminosulfur trifluoride
DAST	*N*,*N*-Dimethylaminosulfur trifluoride
DATMP	Diethylaluminium 2,2,6,6-tetramethylpiperidide
2,4-DB	2,4-Dichlorophenoxybutyric acid
dba	Dibenzylideneacetone
DBA	Dibenz[*a*,*h*]anthracene
DBAD	Di-*tert*-butyl azodicarboxylate
DBC·Br$_2$	Dibenzo-18-crown-6/Br$_2$
DBCP	1,2-Dibromo-3-chloropropane
DBDPO	Decabromodiphenyl ether
DBD-Tmoc	2,7-Di-*tert*-butyl [9-(10,10-dioxo-10,10,10,10-tetrahydrothioxanthyl)]methoxycarbonyl
DBIC	Dibutylindolocarbazole
DBMIB	Dibromomethylisopropylbenzoquinone
DBN	1,5-Diazabicyclo[4.3.0]non-5-ene
DBN	*p*,*p*′-Dinitrobenzhydryl
DBP	Dibutyl phthalate
DBPC	2,6-Di-*tert*-butyl-*p*-cresol
DBPO	Dibenzoyl peroxide
DBS	Dibenzosuberyl
DBS	Dibutyl sebacate
DBU	1,8-Diazabicyclo[5.4.0]undec-7-ene
2,4-DCAD	2,4-Dichlorobenzaldehyde
DCAF	2′,4′-Bis[di(carboxymethyl)aminomethyl]fluorescein
DCB	Dicyanobenzene
2,4-DCBA	2,4-Dichlorobenzoic acid
2,4-DCBC	2,4-Dichlorobenzyl chloride
2,4′-DCBP	2,4′-Dichlorobenzophenone
2,4-DCBTF	2,4-Dichlorobenzotrifluoride
3,4-DCBTF	3,4-Dichlorobenzotrifluoride
DCC	Dicyclohexylcarbodiimide
DCCI	(See DCC)
DCE	Dichloroethane
DCEE	Dichloroethyl ether
DCHA	Dicyclohexylamine
DCHBH	Dicyclohexylborane
DCI-HCl	1-(3′,4′-Dichlorophenyl)-2-isopropylaminoethanol hydrochloride
DCM	Dichloromethane
DCME	Dichloromethyl methyl ether

DCOC	2,4-Dichlorobenzoyl chloride
DCPD	Dicyclopentadiene
DCPhth	4,5-Dichlorophthaloyl
2,4-DCT	2,4-Dichlorotoluene
3,4-DCT	3,4-Dichlorotoluene
2,4-DCTC	2,4-Dichlorobenzotrichloride
3,4-DCTC	3,4-Dichlorobenzotrichloride
DCU	*N,N*-Dichlorourethane
DDA	4,4'-Dichlorodiphenylacetic acid
DDB	2,3-Dimethoxy-1,4-bis(dimethylamino)butane
DDD	2,2'-Dihydroxy-6,6'-dinaphthyl disulfide
o,p'-DDD	1-(*o*-Chlorophenyl)-1-(*p*-chlorophenyl)-2,2-dichloroethane
p,p'-DDD	2,2-Bis(*p*-chlorophenyl)-1,1-dichloroethane
o,p'-DDE	1-(*o*-Chlorophenyl)-1-(*p*-chlorophenyl)-2,2-dichloroethylene
p,p'-DDE	2,2-Bis(*p*-chlorophenyl)-1,1-dichloroethylene
DDH	1,3-Dibromo-5,5-dimethylhydantoin
Ddm	4,4'-Dimethoxydiphenylmethyl [bis-(4-methoxyphenyl)methyl]
DDM	4,4'-Dichlorodiphenylmethane
DDM	Diphenyldiazomethane
DDMU	4,4'-Dichlorodiphenyl-2-chloroethylene [1-Chloro-2,2-bis(4'-chlorophenylethene)]
DDOH	4,4'-Dichlorodiphenylethanol
DDP	Dichlorodiammineplatinum
DDQ	2,3-Dichloro-5,6-dicyano-1,4-benzoquinone
DDS	*p,p'*-Diaminodiphenyl sulfone
DDS	Dihydroxydiphenyl sulfone
DDSA	Dodecenylsuccinic anhydride
o,p'-DDT	1-(*o*-Chlorophenyl)-1-(*p*-chlorophenyl)-2,2,2-trichloroethane
p,p'-DDT	1,1-bis(*p*-Chlorophenyl)-2,2,2-trichloroethane
DDVP	Dimethyl 2,2-dichlorovinyl phosphate
DDZ	α,α-Dimethyl-3,5-dimethoxybenzyloxycarbonyl
DEA	*N,N*-Diethylaniline
DEAA	*N,N*-Diethylacetoacetamide
DEAC	Diethylaluminium chloride
DEAD (or DEADCAT)	Diethyl azodicarboxylate
DEAE-cellulose	Diethylaminoethyl cellulose
DEAH	Diethylaluminium hydride
DEAI	Diethylaluminium iodide
DEAP	2,2-Diethoxyacetophenone
DEASA	*N,N*-Diethylaniline-3-sulfonic acid
DEC	2-Diethylaminoethyl chloride hydrochloride
DEDM	Diethyl diazomalonate
DEII	Diethylindoloindole
DEIPS	Diethylisopropylsilyl
DEP	Diethyl phthalate
DEP	Diethyl pyrocarbonate
DEPC	Diethylphosphoryl cyanide
DEPHA	Di(2-ethylhexyl)phosphoric acid
DESS	Diethyl succinylsuccinate
DET	Diethyl tartrate
DFP	Diisopropyl fluorophosphate

DHA	Dehydroacetic acid
DHA	9,10-Dihydroanthracene
DHBA	3,4-Dihydroxybenzylamine hydrobromide
DHBP	Dihydroxybenzophenone (usually 4,4′)
DHEBA	1,2-Dihydroxyethylenebisacrylamide
DHET	Dihydroergotoxine
DHN	5,12-Dihydronaphthacene
DHP	Diheptyl phthalate
DHP	Dihydropyran
DIAD	Diisopropyl diazodicarboxylate
DIB	1,3-Diphenylisobenzofuran
DIBAC	Diisobutylaluminium chloride
DIBAH	Diisobutylaluminium hydride
DIBAL	(See DIBAH)
DIBAL-H	(See DIBAH)
DIC	Diisopropylcarbodiimide
DIC	(Dimethylamino)isopropyl chloride hydrochloride
DIDP	Diisodecyl phthalate
DIEA	Diisopropylethylamine
DI-ET	*N,N*-Diethyl-*p*-phenylenediamine monohydrochloride
Diglyme	Diethylene glycol dimethyl ether
DiHPhe	2,5-Dihydroxyphenylalanine
Dim	2-(1,3-Dithianyl)methyl
Dimethyl-POPOP	1,4-Bis(4-methyl-5-phenyloxazol-2-yl)benzene
Dimsyl Na	Sodium methylsulfinylmethide
Diop (or DIOP)	2,3-*O*-Isopropylidene-2,3-dihydroxy-1,4-bis(diphenylphosphino)butane
Diox	Dioxane
DIPC	2-Dimethylaminoisopropyl chloride hydrochloride
DIPEA	Diisopropylethylamine
DIPHOS (or diphos)	Ethylenebis(diphenylphosphine); see also dppe
DIPSO	3-[Bis(2-hydroxyethyl)amino]-2-hydroxy-1-propanesulfonic acid
DIPT (or DiPT)	Diisopropyl tartrate
Di-SNADNS	2,7-Bis(4-sulfo-1-naphthylazo)-1,8-dihydroxynaphthalene-3,6-disulfonic acid
DITC	1,4-Phenylene diisocyanate
2,6-DMA	2,6-Dimethylanisole
DMA or DMAc	*N,N*-Dimethylacetamide
DMA	*N,N*-Dimethylaniline
DMAA	*N,N*-Dimethylacetoacetamide
DMAC	(See DMA, dimethylacetamide)
DMAD	dimethyl acetylenedicarboxylate
DMA-DEA	*N,N*-Dimethylacetamide diethyl acetal
DMAEMA	2-Dimethylaminoethyl methacrylate
DMAP	Dimethylaminopropylamine
DMAP	4-(Dimethylamino)pyridine
DMAPMA	Dimethylaminopropyl methacrylamide
DMB	4,4′Dichloro-α-methylbenzhydrol
DMB	2,4- or 3,4-Dimethoxybenzyl
DMC	2-(Dimethylamino)ethyl chloride
dmch	6,6-Dimethylcyclohexadienyl
DMCS	Dimethylchlorosilane

DMDAAC	Dimethyldiallylammonium chloride
DMDO	Dimethyldioxirane
DME	1,2-Dimethoxyethane (glyme)
DMECS	Dimethylethylchlorosilane
DMEU	*N,N′*-Dimethylethyleneurea
DMF	*N,N*-Dimethylformamide
DMF-DMA	Dimethylformamide dimethyl acetal
DMI	1,3-Dimethyl-2-imidazolidinone
DMIPS	Dimethylisopropylsilyl
DMM	Dimethylmaleoyl
Dmoc	Dithianylmethoxycarbonyl
Dmp	Dimethylphosphinyl
2,6-DMP	2,6-Dimethylphenol
DMP	Dimethyl phthalate
DMP	Dimethyl pyrocarbonate
DMP	2,2-Dimethoxypropane
DMP-30	2,4,6-Tris(dimethylaminomethyl)phenol
DMPA	2,2-Dimethoxy-2-phenylacetophenone
DMPC	3-Dimethylaminopropyl chloride hydrochloride
dmpd	2,4-Dimethylpentadienyl
DMPE	1,2-Bis(dimethylphosphino)ethane
DMPM	2,4- or 3,4-Dimethoxybenzyl
DMPO	5,5-Dimethyl-1-pyrroline *N*-oxide
DMPP	1,1-Dimethyl-4-phenylpiperazinium iodide
DMPS	2,3-Dimercapto-1-propanesulfonic acid (sodium salt)
DMPU	1,3-Dimethyl-3,4,5,6-tetrahydropyrimidin-2(1*H*)-one (also named *N,N′*-dimethylpropyleneurea)
DMS	4,6-Dimethoxybenzene-1,3-disulfonyl chloride
DMS	Dimethyl sulfide
DMSO	Dimethyl sulfoxide
DMSS	Dimethyl succinylsuccinate
DMT	Dimethyl tartrate
DMT	Dimethyl terephthalate
DMTD	2,5-Dimercapto-1,3,4-thiadiazole
DMTr	Di(4-methoxyphenyl)phenylmethyl or dimethoxytrityl
DMTSF	Dimethyl(methylthio)sulfonium fluoroborate
DMTST	Dimethyl(methylthio)sulfonium Trifluoromethanesulfonate
DNA	Deoxyribonucleic acid
DNAP	4-(2,4-Dinitrophenylazo)-9-phenanthrol
DNB	*p,p′*-Dinitrobenzhydryl
DNBS	2,4-Dinitrobenzenesulfonic acid
DNBSC	2,4-Dinitrobenzenesulfenyl chloride
DNF	2,4-Dinitrofluorobenzene
DNFA	2,4-Dinitro-5-fluoroaniline (Bergmann's reagent)
DNFB	(See DNF)
DNMBS	4-(4,8-Dimethoxynaphthylmethyl)benzenesulfonyl
DNP	2,4-Dinitrophenyl
DNP	2,4-Dinitrophenylhydrazine
DNP	Dinonyl phthalate
DNPBA	3,5-Dinitroperoxybenzoic acid or 2,4-dinitroperoxybenzoic acid
2,6-DNPC	2,6-Dinitro-*p*-cresol

Dnp-F	(See DNF)
DNPF	(See DNF)
DNS	5-Dimethylamino-1-naphthalenesulfonic acid
DNS	4,4′-Dinitrostilbene-2,2′-disulfonic acid, disodium salt
DNSA	5-Dimethylaminonaphthalene-1-sulfonamide
DNS-BBA	N-Dansyl-3-aminobenzeneboronic acid
DNTC	4-Dimethylamino-1-naphthyl isothiocyanate
DOA	Dioctyl adipate
Dobz	p-(Dihydroxyboryl)benzyloxycarbonyl
DOP	Dioctyl phthalate
DOPET	3,4-Dihydroxyphenethyl alcohol
2,4-DP	2,4-Dichlorophenoxypropionic acid
DPB	1,4-Diphenyl-1,3-butadiene
DPDM	Diphenyl diazomalonate
DPH	1,6-Diphenyl-1,3,5-hexatriene
DPM (or dpm)	Diphenylmethyl
DPMS	Diphenylmethylsilyl
Dpp	Diphenylphosphinyl
DPPA	Diphenylphosphoryl azide
dppb	1,4-Bis(diphenylphosphino)butane
DPPC	Dipalmitoylphophatidylcholine
DPP-Cl	Diphenylphosphinyl chloride
dppe	1,2-Bis(diphenylphosphino)ethane; see also DIPHOS
Dppe	2-(Diphenylphosphino)ethyl
dppf	1,1′-bis(diphenylphosphino)ferrocene
dppm	Bis(diphenylphosphino)methane
Dppm	Diphenyl-4-pyridylmethyl
dppp	1,3-Bis(diphenylphosphino)propane
DPS	trans-p,p′-Diphenylstilbene
DPSME	2-(Methyldiphenylsilyl)ethyl
DPTC	Di-2-pyridyl thionocarbonate
DSAH	Disuccinimidyl (N,N′-diacetylhomocysteine)
DSP	Dithiobis(succinimidyl propionate)
DSS	2,2-Dimethyl-2-silapentane-5-sulfonate
DSS	3-(Trimethylsilyl)-1-propanesulfonic acid (sodium salt)
DSS	Disuccinimidyl suberate
DST	Disuccinimidyl tartrate
DTBB	4,4′-Di-tert-butylbiphenyl
DTBMS	Di-tert-butylmethylsilyl
DTBP	Di-tert-butyl peroxide
DTBS	Di-tert-butylsilylene
DTE	Dithioerythritol
DTMC	4,4′-Dichloro-α-(trichloromethyl)benzhydrol
DTNB	5,5′-Dithiobis(2-nitrobenzoic acid)
DTPA	Diethylenetriaminepentaacetic acid
Dts	Dithiasuccininyl
DTT	Dithiothreitol
DVB	Divinylbenzene
DXE	Dixylylethane
E (or cathyl)	Ethoxycarbonyl

EAA	Ethyl acetoacetate
EAA	*N*-Ethylanthranilic acid
EADC	Ethylaluminium dichloride
EAK	Ethyl amyl ketone
EASC	Ethylaluminium sesquichloride
EBA	*N*-Ethyl-*N*-benzylaniline
EBASA	*N*-Ethyl-*N*-benzylaniline-4-sulfonic acid
EBSA	*p*-Ethylbenzenesulfonic acid
ECEA	*N*-Ethyl-*N*-chloroethylaniline
EDA	Ethyl diazoacetate
EDANS	2-Aminoethylamino-1-naphthalenesulfonic acid (1,5 or 1,8)
EDB	Ethylene dibromide
EDC	Ethylene dichloride
EDCl (or EDC)	1-Ethyl-3-[3-(dimethylamino)propyl]carbodiimide hydrochloride
EDDP	*O*-Ethyl *S,S*-diphenyl dithiophosphate
EDTA (or edta)	Ethylenediaminetetraacetic acid
EDTN	1-Ethoxy-4-(dichloro-*s*-triazinyl)-naphthalene
EDTP	Ethylenediamine tetrapropanol
EE	1-Ethoxyethyl
EEDQ	*N*-Ethoxycarbonyl-2-ethoxy-1,2-dihydroquinoline
EGS	Ethylene glycol bis(succinimidyl succinate)
EGTA	1,2-Bis(2-aminoethoxy)ethane-*N,N,N′,N′*-tetraacetic acid
en	Ethylenediamine
EPN	*O*-Ethyl *O*-(*p*-nitrophenyl)thiobenzenephosphate
EPPS	4-(2-Hydroxyethyl)-1-piperazinepropanesulfonic acid
Et	Ethyl
ETA	(See EDTA)
ETSA	Ethyl trimethylsilylacetate
EVK	Ethyl vinyl ketone
FA	Furfuryl alcohol
FAMSO	Methyl methylsulfinylmethyl sulfide
Fc	Ferrocenyl
FDMA	Perfluoro-*N,N*-dimethylcyclohexylmethylamine
FDNB	(See DNF)
FDNDEA	5-Fluoro-2,4-dinitro-*N,N*-diethylaniline
Fm	9-Fluorenylmethyl
Fmoc	9-Fluorenylmethoxycarbonyl
FNPS	Bis(4-fluoro-3-nitrophenyl) sulfone
For	Formyl
Fp	Cyclopentadienyl(dicarbonyl)ferrate
FS	Fremy's salt (dipotassium nitrosodisulfonate)
FTN	Perfluoro-1,3,7-trimethylbicyclo[3.3.1]nonane
GABA	4-Aminobutyric acid
Glyme (glyme)	1,2-Dimethoxyethane (see DME)
GLYMO	3-Glycidyloxypropyltrimethoxysilane
GUM	Guaiacolmethyl
HABA	2-(*p*-Hydroxyphenylazo)benzoic acid
HABBA	2-(4′-Hydroxyazobenzene)benzoic acid
HBD	Hexabutyldistannoxane
HBT also HOBT	1-Hydroxybenzotriazole

HDCBS	2-Hydroxy-3,5-dichlorobenzenesulfonic acid
HDODA	1,6-Hexanediol diacrylate
HDPE	High-density polyethylene
HEA	*N*-(2-Hydroxyethyl)aziridine
HEDTA	2-Hydroxyethylethylenediaminetriacetic acid
HEEI	*N*-(2-Hydroxyethyl)ethyleneimine
HEMA	2-Hydroxyethyl methacrylate
HEPES	4-(2-Hydroxyethyl)-1-piperazineethanesulfonic acid
HEPSO	*N*-Hydroxyethylpiperazine-*N*′-2-hydroxypropanesulfinic acid
HETE	Hydroxy(e)icosatetraenoic acid
Hex	Hexane (or hexyl)
HFA	Hexafluoroacetone
HFBA	Heptafluorobutyric acid
HFIP	hexafluoroisopropyl alcohol
HFP	hexafluoropropene
HFTA	hexafluorothioacetone
HHPA	Hexahydrophthalic anhydride
HMAT	Hexa[1-(2-methyl)aziridinyl]-1,3,5-triphorphatriazine
HMB	2-Hydroxy-5-methoxybenzaldehyde
HMB	2-Hydroxy-4-methoxybenzophenone
HMDS	1,1,1,3,3,3-Hexamethyldisilazane
HMDSO	Hexamethyldisiloxane
HMI	Hexamethyleneimine
HMN	2,2,4,4,6,8,8-Heptamethylnonane
HMPA	Hexamethylphosphoramide (hexamethylphosphoric triamide)
HMPT	Hexamethylphosphorous triamide
HMPTA	(See HMPA)
HMTT	3-Hexadecanoyl-4-methoxycarbonyl-1,3-thiazolidine-2-thione
HOAt	1-Hydroxy-7-azabenzotriazole
HOBT also HBT	1-Hydroxybenzotriazole
HONB	*N*-Hydroxy-5-norbornene-2,3-dicarboxylic acid imide
HOSA	Hydroxylamine-*O*-sulfonic acid
HPETE	Hydroperoxy(e)icosatetraenoic acid
HPPH	5-Hydroxyphenyl-5-phenylhydantoin
HQ	Hydroquinone
HTMP	4-Hydroxy-2,2,6,6-tetramethylpiperidine
HVA	Homovanillic acid (4-hydroxy-3-methoxyphenylacetic acid)
Hyiv	α-Hydroxyisovaleric acid
Hz	Homobenzyloxycarbonyl
I-AEDANS	*N*-Iodoacetyl-*N*′-(X-sulfo-1-naphthyl)ethylenediamine (X = 5, 1,5-I-AEDANS; X = 8, 1,8-I-AEDANS)
IBD	Iodobenzene dichloride
IBMX	3-Isobutyl-1-methylxanthine
IBTMO	Isobutyltrimethoxysilane
IBX	2-Iodobenzoic acid
ICl	Isophthaloyl choride
IDTr	3-(Imidazol-1-ylmethyl)-4,4′-dimethoxytriphenylmethyl
IIDQ	2-Isobutoxy-1-isobutoxycarbonyl-1,2-dihydroquinoline
Im	1-Imidazolyl
IMds	2,6-Dimethoxy-4-methylbenzenesulfonyl

IMEO	Imidazolinepropyltriethoxysilane
INAH	Isonicotinic acid hydrazide
INH	(See INAH)
INT	2-(*p*-Iodophenyl)-3-(*p*-nitrophenyl)-5-phenyltetrazolium chloride
IPA	Isopropyl alcohol
Ipaoc	1-Isopropylallyloxycarbonyl
Ipc	Isopinocampheyl
IPC	Isopropyl *N*-phenylcarbamate
IpcBH$_2$	Isopinocampheylborane
Ipc$_2$BH	Bisisopinocampheylborane
IPDI	Isophorone diisocyanate (3-isocyanatomethyl-3,4,4-trimethylcyclohexyl isocyanate
IPDMS	Isopropyldimethylsilyl
IPN	Isophthalonitrile
IPOTMS	Isopropenyloxytrimethylsilane
Ips	[(4-Iodophenyl)sulfonyl]
ITA	Itaconic anhydride
IZAA	5-Chloroindazol-3-acetic acid ethyl ester
KAPA	Potassium 3-aminopropylamide
KBA	3-Ketobutyraldehyde dimethyl acetal
KBT	4-Ketobenztriazine
KDA	Potassium diisopropylamide
KDO	2-Keto-3-deoxyoctonate
KHMDS	Potassium hexamethyldisilazanide
K-Selectride®	Potassium tri-*sec*-butylborohydride
KS-Selectride®	Potassium triisoamylborohydride
LAH	Lithium aluminium hydride
LDA	Lithium diisopropylamide
LDBB (or LiDBB)	Lithium 4,4′-di-*tert*-butylbiphenylide
LDPE	Low-density polyethylene
Lev	Levulinoyl (4-oxopentanoyl)
LevS	[4,4-(Ethylenedithio)pentanoyl]
Lgf$_2$BH	Dilongifolylborane
LHMDS	Lithium hexamethyldisilazane
LICA	Lithium isopropylcyclohexylamide
LiHMDS	Lithium hexamethyldisilazanide
LiTMP	Lithium tetramethylpiperidide
LPO	Lauroyl peroxide
L-Selectride®	Lithium tri-*sec*-butylborohydride
LS-Selectride®	Lithium triisoamylborohydride
LTA	Lead tetraacetate
LTMAC	Dodecyltrimethylammonium chloride
LTMP	Lithium 2,2,6,6-tetramethylpiperidide
lut	Lutidine
M	Metal
MA	Maleic anhydride
MAA	Menthoxyacetic acid
MAA	Methyl acetoacetate
MABR	Methylaluminium bis(4-bromo-2,6-di-*tert*-butylphenoxide)
MAD	Methylaluminium bis(2,6-di-*tert*-butyl-4-methylphenoxide)
Mal	Maleyl

-Mal-	Maleoyl
MAM-acetate	Methylazoxymethyl acetate
MAPO	Tris[1-(2-methyl)aziridinyl]phosphine
MAPS	Tris[1-(2-methyl)aziridinyl]phosphine sulfide
MAPTAC	Methacrylamidopropyltrimethylammonium chloride
MASC	Methylaluminium sesquichloride
MBA	*N,N'*-Methylenebisacrylamide
MBBA	*N*-(*p*-Methoxybenzylidene)-*p*-butylaniline
MBE	1-Methyl-1-benzyloxyethyl
MBF	2,3,3*a*,4,5,6,7,7*a*-Octahydrotrimethyl-4,7-methanobenzofuran-2-yl
MBS	*m*-Maleimidobenzoyl-*N*-hydroxysuccinimide ester
MBS	*p*-Methoxybenzenesulfonyl
MBTH	3-Methyl-2-benzothiazolinone hydrazone
3-MC	3-Methylcholanthrene
MCA	Monochloroacetic acid
MCAA	(See MCA)
3,3-MCH	3-Methyl-3-cyclohexen-1-one
MCPBA (or m-CPBA)	3-Chloroperoxybenzoic acid (*m*-chloroperoxybenzoic acid)
MCPCA	2-Methyl-4-chlorophenoxyaceto-*o*-chloroanilide
MCPDEA	*N,N*-Di(2-hydroxyethyl)-*m*-chloroaniline
MCPP	4-Chloro-3-methylphenoxypropionic acid
MDA	1,8-*p*-Menthanediamine
MDEB	*N*-Methyl-*N*-dodecylephedrinium bromide
Mds	2,6-Dimethyl-4-methoxybenzenesulfonyl
Me	Methyl
MeCCNU	1-(2-Chloroethyl)-3-(4-*trans*-methylcyclohexyl)-1-nitrosourea
MEI	2-Morpholinoethyl isocyanide
MEK	Methyl ethyl ketone
MEM	2-Methoxyethoxymethyl
MEMCl	2-Methoxyethoxymethyl chloride
MEMO	3-Methacryloxypropyltrimethoxysilane
MeOTf	Methyl trifluoromethanesulfonate
1-MEO-PMS	1-Methoxy-5-methylphenazinium methyl sulfate
MeOZ	*p*-Methoxybenzyloxycarbonyl
MEP	*O,O*-Dimethyl *O*-(3-methyl-4-nitrophenyl) phosphorothioate
Mes	Mesityl (2,4,6-trimethylphenyl)
MES-hydrate	4-Morpholineethanesulfonic acid
Meth	2-Mercaptoethanol
MG-Ch	Methyl glycol chitosan
MHHPA	4-Methylhexahydrophthalic anhydride
MIA	*N*-Methylisatoic anhydride
MIBK	Methyl isobutyl ketone
MICA	Magnesium isopropyl cyclohexamide
MIPK	Methyl isopropyl ketone
MIX	3-Isobutyl-1-methylxanthine
MMA	Methyl methacrylate
MMAA	Mono-*N*-methylacetoacetamide
MMC	Methyl magnesium carbonate
MMF	*N*-Monomethylformamide
MMH	Methyl mercuric hydroxide

MMS	Methyl methanesulfonate
MMTr	Monomethoxytrityl (4-methoxyphenyldiphenylmethyl)
MMTrCl	Monomethoxytrityl chloride
MMTS	(See FAMSO)
MNA	Methylnadic anhydride (methylnorbornene-2,3-dicarboxylic acid anhydride)
MNNG	*N*-Methyl-*N'*-nitro-*N*-nitrosoguanidine
MNPT	*m*-Nitro-*p*-toluidine
MOM	Methoxymethyl
MOMCl	Chloromethyl methyl ether
MoOPH	Oxodiperoxymolybdenum(pyridine) hexamethylphosphoramide ($MoO_5 \cdot Py \cdot HMPA$)
MOP	2-Methoxy-2-propyl
MOPS	4-Morpholinepropanesulfonic acid
MOPSO	3-(*N*-Morpholino)-2-hydroxypropanesulfonic acid
Moz	4-Methoxybenzyloxycarbonyl
MP	4-Methoxyphenyl
MPEMA	2-Ethyl-2-(*p*-tolyl)malonamide
MPM (or PMB)	(4-Methoxyphenyl)methyl (*p*-methoxybenzyl)
MPP	*O,O*-Dimethyl *O*-(4-methylmercapto-3-methylphenyl) thiophosphate
MPPH	5-(*p*-Methylphenyl)-5-phenylhydantoin
Mps	4-Methoxyphenylsulfonyl
MPS	Methyl phenyl sulfide
Mpt	Dimethylthiophosphinyl
Mpt-Cl	Methylphosphinothionyl chloride
MRITC	Methylrhodamine isothiocyanate
Ms (or MS)	Mesyl (methanesulfonyl)
MSA	Methanesulfonic acid
bis-MSB	4-Bis(2-methylstyryl)benzene
MsCl	Methanesulfonyl chloride
MSE	2-(Methylsulfonyl)ethyl
MSH	2,4,6-Trimethylbenzenesulfonyl hydrazide
Msib	4-(Methylsulfinyl)benzyl
MSMA	Monosodium methanearsonate
MSO	4-Cresyl methyl ether
MSOC	*N*-(2-Methylsulfonyl)ethyloxycarbonyl
MsOH	Methanesulfonic acid
MST	Mesitylenesulfonyltetrazolide
MSTFA	*N*-Methyl-*N*-trimethylsilyltrifluoroacetamide
Msz	4-Methylsulfonylbenzyloxycarbonyl
Mtb	2,4,6-Trimethoxybenzenesulfonyl
MTBE	Methyl *tert*-butyl ether (*tert*-butyl methyl ether)
MTBSTFA	*N*-(*tert*-Butyldimethylsilyl)-*N*-methyltrifluoroacetamide
MTCA	2-Methylthiazolidine-4-carboxylic acid
MTD	*m*-Toluenediamine
MTDEA	*N,N*-Di(2-hydroxyethyl)-*m*-toluidine (*m*-toluidine-*N,N*-diethanol)
Mte	2,3,5,6-Tetramethyl-4-methoxybenzenesulfonyl
MTES	Methyltriethoxysilane
MTH	Methylthiohydantoin
MTHP	4-Methoxytetrahydropyranyl
MTHPA	Methyltetrahydrophthalic anhydride
MTM	Methylthiomethyl

MTMB	4-(Methylthiomethoxy)butanoyl
MTMC	4-(Methylthio)-*m*-cresol
MTMECO	2-(Methylthiomethoxy)ethoxycarbonyl
MTMS	Methyltrimethoxysilane
MTMT	2-(Methylthiomethoxymethyl)benzoyl
MTN	*m*-Tolunitrile
MTP	4-(Methylthio)phenol
MTPA	α-Methoxy-α-trifluoromethylphenylacetic acid
Mtpc	4-Methylthiophenoxycarbonyl
Mtr	4-Methoxy-2,3,6-trimethylphenylsulfonyl
Mts	2,4,6-Trimethylbenzenesulfonyl
MTT	3-(4,5-Dimethylthiazol-2-yl)-2,5-diphenyl-2*H*-tetrazolium bromide
MTX	Methotrexate
MUGB	4-Methylumbelliferyl *p*-guanidinobenzoate
MVK	Methyl vinyl ketone
MVP	2-Methyl-5-vinylpyridine
MXDA	*m*-Xylylenediamine
5-NAA	5-Nitroanthranilic acid
NAC	1-Naphthyl *N*-methylcarbamate
NaHMDS	Sodium hexamethyldisilazanide
NAP	2-Naphthylmethyl
Naph	2-Naphthyl
NB	*p*-Nitrobenzyl
NBA	*N*-Bromoacetamide
nbd	Norbornadiene (bicyclo[2.2.1]hepta-2,5-diene)
NBDCl	4-Chloro-7-nitro-2,1,3-benzoxadiazole
NBD-F	7-Fluoro-4-nitro-2,1,3-diazole
NBMPR	*S*-(*p*-Nitrobenzyl)-6-thioinosine
NBS	*N*-Bromosuccinimide
Nbs	[(3-Carboxy-4-nitrophenyl)thio]
NBSac	*N*-Bromosaccharin
NBSC	2-Nitrobenzenesulfenyl chloride
NCA	*N*-Chloroacetamide
NCDC	2-Nitro-4-carboxyphenyl *N,N*-diphenylcarbamate
NCN	Cyanonaphthalene
NCS	*N*-Chlorosuccinimide
NEM	*N*-Ethylmaleimide
NEP	*N*-Ethyl-2-pyrrolidinone
NEPIS	*N*-Ethyl-5-phenylisoxazolium-3′-sulfonate
NesMIC	(+)-(Neomenthylsulfonyl)methyl isocyanide
Nf	Nonaflyl (perfluoro-1-butanesulfonyl) or nonaflate
5-NIA	5-Nitroisatoic anhydride
NHS	*N*-Hydroxysuccinimide
NIP	2,4-Dichlorophenyl 4′-nitrophenyl ether
NIP	4-Hydroxy-5-nitro-3-iodophenyl acetic acid
NIS	*N*-Iodosuccinimide
NM	Nitromethane
NMA	*N*-Methylolacrylamide
NMM	*N*-Methylmaleimide
NMM	*N*-Methylmorpholine

NMO (or NMMO)	*N*-Methylmorpholine N-oxide
NMP	*N*-Methylphthalimide
NMP	*N*-Methyl-2-pyrrolidone
NMP	*N*-Methylpyrrolidin-2-one
NMSO	4-Methyl-2-nitroanisole
Noc	4-Nitrocinnamyloxcarbonyl
NORPHOS	Bis(diphenylphosphino)bicyclo[2.2.1]hept-5-ene
NP	2-(or 4-)Nitrophenyl
Npe	2-(4-Nitrophenyl)ethyl
NPM	*N*-Phenylmaleimide
α-NPO	2-(1-Naphthyl)-5-phenyloxazole
NPP	2-Nitro-2-propenyl pivalate
NPS	*o*-Nitrophenylsulfenyl
NPSP	*N*-Phenylselenylphthalimide
Npys-Cl	3-Nitro-2-pyridinesulfenyl chloride
Ns	2-(or 4-)Nitrophenylsulfonyl
N-Selectride®	Sodium tri-*sec*-butylborohydride
NTA	Nitrilotriacetic acid
N-t-B	2-Methyl-2-nitropropane
OBO	4-Methyl-2,6,7-trioxabicyclo[2.2.2]octane
OCAD	*o*-Chlorobenzaldehyde
OCBA	*o*-Chlorobenzoic acid
OCBC	*o*-Chlorobenzyl chloride
OCBN	*o*-Chlorobenzonitrile
OCCN	*o*-Chlorobenzyl cyanide
OCDC	*o*-Chlorodichlorotoluene
OCOC	*o*-Chlorobenzoyl chloride
OCPA	*o*-Chlorophenylacetic acid
OCPT	2-Chloro-4-aminotoluene (*o*-chloro-*p*-aminotoluene)
OCT	*o*-Chlorotoluene
OCTC	*o*-Chlorobenzotrichloride
OCTEO	Octyltriethoxysilane
ODA	4,4′-Oxydianiline
OMH-1	Sodium diethylhydroaluminate
ONB	*o*-Nitrobenzyl
OTB	*o*-Toluidine boric acid
OTD	*o*-Toluenediamine
PABA	*p*-Aminobenzoic acid
PADA	Poly(adipic anhydride)
PADA	Pyridine-2-azo-*p*-dimethylaniline
PAH	*p*-Aminohippuric acid
PAH	Polycyclic aromatic hydrocarbon
PAM	Pyridine-2-aldoxime methiodide
2-PAM	(See PAM)
2-PAMCl	2-Pyridinealdoxime methochloride
PAN	1-(2-Pyridylazo)-2-naphthol
PAP	*O,O*-Dimethyl *S*-α-(ethoxycarbonyl)benzyl phosphorothiolothioate
PAPA	Poly(azelaic anhydride)
p-APMSF	(*p*-Amidinophenyl)methylsulfonylfluoride
PAS	*p*-Aminosalicylic acid

PASAM	*p*-Toluenesulfonamide
PBA	*p*-Benzoquinone-2,3-dicarboxylic anhydride
PBB	*p*-Bromobenzyl
PBBO	2-(4-Biphenylyl)-6-phenylbenzoxazole
PBD	2-(4-Biphenylyl)-5-phenyl-1,3,4-oxadiazole
PBI	*p*-Benzoquinone-2,3-dicarboxylic imide
PBN	*N-tert*-Butyl-α-phenylnitrone
PBP	*p*-(Benzyloxy)phenol
PBS	Poly(butene-1-sulfone)
PBz	*p*-Phenylbenzoyl
PC	Propylene carbonate
PCAD	*p*-Chlorobenzaldehyde
PCB	*p*-Chlorobenzyl
p-CBA	*p*-Carboxybenzaldehyde
PCBA	*p*-Chlorobenzoic acid
PCBC	*p*-Chlorobenzyl chloride
PCBN	*p*-Chlorobenzonitrile
PCBTF	*p*-Chlorobenzotrifluoride
PCC	Pyridinium chlorochromate
PCCN	*p*-Chlorobenzyl cyanide
PCDC	*p*-Chlorodichlorotoluene
P-Cellulose	Cellulose phosphate
PCMB	*p*-Chloromercuribenzoic acid
PCMX	*p*-Chloro-*m*-xylenol
PCNB	Pentachloronitrobenzene
PCOC	*p*-Chlorobenzoyl chloride
PCONA	*p*-Chloro-*o*-nitroaniline
PCOT	4-Chloro-2-aminotoluene (*p*-chloro-*o*-aminotoluene)
PCP	Pentachlorophenol
PCPA	*p*-Chlorophenylacetic acid
PCT	*p*-Chlorotoluene
PCT	Polychloroterphenyl
PCTC	*p*-Chlorobenzotrichloride
PDC	Pyridinium dichromate
PDEA	*N*-Phenyldiethanolamine
PDQ	Sodium (2-methyl-4-chlorophenoxy)butyrate
PDT	3-(2-Pyridyl)-5,6-diphenyl-1,2,4-triazine
PEA	*N*-(2-Hydroxyethyl)aniline (*N*-phenylethanolamine)
PEEA	*N*-(2-Hydroxyethyl)-*N*-ethylaniline (*N*-phenyl-*N*-ethylethanolamine)
PEEK	Poly(ether ether ketone)
PEG	Poly(ethylene glycol)
PEI-cellulose	Polyethyleneimine-impregnated cellulose
PEMA	2-Ethyl-2-phenylmalonamide
Peoc	2-Phosphonioethoxycarbonyl
Peoc	2-(Triphenylphosphonio)ethoxycarbonyl
PEP	Phosphoenolpyruvic acid
Pet	2-(2′-Pyridyl)ethyl
PET	Poly(ethylene terephthalate)
PETA	Pentaerythritol triacrylate
Pfp	Pentafluorophenyl

PG	Protective group
PGE	Phenyl glycidyl ether
Ph	Phenyl
Phenoc	4-Methoxyphenacyloxycarbonyl
Phenyl-MAPO	Bis[1-(2-methyl)aziridinyl]phenylphosphine oxide
Pht	Phthalyl
Phth	Phthaloyl
PhthN	Phthalimido
PIA	Phenyliodoso diacetate
PIPES	1,4-Piperazinebis(ethanesulfonic acid)
Pixyl (or Px)	9-Phenyl-9-xanthenyl
PMA	Phenylmercuric acetate
PMB (or MPM)	4-Methoxybenzyl (*p*-methoxybenzyl)
PMBCl	*p*-Methoxybenzyl chloride
PMBM	*p*-Methoxybenzyloxymethyl
PMBOH	*p*-Methoxybenzyl alcohol
Pmc	2,2,5,7,8-Pentamethylchroman-6-sulfonyl
PMDTA	Pentamethyldiethylenetriamine
Pme	Pentamethylbenzenesulfonyl
PMEA	*N*-(2-Hydroxyethyl)-*N*-methylaniline (*N*-phenyl-*N*-methylethanolamine)
PMH	Phenylmercuric hydroxide
PMHS	Polymethylhydrosiloxane
PMI	3-Phenyl-5-methylisoxazole
PMI-ACID	3-Phenyl-5-methylisoxazole-4-carboxylic acid
PMP	*p*-Methoxyphenyl
PMS	*p*-Methylbenzylsulfonyl
PMS	Phenazine methosulfate
PNASA	*p*-Nitroaniline-*o*-sulfonic acid
PNB	*p*-Nitrobenzyl
PNMT	Phenylethanolamine-*N*-methyltransferase
PNOT	*p*-Nitro-*o*-toluidine
PNPDPP (*p*-NPDPP)	*p*-Nitrophenyl diphenyl phosphate
PNPG	α-*p*-Nitrophenylglycerine
PNPP	*p*-Nitrophenyl phosphate
PNZ	*p*-Nitrobenzyloxycarbonyl
4-POBN	(See POBN)
POBN	α-(4-Pyridyl-1-oxide)-*N*-*tert*-butylnitrone
POC	Cyclopentyloxycarbonyl
POM	Chloromethyl pivalate
POM	4-Pentenyloxymethyl
POM (or Pom)	Pivaloyloxymethyl
POPOP	1,4-Bis(5-phenyloxazol-2-yl)benzene
POPSO	Piperazine-*N*,*N*′-bis(2-hydroxypropanesulfonic acid)
PPA	Polyphosphoric acid
PPDA	Phenyl phosphorodiamidate
PPDP	*p*,*p*′-Diphenol
PPE	Polyphosphate ester
PPNCl	Bis(triphenylphosphoranylidene)ammonium chloride
PPO	2,5-Diphenyloxazole
Ppoc	2-Triphenylphosphonioisopropoxycarbonyl

Ppt	Diphenylthiophosphinyl
PPTS	Pyridinium 4-toluenesulfonate
4-Ppy	4-Pyrrolidinopyridine
Pr	Propyl
iPr	Isopropyl
Proton sponge	1,8-Bis(dimethylamino)naphthalene
P2S	2-Pyridinealdoxime methyl methanesulfonate
PS-Cl	2-Pyridinesulfenyl chloride
Psec	2-(Phenylsulfonyl)ethoxycarbonyl
Psoc	2-Phenyl-2-(trimethylsilyl)ethoxycarbonyl
PSPA	Poly(sebacic anhydride)
PTAD	*N*-Phenyl-1,2,4-triazoline-3,5-dione
PTAP	Phenyltrimethylammonium perbromide
PTBBA	*p-tert*-Butylbenzoic acid
Ptc	Phenyl(thiocarbamoyl)
PTC	Phase transfer catalyst
PTC	Phenyl isothiocyanate
PTH	Phenylthiohydantoin
PTM	Phenylthiomethyl
PTMO	Propyltrimethoxysilane
PTSA	*p*-Toluenesulfonic acid
PTSI	*p*-Toluenesulfonyl isocyanate
Pv	Pivaloyl
PVA	Poly(vinyl alcohol)
PVC	Poly(vinyl chloride)
PVDF	Poly(vinylidene fluoride)
PVP	Polyvinylpyrrolidone
PVPDC	Poly(4-vinylpyridinium) dichromate
PVP-I	Polyvinylpyrrolidone-iodine complex
PVSK	Potassium poly(vinyl sulfate)
Px	(See Pixyl)
py (or Py or Pyr)	Pyridine
Pyoc	2-(Pyridyl)ethoxycarbonyl
PyOTs	(See PPTS)
Pz	4-Phenylazobenzyloxycarbonyl
Qu	8-Quinolinyl
QUIBEC	Benzylquinidinium chloride
RAMP	(*R*)-1-Amino-2-(methoxymethyl)pyrrolidine
RDB	Sodium dihydrobis(2-methoxyethoxy)aluminate (sodium bis(2-methoxyethoxy)aluminium hydride)
Red-Al	Sodium bis(2-methoxyethoxy)aluminium hydride
RNA	Ribonucleic acid
SAA	Succinic anhydride
SADP	*N*-Succinimidyl (4-azidophenyldithio)propionate
salen	Bis(salicylidene)ethylenediamine
SAMP	(*S*)-1-Amino-2-(methoxymethyl)pyrrolidine
SBH	Sodium borohydride
Scm	*S*-Carboxymethylsulfenyl
SDP	4,4′-Sulfonyldiphenol
SDPP	*N*-Succinimidyl diphenyl phosphate

SDS	Sodium dodecyl benzenesulfonate
SDS	Sodium dodecyl sulfate
SEM	2-(Trimethylsilyl)ethoxymethyl
SEMCl	2-(Trimethylsilyl)ethoxymethyl chloride
SES	2-(Trimethylsilyl)ethylsulfonyl
SESNHBoc	*tert*-Butyl 2-(trimethylsilyl)ethanesulfonyl carbamate
SEX	Sodium ethyl xanthate
Sia$_2$BH	Disiamylborane
SLS	Sodium lauryl sulfate
SMCC	Succinimidyl 4-(*N*-maleimidomethylcyclohexane)-1-carboxylate
SMOM	(Phenyldimethylsilyl)ethoxymethyl
SMPB	Succinimidyl 4-(*p*-maleimidophenyl)butyrate
Snm	*S*-(*N*-Methyl-*N*-phenylcarbamoyl)sulfenyl
SPA	Superphosphoric acid
SPADNS	2-(*p*-Sulfophenylazo)-1,8-dihydroxy-3,6-naphthalenedisulfonic acid (trisodium salt)
SPDP	*N*-Succinimidyl 3-(2-pyridyldithio)propionate
SSP	1,2-Distearoylpalmitin
STABASE	1,1,4,4-Tetramethyldisilylazacyclopentane
STPP	Sodium tripolyphosphate
STr	Triphenylmethanesulfenyl
Su	Succinimido
Suc	3-Carboxypropanoyl
-Suc-	Succinyl
Super-Hydride®	Lithium triethylborohydride
2,4,5-T	2,4,5-Trichlorophenoxyacetic acid
TAC	Triallyl cyanurate
Tacm	Trimethylacetamidomethyl
TAMA	*N*-Methylanilinium trifluoroacetate
TAME	*N*-α-*p*-Tosyl-L-arginine methyl ester hydrochloride
TAMM	tetrakis(acetoxymercuri)methane
TAPA	α-(2,4,5,7-Tetranitro-9-fluorenylideneaminooxy)propionic acid
TAPS	3-[Tris(hydroxymethyl)methylamino]-1-propanesulfonic acid
TAPSO	3-[*N*-(Tris(hydroxymethyl)methylamino]-2-hydroxypropanesulfonic acid
TAS	Tris(diethylamino)sulfonium
TASF (or TAS-F)	Tris(dimethylamino)sulfonium (trimethylsilyl)difluoride
TB	Thexylborane
2,3,6-TBA	2,3,6-Trichlorobenzoic acid
TBAB	Tetrabutylammonium bromide
TBAC	*tert*-Butylacetyl chloride
TBACl	Tetrabutylammonium chloride
TBAF	Tetrabutylammonium fluoride
TBAHS	Tetrabutylammonium hydrogen sulfate
TBAI	Tetrabutylammonium iodide
TBAP	Tetra-*n*-butylammonium perchlorate
TBAS	Tetra-*n*-butylammonium succinimide
TBC	*p-tert*-Butylcatechol
TBDA	Thexylborane-*N*,*N*-diethylaniline
t-BDEA	*tert*-Butyldiethanolamine
TBDMS (or TBS)	*tert*-Butyldimethylsilyl
TBDMSCl (or TBSCl)	*tert*-Butyldimethylsilyl chloride

TBDMSI	1-(*tert*-Butyldimethylsilyl)imidazole
TBDPS	*tert*-Butyldiphenylsilyl
TBDS	Tetra-*tert*-butoxydisilane-1,3-diylidene
TBE	1,1,2,2-Tetrabromoethane
TBHC	*tert*-Butyl hypochlorite
TBHP	*tert*-Butyl hydroperoxide
TBMPS	*tert*-Butylmethoxyphenylsilyl
TBO	3-[(Trimethylsilyl)oxy]-3-buten-2-one
TBP	Tri-*n*-butyl phosphate
TBP	Triphenylbutylphosphonium bromide
TBPB	*tert*-Butylbenzoyl peroxide
TBS	(See TBDMS)
TBSCl	(See TBDMSCl)
TBSOTf	*tert*-Butyldimethylsilyl triflate
TBTD	Tetrabutylthiuram disulfide
TBTr	4,4′,4″-Tris(benzyloxy)triphenylmethyl
tBu	*tert*-Butyl
t-BuOK	Potassium *tert*-butoxide
TBUP	Tri-*n*-butylphosphine
TC	2,3,4,5-Tetraphenylcyclopentadienone
TCA	Trichloroacetic acid
TCB	Trichlorobenzene (usually 1,3,5)
TCB	2,2,2-Trichloro-1,1-dimethylethyl
TcBoc	1,1-Dimethyl-2,2,2-trichloroethoxycarbonyl
TCE (or Tce)	2,2,2-Trichloroethyl
Tcec also Troc	2,2,2-Trichloroethoxycarbonyl
TcecCl also TrocCl	2,2,2-Trichloroethoxycarbonyl chloride (2,2,2-trichloroethyl chloroformate)
TCl	Terephthaloyl chloride
TCNE	Tetracyanoethene (tetracyanoethylene)
TCNP	11,11,12,12-Tetracyanopyreno-2,7-quinodimethane
TCNQ	7,7,8,8-Tetracyanoquinodimethane
TCP	Tetrachlorophthaloyl
TCP (or Tcp)	Trichlorophenol (usually 2,4,5 or 2,4,6)
TCP	Tricresyl phosphate
Tcroc	2-(Trifluoromethyl)-6-chromonylmethylenecarbonyl
Tcrom	2-(Trifluoromethyl)-6-chromonylmethylene
TCTFP	1,1,2,2-Tetrachloro-3,3,4,4-tetrafluorocyclobutane
TDI	Tolylene diisocyanate
TDP	4,4′-Thiodiphenol
TDS	Thexyldimethylsilyl
TEA	Triethanolamine
TEA	Triethylaluminium
TEA	Triethylamine
TEAB	Triethylammonium bicarbonate
TEAE-cellulose	Triethylaminoethyl cellulose
TEAS	Tetraethylammonium succinimide
TEBA (or TEBAC)	Benzyltriethylammonium chloride
TEBAB	Triethylbenzylammonium bromide
TED	(See DABCO)
TEG	Triethylene glycol

TEM	Triethylenediamine (1,4-diazabicyclo[2.2.2]octane)
TEMPO	2,2,6,6-Tetramethylpiperidinyloxy
Teoc	2-(Trimethylsilyl)ethoxycarbonyl
TES	N,N,N',N'-Tetraethylsulfamide
TES	Triethylsilyl
TES	2-[Tris(hydroxymethyl)methylamino]-1-ethanesulfonic acid
TESOTf	Triethylsilyl triflate
TETD	Tetraethylthiuram disulfide
TETM	Tetraethylthiuram monosulfide
Tf	Trifluoromethanesulfonyl (triflyl)
TFA	Trifluoroacetic acid
TFA	Trifluoroacetyl
TFAA	Trifluoroacetic anhydride
TFA-ME	Methyl trifluoroacetate
TFE	2,2,2-Trifluoroethanol
TFMC-Eu	Tris[3-(trifluoromethylhydroxymethylene)-d-camphorato]·Eu(III)
TFMC-Pr	Tris[3-(trifluoromethylhydroxymethylene)-d-camphorato]·Pr(III)
TfOH	Trifluoromethanesulfonic acid
THAM	Tris(hydroxymethyl)aminomethane
THF	Tetrahydrofuran, tetrahydrofuranyl
THFA	Tetrahydrofurfuryl alcohol
THFC-Eu	Tris[3-(heptafluoropropylhydroxymethylene)-d-camphorato]·Eu(III)
THIP	4,5,6,7-Tetrahydroisoxazolo[5,4-c]pyrimidin-3($2H$)-one
THP	Tetrahydropyran (or tetrahydropyranyl)
Thx	Thexyl (2,3-dimethyl-2-butyl)
TIBA	Triiodobenzoic acid (usually 2,3,5)
TIBA	Triisobutylaluminium
TIPDS	1,3-(1,1,3,3-Tetraisopropyldisilanoxylidene)
TIPS	Triisopropylsilyl
TLCK	1-Chloro-3-tosylamido-7-amino-2-heptanone hydrochloride
TLTr (or TLT)	4,4',4''-Tris(levulinoyloxy)triphenylmethyl
TMA	Trimethylaluminium
TMAC	Trimellitic anhydride monoacid chloride
TMAEMC	2-Trimethylammoniumethylmethacrylic chloride
TMANO	Trimethylamine N-oxide
TMAT	Tetramethylammonium tribromide
TMAT	Tris-2,4,6-[1-(2-methyl)aziridinyl]-1,3,5-triazine
TMB	3,3',5,5'-Tetramethylbenzidine
TMB	N,N,N',N'-Tetramethylbenzidine
TMB (or Tmob)	2,4,6-Trimethoxybenzyl
TMB-4	1,1'-Trimethylenebis[4-(hydroxyiminomethyl)pyridinium bromide]
TMBA	3,4,5-Trimethylbenzaldehyde
TMC	3,3,5-Trimethylcyclohexanol
TMCS	(See TMSCl)
TMEDA	N,N,N',N'-Tetramethylethylenediamine
TMM	Trimethylenemethane
TMO	Trimethylamine N-oxide
TMP	2,2,6,6-Tetramethylpiperidine
TMPM	Trimethoxyphenylmethyl
TMPTA	Trimethylolpropane triacrylate

TMPTMA	Trimethylolpropane trimethacrylate
TMS	Tetramethylsilane
TMS	Trimethylsilyl
TMSCl	Trimethylsilyl chloride
TMSCN	Trimethylsilyl cyanide
TMSDEA	N,N-Diethyl-1,1,1-trimethylsilylamine
TMSE	2-(Trimethylsilyl)ethyl
TMSEC	2-(Trimethylsilyl)ethoxycarbonyl
TMSI	Trimethylsilyl iodide
TMSIM	1-(Trimethylsilyl)imidazole
TMSOTf	Trimethylsilyl trifluoromethanesulfonate (triflate)
TMTD	Tetramethylthiuram disulfide
TMTM	Tetramethylthiuram monosulfide
TMTr (or TMT)	Tris(p-methoxyphenyl)methyl (trimethoxytrityl)
TNBA	Tri-n-butylaluminium
TNF	2,4,7-Trinitrofluorenone
TNM	Tetranitromethane
TNPA	Tri-n-propylaluminium
TNS	6-(p-Toluidino)-2-naphthalenesulfonic acid, potassium salt
TNT	2,4,6-Trinitrotoluene
Tol	4-Tolyl (4-methylphenyl)
TOPO	Tri-n-octylphosphine oxide
TOS	p-Toluenesulfonyl (tosyl)
TosMIC (or TOSMIC)	Tosylmethyl isocyanide
TPAP	Tetra-n-propylammonium perruthenate
TPB	1,1,4,4-Tetraphenyl-1,3-butadiene
TPCD	Tetraphenylcyclopentadienone
TPCK	L-1-p-Tosylamino-2-phenylethyl chloromethyl ketone
TPE	Tetraphenylethylene
TPP	Tetraphenylporphyrin
TPP	Triphenyl phosphate
TPP	Triphenylphosphine
TPPTS	Trisodium 3,3′,3″-phosphinetriyltribenzenesulfonate
TPS	2,4,6-Triisopropylbenzenesulfonyl
TPS	Triphenylsilyl
TPS	Triphenylsulfonium chloride
TPSCl	1,3-Dichloro-1,1,3,3-tetraisopropyldisiloxane
TPSCl (or TPS)	2,4,6-Triisopropylbenzenesulfonyl chloride
TPTZ	2,4,6-Tris(2-pyridyl)-s-triazine triaminosilane
Tr	Trityl (triphenylmethyl)
TRIAMO	Triaminosilane
Tricine	N-[Tris(hydroxymethyl)methyl]glycine
Triglyme	Triethylene glycol dimethyl ether
Tris	Tris(hydroxymethyl)aminomethane
trien	Triethylenetetramine
TRITC	Tetramethylrhodamine isothiocyanate
Troc	2,2,2-Trichloroethyloxycarbonyl
TrocCl	2,2,2-Trichloroethyl chloroformate; see also TcecCl
TRPGDA	Tripropylene glycol diacrylate
TrS	Triphenylmethanesulfenyl

TrtF$_7$	2,3,4,4′,4″,5,6-Heptafluorotriphenylmethyl
Ts	Tosyl (or *p*-toluenesulfonyl)
Tse	2-*p*-Toluenesulfonylethyl
Tsoc	2-(*p*-Toluenesulfonyl)ethoxycarbonyl
TSIM	*N*-Trimethylsilylimidazole
TSNI	1-(*p*-Toluenesulfonyl)-4-nitroimidazole
TsOH	4-Toluenesulfonic acid
TTC	2,3,5-Triphenyltetrazolium chloride
TTEGDA	Tetraethylene glycol diacrylate
TTF	Tetrathiafulvalene
TTFA	Thallium(*III*) trifluoroacetate
TTN	Thallium(*III*) nitrate
UDMH	*unsym*-Dimethylhydrazine
VMA	4-Hydroxy-3-methoxymandelic acid (vanillomandelic acid)
Voc	Vinyloxycarbonyl
VTC	Vinyltrichlorosilane
VTEO	Vinyltriethoxysilane
VTMO	Vinyltrimethoxysilane
VTMOEO	Vinyltris(2-methoxyethoxy)silane
Xan	9*H*-Xanthen-9-yl
Xy	Xylene
Z	Benzyloxycarbonyl; see also CBz and CBn
Z(Br)	4-Bromobenzyloxycarbonyl
Z(NO$_2$)	4-Nitrobenzyloxycarbonyl
Z(OMe)	4-Methoxybenzyloxycarbonyl
ZDBC	Zinc dibutyldithiocarbamate
ZDEC	Zinc diethyldithiocarbamate
ZDMC	Zinc dimethyldithiocarbamate
ZPCK	*N*-CBZ-L-Phenylalanine chloromethyl ketone

6.2   GLOSSARY OF MISCELLANEOUS TERMS AND TECHNIQUES USED IN NOMENCLATURE, INCLUDING COLLOQUIAL TERMS

abeo-: Used in terpenoid and steroid nomenclature to indicate that a bond has migrated. For example, in a 5(4→3)*abeo*-terpene, the 5–4 bond has been replaced by a 5–3 bond contracting ring A from six to five members.

normal triterpene　　　5(4→3)-*abeo*-triterpene

-acene: The names of polycyclic aromatic hydrocarbons containing five or more fused benzene rings in a straight linear arrangement are formed by a numerical prefix followed by -*acene*.

hexacene

acetals: Diethers of *gem*-diols $R_2C(OR)_2$ (R can be the same or different). Often named as derivatives of aldehydes or ketones. Thus, acetaldehyde dimethyl acetal is $H_3CCH(OMe)_2$. It is now more usual to name them as dialkoxy compounds, e.g., 1,1-dimethoxyethane. The term *acetal* is sometimes extended to compounds containing heteroatoms other than oxygen, as in *N,O*-acetals $R_2C(OR)(NR_2)$. Derivatives of ketones can be called ketals. This term was abandoned by IUPAC but has been reinstated.

acetonides: Cyclic acetals derived from acetone and diols. Better described as isopropylidene derivatives.

glycerol acetonide =
1,2-isopropylidene glycerol =
2,2-dimethyl-1,3-dioxolane-4-methanol(CAS)

acetylenes: A general term for hydrocarbons having one or more triple bonds. *Alkynes* is now the more usual term. Acetylene itself is $HC{\equiv}CH$.

acetylides: Metal derivatives of acetylene. Sodium acetylide is $HC{\equiv}CNa$.

aci-: The acid form of (prefix).

acid anhydrides: *See* anhydrides.

acid halides: *See* acyl halides.

acylals: General term for diesters of *gem*-diols. They are named as esters. Thus, $H_3CCH(OAc)_2$ is ethylidene diacetate.

acyl halides (acid halides): General term for compounds in which the hydroxy group of an acid is replaced by a halogen atom, e.g., H_3CCOCl, $PhSO_2Br$. They are named by placing the name of the halide after the name of the acyl radical, e.g., acetyl chloride, benzenesulfonyl bromide.

acyloins: α-Hydroxy ketones RCH(OH)COR. An acyloin name is formed by changing the *-ic acid* or *-oic acid* of the trivial name of the acid RCOOH to *-oin*. Thus, $H_3CCH(OH)COCH_3$ is acetoin. They are now usually given normal substitutive names, e.g., 3-hydroxy-2-butanone.

aetio-: *See* etio.

aglycones (aglycons): Nonsugar compounds remaining after hydrolysis of the glycosyl groups from glycosides.

aldazines: Azines of aldehydes.

aldehydo-: Occasionally used in place of a locant in order to denote unambiguously the position of a functional derivative. For example, α-oxo-benzeneacetaldehyde *aldehydo*-hydrazone is $PhC(O)CH{=}NHNH_2$.

aldimines: Imines derived from aldehydes, $R^1CH{=}NR^2$.

aldoximes: Oximes derived from aldehydes, $RCH{=}NOH$.

allenes: General term for substances containing $C{=}C{=}C$. The lowest member, propadiene ($H_2C{=}C{=}CH_2$), is known as allene.

allo- (Greek "other"): A configurational prefix used in carbohydrate nomenclature. *See* carbohydrates. Also as a general prefix to denote close relationship, e.g., alloaromadendrene or the more stable of a pair of geometric isomers, e.g., allomaleic acid (obsol.) = fumaric acid.

-amic acid: Denotes that one COOH group of a trivially named dicarboxylic acid has been replaced by a $CONH_2$ group. Thus, succinamic acid is $H_2NCOCH_2CH_2COOH$.

amidines: Compounds of the type $RC({=}NH)NH_2$. The ending *-amidine* can replace the *-ic acid* or *-oic acid* of the name of the acid RCOOH. Thus, acetamidine is $H_3CC({=}NH)NH_2$.

amidoximes (amide oximes): Oximes of carboxamides or amides derived from hydroximic acids, i.e., $RC(NH_2){=}NOH$ or $RC({=}NH)NHOH$.

amidrazones (amide hydrazones): Hydrazones of carboxamides or hydrazides of hydroximic acids, i.e., $RC(NH_2)=NNH_2$ or $RC(=NH)NHNH_2$.

aminals: *gem*-Diamines, i.e., $R_2C(NR_2)_2$ (R is the same or different).

-amoyl: Denotes a radical derived by loss of a hydroxy group from an amic acid. Thus, succinamoyl is $H_2NCOCH_2CH_2CO-$.

amphi- **(Greek "around"):** For example, *amphi*-naphthoquinone (obsol.) = 2,6-naphthoquinone.

ang-: Prefix for angular, i.e., referring to an angular isomer (obsol.).

anhydrides: Compounds derived by the elimination of the elements of water from two acid molecules. Thus, acetic anhydride is $(H_3CCO)_2O$ and acetic benzoic anhydride is $H_3CCOOCOPh$. Cyclic anhydrides, e.g., succinic anhydride are formed by the elimination of the elements of water from a dibasic acid.

anhydro: A subtractive prefix denoting the loss of the elements of water within one molecule.

D-gulonic acid   2,3-anhydro-D-gulonic acid

anhydrosulfide: An analogue of an anhydride in which the oxygen atom connecting the two acyl residues has been replaced by a sulfur atom. Anhydroselenides are the Se analogues.

-anilic acid: Denotes that one COOH group of a trivially named dicarboxylic acid has been replaced by a CONHPh group. Thus, succinanilic acid is $PhNHCOCH_2CH_2COOH$.

anilides: *N*-Phenyl amides RCONHPh. They may be named by replacing the *-ic acid* or *-oic acid* in the name of the acid RCOOH by *-anilide*. Thus, acetanilide is $H_3CCONHPh$. Primed locants are used for the phenyl ring.

anils: Another term for azomethine compounds or Schiff bases. Sometimes restricted to *N*-phenylimines $PhN=CR_2$.

annulenes: Monocyclic conjugated hydrocarbons with the general formula $(CH)_n$. Thus [8]annulene is cyclooctatetraene.

ansa compounds (Latin "handle"): Compounds containing a ring system bridged by an aliphatic chain. The simplest type consists of a benzene ring with the *para* positions bridged by a methylene chain ten to twelve atoms long.

anthocyanins: Flavonoid pigments of glycosidic nature. On hydrolysis they give anthocyanidins, which are oxygenated derivatives of flavylium salts.

anthra: The ring fusion prefix derived from anthracene.

apo (Greek "from"): In general means "derived from," e.g., apomorphine. Oxidative degradation products of carotenoids can be named as apocarotenoids. The prefix *apo-* preceded by a locant is used to indicate that all of the molecule beyond the carbon atom corresponding to that locant has been replaced by a hydrogen atom. The prefix *diapo-* indicates removal of fragments from both ends of the molecule.

ar-: Abbreviation for "aromatic," used as a locant to indicate an attachment at an unspecified position on an aromatic ring. Thus, in *ar*-methylaniline the methyl group is attached to the aromatic ring and not to the amine *N* atom.

Ar: Denotes an unspecified aryl group.

arenes: A general name for monocyclic and polycyclic aromatic hydrocarbons.

arynes: Hydrocarbons derived formally from arenes by removal of a hydrogen atom from two-ring carbons, e.g., benzyne.

as-: Abbreviation for asymmetric, as in *as*-triazine (1,2,4-triazine). Sometimes used to indicate 1,2,4-substitution on an aryl ring, e.g., *as*-trichlorobenzene is $1,2,4-Cl_3C_6H_3$.

-azane: With a numerical prefix, *-azane* denotes a chain of nitrogen atoms. Thus, triazane is H_2NNHNH_2, tetrazane is $H_2NNHNHNH_2$, etc.

-azene: With a numerical prefix, *-azene* denotes a chain of nitrogen atoms containing one double bond. Thus, triazene is $N_2NN=NH$, tetrazene is $H_2NN=NNH_2$, etc.

azi: $-N=N-$. Usually used when both free valencies are attached to the same atom.

azines: Compounds containing the azino group. They may be named by adding the word *azine* after the name of the corresponding aldehyde or ketone. Thus, acetone azine is $(H_3C)_2C=N-N=C(CH_3)_2$. *Azines* is sometimes used as a general term to refer to six-membered heterocycles containing nitrogen in the ring.

azoles: *Azoles* is sometimes used as a general term to refer to five-membered heterocycles containing nitrogen in the ring.

azomethines: Compounds with the formula $R_2C=NR'$. When the N atom is substituted ($R' \neq H$), they are known as Schiff bases. Azomethine itself is methanimine, $H_2C=NH$.

azonic acids: Compounds with structure $R_2N(O)OH$.

benzeno: $-(C_6H_4)-$. Bridge name used in naming bridged fused ring systems.

benzo: The ring fusion prefix from benzene. See Chapter 4.

betaine: Trivial name for zwitterionic compounds characterised by $Me_3N^+CH_2COO^-$. Also used as a class name for similar compounds containing a cationic centre and an anionic centre; they are also called inner salts and zwitterionic compounds. Named as hydroxide, inner salts in CAS.

biimino: $-NH-NH-$. Used in naming bridged fused ring systems.

bisnor: *See* nor.

Bunte salts: Salts of *S*-alkyl thiosulfates with structure $RSS(O)_2O^-M^+$.

calixarenes: Cyclic oligomers formed from *para*-substituted phenols and formaldehyde.

calixarenes

> *See* Shinkai, S., *Tetrahedron,* 49, 8933, 1993. Gutsche, C. D., *Calixarenes: An Introduction (Monographs in Supramolecular Chemistry)* (Cambridge: Royal Society of Chemistry, 2008).

carba: Occasionally used as a replacement prefix indicating that a carbon atom has replaced a heteroatom.

carbamates: Salt or esters of carbamic acid H_2NCOOH or of N-substituted carbamic acids R_2NCOOH.

carbenes: Used as a general name for a type of neutral species in which the carbon atom is covalently bonded to two groups and also bears two nonbonding electrons, i.e., derivatives of methylene, $:CH_2$.

carbinol: Old name for the parent H_3OCH in naming substituted alcohols. Thus, diphenylcarbinol is Ph_2CHOH and triethylcarbinol is $(H_3CCH_2)_3COH$

-carbolactone: Suffix denoting the presence of a lactone ring fused to a ring system.

1,10-phenanthrenecarbolactone

-carbonitrile: Suffix denoting $-C\equiv N$.

carbocations: Electron-deficient, positively charged, tricoordinate carbon atoms. For example, H_3C^+ is methylium, $C_6H_5^+$ is phenylium.

carboranes: A contraction of carbaboranes. Compounds in which a boron atom in a polyboron hydride is replaced by a carbon atom.

carboximide (dicarboximide): Suffix denoting an imide of a dicarboxylic acid. *See also* imides.

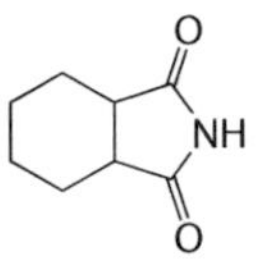

1,2-Cyclohexanedicarboximide

carbylamines: Isocyanides.

carbynes: Neutral species, R–C, in which the carbon atom is covalently bonded to one group and also bears three nonbonding electrons.

carceplex: A complex formed by a carcerand. *See* Cram, D. J., et al. *JACS*, 116, 111, 1994. Chapman, R. G., et al., *JACS*, 116, 369, 1994.

carcerand: A globular molecule capable of encapsulating smaller molecules in its interior cavity.

catecholamines: Derivatives of 4-(2-aminoethyl)-1,2-benzenediol.

catenanes: Compounds having two or more rings connected in the manner of the links of a chain, without a covalent bond between the rings.

cavitand: A compound containing a geometrically enforced cavity large enough to accommodate simple molecules or ions. *See* Cram, D. J., et al., *Container Molecules and Their Guests* (Cambridge: Royal Society of Chemistry, 1997).

ceramides: *N*-Acylated sphingoids. *See* sphingoids.

chalcones (chalkones): Substituted derivatives of the parent compound 1,3-diphenyl-2-propen-1-one, PhCH=CHCOPh.

chelates: Compounds in which a multidentate ligand is bound to a receptor centre, i.e., the central atom of a coordination complex.

clathrates: Inclusion compounds in which the guest molecule is in a cage formed by the host molecule or by a lattice of host molecules.

corrinoids: Compounds containing the corrin nucleus.

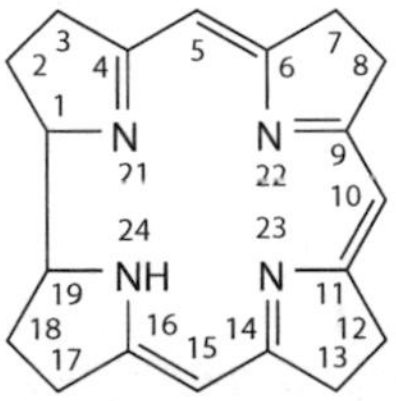

The number 20 is omitted when numbering the corrin nucleus so that the numbering system will correspond to that of the porphyrin nucleus.

See Pure Appl. Chem., 48, 495, 1976.

crown ethers: A class of macrocyclic ethers that form chelates with cations.

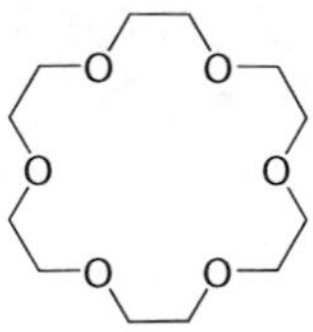

18-crown-6

The name 18-crown-6 indicates a total of eighteen ring atoms including six oxygens.

cumulenes: Compounds having three or more cumulative double bonds; $R_2C=C=C=CR_2$.

cyanates: Compounds containing the –OCN group. Thus, methyl cyanate is MeOCN.

cyanides: Compounds containing the –CN group. Thus, ethyl cyanide is EtCN. The more usual name is nitriles. Note that EtCN is propanenitrile.

cyanohydrins: Cyanoalcohols. Acetone cyanohydrin is $(H_3C)_2C(OH)(CN)$; ethylene cyanohydrin is $HOCH_2CH_2CN$.

cyclitols: Cycloalkanes in which the hydroxyl group is attached to each ring atom. See Chapter 5.

cyclo: Denotes the formation of a ring by means of a direct link between two atoms with loss of one hydrogen from each, e.g., cyclohexane, cyclotrisilane. In terpene and steroid names *cyclo-* indicates that an additional ring has been formed by means of a direct link between atoms of the fundamental skeleton.

3,5-cyclopregnane

cyclodextrins: Cyclic oligosaccharides consisting of α-D-(1→4)-linked D-glucose residues.

cyclophanes: Cyclic compounds having two or more aromatic rings with aliphatic bridging chains.

2,2-[1,4]cyclophane

de: The prefix *de-* followed by the name of a group or atom denotes replacement of that group or atom by hydrogen. Thus, in de-*N*-methylmorphine, the N–Me group of morphine has been replaced by N–H. Sometimes used in steroid nomenclature to denote the loss of an entire ring as in de-*A*-cholestane. *Des-* is more frequently used instead.

dehydro: Loss of two hydrogen atoms from a compound designated by a trivial name can be denoted by the prefix *didehydro*. Thus, 7,8-didehydrocholesterol is cholesterol with an additional double bond between atoms 7 and 8. In common usage, *dehydro* is sometimes used instead of *didehydro*. *Dehydro* can also mean removal of water, e.g., dehydromorphine.

dendrimer: Highly branched oligo- and polymeric compounds formed by reiterative reaction sequences. Also called starburst dendrimers, cascade molecules, and arborols.
    See Tomalia, D. A., et al., *Angew. Chem. Int. Ed. Engl.*, 29, 138 (rev.), 1990.

depsides: Esters formed from two or more molecules of the same or different phenolic acids.

depsipeptides: Compounds containing amino acids and hydroxy acids (not necessarily α-hydroxy acids) and having both esters and peptide bonds.

des-: Occasionally used in steroid/terpenoid nomenclature to describe loss of an entire ring, as in des-*A*-cholestane.

diazoate: Metal diazoates are compounds with the formula RN=N–OM (M = metal). Thus, PhN=NONa is sodium benzenediazoate.

-diazonium: Ions RN_2^+. Named by adding the suffix *-diazonium* to the name of the parent substance RH. Thus, $PhN_2^+Cl^-$ is benzenediazonium chloride.

didehydro: *See* dehydro.

dinor: *See* nor.

dioxy: –O–O–. Used when the free valencies are attached to different atoms that are not otherwise connected. Also called epidioxy.

diterpenoids: Terpenes having a C_{20} skeleton.

dithio: −S−S−. Usually used when the free valencies are attached to different atoms that are not otherwise connected.

dithioacetals: Sulfur analogues of acetals $R_2C(SR)_2$ (R is the same or different).

eicosanoids: *See* icosanoids.

enamines: Vinylic amines containing the unit N−C=C−. *Enamino* is a general term for a radical derived from an enamine by removal of a hydrogen from the nitrogen atom.

enols: Vinylic alcohols, tautomeric with aldehydes and ketones, containing the unit HO−C=.

epi (Greek "upon"): In carbohydrate chemistry, denotes an isomer differing in configuration at the α-carbon. Generally, to denote the opposite configuration at a chiral centre (e.g., 4-epiabietic acid). Also denotes a 1,6-disubstituted naphthalene (obsol.).

epoxides: Cyclic ethers. Usually restricted to three-membered cyclic ethers (oxiranes).

etheno: −CH=CH−. Used as a bridge in naming bridged fused ring systems.

ethers: Compounds R^1OR^2. The word *ether* is used in radicofunctional nomenclature. Thus, diethyl ether is Et_2O (sometimes called ethyl ether), methyl phenyl ether is MeOPh, and ethylene glycol monomethyl ether is $MeOCH_2CH_2OH$.

ethiodide, ethobromide, ethochloride: Denotes a base quaternised with ethyl iodide, ethyl bromide, or ethyl chloride.

ethoxide: The anion EtO^-. Thus, sodium ethoxide is EtONa.

etio (aetio) (Greek *aitia*, "cause"): Denotes a degradation product, e.g., etiocholanic acid.

fatty acids: Carboxylic acids derived from animal or vegetable fat or oil. The term is sometimes used to denote all acyclic aliphatic carboxylic acids. See Chapter 5.

flavonoids: A large group of natural products that are widespread in higher plants, derived by cyclisation of a chalcone precursor

friedo-: In a triterpene name, *friedo-* denotes that a methyl group has migrated from one position to another.

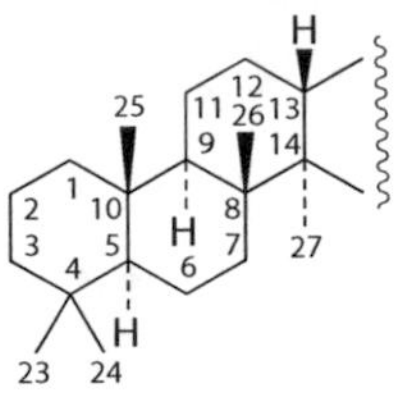

normal triterpene

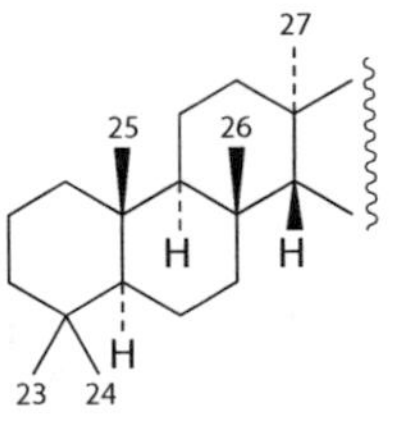

D-friedo-

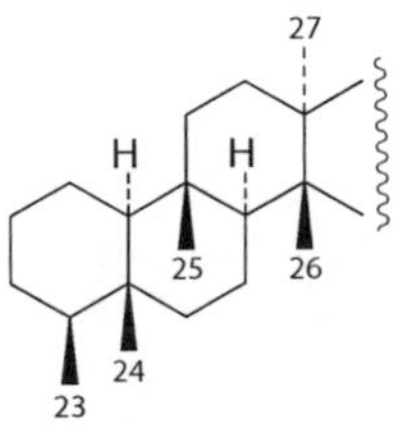

D:A-friedo-

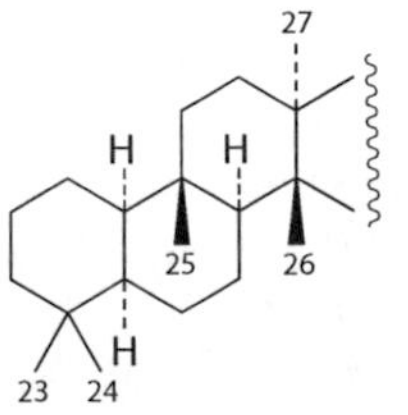

D:B-friedo-

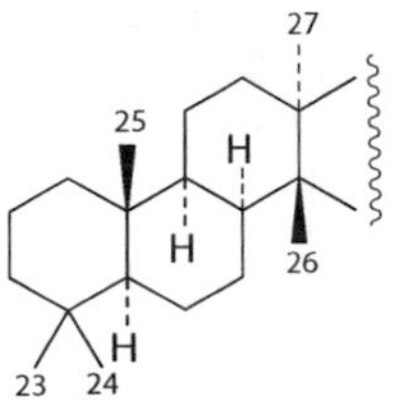

D:C-friedo-

fullerenes: Compounds composed of an even number of carbon atoms forming a cage-like fused structure with twelve five-membered rings and the rest six-membered rings, e.g., [60]-fullerene.

fulminate: An ester of fulminic acid (HONC). Thus, methyl fulminate is MeONC.

functional group: A group characterised by the presence of heteroatoms or unsaturation, which can take part in chemical reactions, e.g., –COOH, –SH.

furanoses: Cyclic acetal or hemiacetal forms of saccharides in which the ring is five-membered. See Chapter 5.

furfural: As a radical name, *furfural* denotes 2-furanylmethylene. *Furfural* usually refers to 2-furancarboxaldehyde.

gem(inal): Used to denote that two groups are attached to the same atom, as in *gem*-diol and *gem*-dimethyl groups.

glucosinolates: Mustard oil glycosides.

glycans: Polysaccharides made up of monosaccharide units linked glycosidically.

glycaric acids: Another name for aldaric acids.

glycerides: Esters of glycerol with fatty acids.

glycols: Olefinic sugars with a double bond between positions 1 and 2.

glycols: Diols. For example, ethylene glycol is $HOCH_2CH_2OH$ and propylene glycol is $H_3CCH(OH)CH_2OH$.

glycopeptides, glycoproteins: Substances in which a carbohydrate component is linked to a peptide or protein.
See *J. Biol. Chem.*, **262,** 13, 1987.

Grignard reagents: Organomagnesium halides RMgX having a C–Mg bond.

halohydrins: Halo alcohols. For example, ethylene bromohydrin is $BrCH_2CH_2OH$.

helicenes: Ortho-fused polycyclic aromatic compounds that have a helical structure.

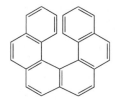

hexahelicene

hemiacetal: A compound with formula $R^1CH(OH)OR^2$ or $R^1R^2C(OH)OR^3$.

hemicarcerand: A bow-shaped molecule capable of complexing small molecules in its cavity. *See* carcerand.

hemiketal: A hemiacetal derived from a ketone.

hemimercaptals, hemimercaptoles: Compounds $R^1R^2C(SH)(SR^3)$.

hetero (Greek *heteros*, "other"): Prefix meaning "different," e.g., heteroxanthine, heterocycle.

homo: Denotes incorporation of CH_2 as an additional member in a ring in a steroid or a terpene; also, for example, in homophthalic acid.

A-homoandrostane

hydrazide: A compound formed by the replacement of the hydroxy group of an acid by $-NHNH_2$. Thus, acetohydrazide is $H_2CCONHNH_2$ and benzenesulfonohydrazide is $PhSO_2NHNH_2$

hydrazidines: Compounds $RC(=NNH_2)NHNH_2$. The term has also been applied to $RC(=NH)$ $NHNH_2$, $RC(=NH)NH_2$, and $RC(NH_2)=NN=C(NH_2)R$.

hydrazo: $-NHNH-$. Usually used when the free valencies are attached to different atoms that are usually otherwise connected. Hydrazo compounds are compounds RNHNHR. For example, hydrazobenzene is PhNHNHPh.

hydrazone: A compound derived from an aldehyde or ketone by replacement of the carbonyl oxygen by $=NNH_2$. Thus, acetone hydrazone is $(H_3C)_2=NNH_2$.

hydrazonyl: Suffix denoting a radical formed by loss of OH from a hydrazonic acid.

hydro: Denotes an added hydrogen atom. Thus, *dihydro* denotes saturation of one double bond.

hydrodisulfides: Compounds $R-S-SH$.

hydrogen: The word *hydrogen* is used to indicate an acid salt or ester of a dibasic acid. Thus, potassium hydrogen heptanedioate is $HOOC(CH_2)_5COOK$.

hydroperoxides: Compounds $R-O-OH$. Thus, ethyl hydroperoxide is EtOOH.

hydrosulfides: Old name for thiols. Thus, ethyl hydrosulfide is EtSH.

hydroxamamides: Another name for amidoximes.

-hydroximoyl: Suffix denoting an acyl radical formed by removal of OH from a hydroximic acid.

hypo (Greek "under"): Indicates a lower state of oxidation, e.g., hypoxanthine.

hypochlorite: A salt or ester of hypochlorous acid (HOCl). Thus, methyl hypochlorite is MeOCl.

i-: Obsolete form of *iso-*, as in *i*-pentane.

icosanoids: Unsaturated C_{20} fatty acids and related compounds such as leukotrienes.

imides: A class of compounds derived by replacement of two OH groups of a dibasic acid by $-NH-$ or $-N(R)-$. *See also* carboximides.

succinic acid   succinimide

imidogen: HN:, a neutral monovalent nitrogen species (*see* nitrenes).

imidoyl: Suffix denoting a radical formed by removal of OH from an imidic acid.

imines: Compounds $R^1R^2C=NH$. They can be named by adding the suffix *-imine* either to a parent name or to an *-ylidene* radical. Thus, $H_3C(CH_2)_4CH=NH$ is 1-hexanimine or hexylideneimine.

inclusion compounds: Compounds in which one kind of molecule (the guest compound) is embedded in the matrix of another (the host compound).

indane: A hydrocarbon, C_9H_{10}. Should not be used for InH_3, the CAS name for which is indium hydride (InH_3).

-inium: Denotes a positively charged species derived from a base with a name ending in *-ine*. Thus, anilinium is $PhNH_3^+$.

inner salts: *Chemical Abstracts* considers compounds such as betaines to be formed by the loss of water from the corresponding hydroxides and names them by use of the expression "hydroxide, inner salt."

(2-carboxyphenyl)phenyliodonium,
hydroxide, inner salt

inosamines: Aminodeoxyinositols, i.e., 6-amino-1,2,3,4,5-cyclohexanepentols.

inositols: 1,2,3,4,5,6-Cyclohexanehexols. See Section 5.2.

inososes: 2,3,4,5,6-Pentahydroxycyclohexanones.

iso: Prefix denoting isomerism, especially carbon chain branching (isohexanoic acid = 4-methylpentanoic acid). In the old literature it can be treated as a separable prefix, e.g., *iso*-propyl; in the modern literature it is usually treated as an inseparable prefix, e.g., isopropyl.

isocyanates: Compounds RNCO. Thus, methyl isocyanate is MeNCO.

isocyanides: Compounds RNC. Thus, methyl isocyanide is MeNC.

isonitriles: *See* isocyanides.

isoprenoids: Compounds such as terpenes that are derived from isoprene units. Isoprene is 2-methyl-1,3-butadiene, $H_2C=C(CH_3)CH=CH_2$.

isothiocyanates: Compounds RNCS. Thus, methyl isothiocyanate is MeNCS.

-ium: Suffix denoting a positively charged species.

ketals: Acetals derived from ketones.

ketazines: Azines derived from ketones.

ketene: A general term for compounds $R^1R^2C=C=O$. Ketene itself is ethenone, $H_2C=C=O$.

keto: oxo O=. Now used only in a generic sense, as in "ketoesters."

ketones: Compounds R^1COR^2. Usually named by use of the suffix *-one* or the prefix *oxo-*. Radicofunctional names are sometimes used. Thus, dimethyl ketone is H_3CCOCH_3 and ethyl methyl ketone is $H_3CCH_2COCH_3$.

ketoximes: Oximes of ketones.

lactams: Compounds containing a group of –CO–NH– as part of a ring. β-Lactams have four-membered rings, γ-lactams have five-membered rings, δ-lactams have six-membered rings, etc.

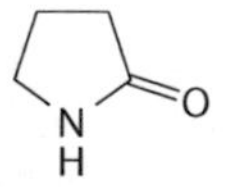

γ-butyrolactam or 4-butanelactam

lactides: Intramolecular cyclic esters formed by self-esterification from two or more molecules of a hydroxy acid.

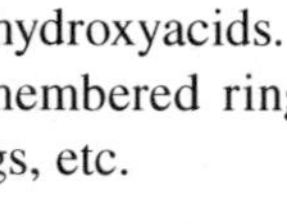

dilactide
(from lactic acid)

lactims: Tautomers of lactams containing a group –C(OH)=N– as part of a ring.

lactones: Intramolecular cyclic esters of hydroxyacids. They contain a group –CO–O– as part of a ring. β-Lactones have four-membered rings, γ-lactones have five-membered tings, δ-lactones have six-membered rings, etc.

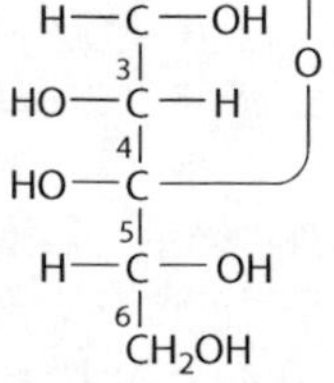

D-glucono-1,4-lactone

lambda (λ): Italicised prefix indicating abnormal (higher) valency of a ring heteroatom, e.g., S, Se, Te. For such compounds, the 2006 CAS nomenclature changes introduce this system to replace roman numeral valency suffixes used in 9CI.

1,2,3-Thia-(*SIV*)diazole, 9CI → 1λ⁴δ²-thiadiazole

leuco- (Greek "white"): Prefix denoting usually the reduced colourless form of a dye.

lin-: Denoting a linear arrangement of rings (obsol.).

m-: Abbreviation of *meta-*.

macrolides: Macrocyclic lactones.

mercaptals: Dithioacetals.

mercaptans: An old name for thiols. Thus, ethyl mercaptan is ethanethiol, EtSH.

mercaptoles: Mercaptals derived from ketones.

meso-: The middle position of substitution, e.g., the 9-position in anthracene (obsol.; the normal meaning of *meso-* is described in Chapter 7).

mesoionic compounds: Polyheteroatom five-membered ring betaines stabilised by electron delocalisation, having dipole moments not less than 5D, and in which electrons and positive charge are delocalised over a part of the ring and attached groups, and in which electrons and a negative charge, formally on an α-atom (normally a heteroatom), are delocalised over the remaining part of the ring. *See* munchnones and sydnones.
Cheung, K., et al., *Acta Cryst. Sect. C*, 49, 1092, 1993. Ollis, W. D., et al., *Tetrahedron,* 41, 2239, 1985.

mes(yl)ate: A salt or ester of methanesulfonic acid, $MeSO_3H$.

meta-: Denotes 1,3-substitution on a benzene ring.

metacyclophanes: Cyclophanes in which the benzene rings are *meta*-substituted by the aliphatic bridging chains.

methine: =C–.

methiodide, methobromide, methochloride, methoperchlorate, methopicrate, etc.: Indicates a base quaternised with methyl iodide, etc.

monoterpenoids: Terpenoids having a C_{10} skeleton.

morpholides: Anions formed from morpholine by loss of the hydrogen attached to the nitrogen.

munchnones: Mesoionic oxazolin-5-ones.

munchnones

mustard oils: An old term for isothiocyanates.

mustards: $(SCH_2CHRX)_2$, X = halogen.

n-: Abbreviation for normal (unbranched), as in *n*-butane.

naphtho: The ring fusion prefix derived from naphthalene.

-naphthone: Suffix denoting a ketone with formula $RCOC_{10}H_7$ ($C_{10}H_7$ = 1- or 2- naphthyl).

neo (Greek "new"): (1) A newly characterised stereoisomer (e.g., neomenthol). (2) A quaternary branched hydrocarbon. (3) In terpenes, the prefix *neo-* indicates the bond migration that converts a *gem*-dimethyl grouping directly attached to a ring carbon into an isopropyl group.

neosteroids: Occasionally used to refer to ring B aromatic steroids.

nitrenes: Neutral derivatives of monovalent nitrogen, including the parent compound HN: (nitrene or imidogen).

nitrile oxides: Compounds RCN(O). Thus, benzonitrile oxide is PhCNO.

nitriles: Compounds RCN. The suffix *-nitrile* denotes a –CN group at the end of an aliphatic chain. Thus, butanenitrile is $H_3CCH_2CH_2CN$. Nitriles can also be named as cyano-substituted compounds.

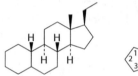

2-furannitrile or 2-cyanofuran

nitrilimines: $HC\equiv N^+–N^-H$.

nitr(o)imines: $RR^1C=NNO_2$.

nitrogen mustards: $RN(CH_2CHRX)_2$ X = halogen.

nitrones: *N*-Oxides of imines. Compounds containing the grouping C=N(O)R.

nitronic acids: *aci*-Nitro compounds, $R^1R^2C=N(O)OH$.

nitroxides: Free radicals derived from *N*-hydroxy amines by loss of the hydrogen from the oxygen atom, i.e., $R^1R^2N–O$. Thus, dimethyl nitroxide is $Me_2N–O\cdot$

nor-: Used mainly in naming steroids and terpenes, *nor* denotes elimination of one CH_2 group from a chain or contraction of a ring by one CH_2 unit.

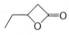

19-norpregnane   *A*-norandrostane

In older usage, particularly for monoterpenes, *nor* denotes loss of all methyl groups attached to a ring system, e.g., norborane, norpinane. The plural form should be *bisnor* when two carbon atoms are lost from the same site and *dinor* where they are lost from different sites, but in practice the terms are used interchangeably.

***o-*:** Abbreviation of *ortho-*.

-oin: Suffix denoting an acyloin RCH(OH)COR.

-olate: Suffix denoting a salt of an alcohol. Thus, sodium methanolate is MeONa.

olefins: Old term for alkenes.

-olide: Suffix denoting a lactone.

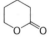

5-pentanolide   4-pentanolide   3-pentanolide

oligo-: Prefix meaning "a few," as in oligosaccharides, oligopeptides.

-olium: Denotes a positively charged species derived from a base with a name ending in *-ole*, e.g., pyrrolium.

-onium: Indicates a positively charged species such as ammonium, phosphonium, sulfonium, oxonium, etc.

***ortho-*:** Denotes 1,2-substitution in a benzene ring (abbreviated to *o-*).

ortho-: The highest-hydrated form of an acid, e.g., orthocarbonic acid, $C(OH)_4$.

orthoesters: Compounds $R^1C(OR^2)_3$, esters of the hypothetical ortho acids $R^1C(OH)_3$. Thus, ethyl orthoacetate is $H_3CC(OEt)_3$; orthoacetic acid is $H_3CC(OH)_3$.

osazones: Dihydrazones having the two hydrazone groups attached to adjacent carbon atoms. They are formed from compounds having the grouping –COCO– or –CH(OH)CO–, in the latter case with formal oxidation of the hydroxy group.

oxides: (1) Ethers have sometimes been named as oxides. Compounds R^1OOR^2 are dioxides, R^1OOOR^3 are trioxides, etc. Thus, dimethyl oxide is Me_2O, dimethyl dioxide is MeOOMe, dimethyl trioxide is MeOOOMe. (2) An alkene oxide is the epoxide derived from that alkene. Thus, styrene oxide is phenyloxirane. (3) Denotes the salt of an alcohol. Thus, sodium ethoxide is EtONa. (4) Indicates addition of O= at a heteroatom, as in trimethyl-amine *N*-oxide (Me_3NO), phosphine oxide ($H_3P{=}O$), and pyridine *N*-oxide.

oxido: Sometimes used to mean "epoxy." Also used as a substituent prefix to denote O = attached to a heteroatom, as in amine oxides; thus, 1-oxidopyridine is pyridine *N*-oxide.

oximes: Compounds RCH=NOH and $R^1R^2C{=}NOH$ considered to derive from carbonyl compounds. Thus, acetaldehyde oxime is $H_3CCH{=}NOH$ and acetamide oxime is $H_3CC({=}NOH)NH_2$.

oxonium: H_3O^+.

ozonides: 1,2,4-Trioxolanes formed by reaction of ozone at a C=C double bond.

***p-*:** Abbreviation of *para-*.

paddlane: A tricyclo[*m,n,o,p*$^{1,\ m+2}$]alkane, commonly called an [*m,n,o,p*]paddlane.

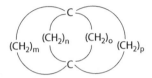

para- (Greek "beside," "beyond"): Denotes 1,4-substitution in a benzene ring.

paracyclophanes: Cyclophanes in which the benzene rings are *para*-substituted by the aliphatic bridging chains.

paraffins: Alkanes (obsol.).

per: (1) The highest state of oxidation, e.g., perchloric acid. (2) Presence of a peroxide (–O–O–) group, e.g., perbenzoic acid. (3) Exhaustive substitution or addition, e.g., perhydronaphthalene.

perbromo, perchloro, perfluoro, etc.: Denotes that all hydrogen atoms (except those that are part of functional groups, e.g., CHO, COOH) have been replaced by halogen atoms. Use can cause ambiguity.

perhydro: Denotes full hydrogenation of a fused polycyclic system.

peri: The 1,8-substitution pattern in napthalene (obsol.). Also, fusion of a ring to two or more adjoining rings, e.g., perinaphthindene.

peroxides: Compounds $R^1O{-}OR^2$. Thus, ethyl phenyl peroxide is EtOOPh and dibenzoyl peroxide is PhCO–O–O–COPh.

peroxy acids: Acids containing the group –C(O)OOH. Thus, peroxypropanoic acid is $H_3CCH_2C(O)$ OOH (also named as propaneperoxoic acid).

phenanthrylene: Phenanthrenediyl.

phenetidides: *N*-(Ethoxyphenyl) amides. They may be named analogously to anilides. Thus, aceto-*p*-phenetidide is *N*-(4-ethoxyphenyl)acetamide, $H_3CCONHC_6H_4OEt$-4 (obsol.).

pheniodide, phenobromide, phenochloride: Indicates a base that has been (formally) quaternised with phenyl iodide, phenyl bromide, or phenyl chloride (reaction not usually feasible in practice).

-phenone: Suffix denoting a ketone with formula RCOPh.

acetophenone   benzophenone

phenoxide: The anion PhO^-. Thus, potassium phenoxide is PhOK.

phosphatidic acids: Derivatives of glycerol in which one primary OH group is esterified with phosphoric acid and the other two OH groups are esterified with fatty acids.

phosphazenes: Compounds containing the group $=C=N-N=P\equiv$, e.g., $(H_3C)_2C=N-N=PPh_3$.

phosphine: PH_3. Phosphine imine is $H_3P=NH$, phosphine oxide is $H_3P=O$, phosphine sulfide is $H_3P=S$. Diphosphine is H_2P-PH_2, triphosphine is H_2PPHPH_2.

phosphite: Denotes a salt or ester of phosphorous acid.

phosphonium: H_4P^+-.

phosphorane: PH_5.

phosphoric acid: $(HO)_3PO$. Diphosphoric acid is $(HO)_2P(O)-OP-(O)(OH)_2$, triphosphoric acid is $(HO)_2P(O)-O-P(O)(OH)-OP-(O)(OH)_2$.

phthalocyanines: Compounds based on the polycyclic phthalocyanine ring system (IUPAC), as shown.

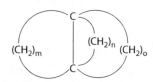

picrate: An ester, salt, or addition compound of picric acid (2,4,6-trinitrophenol).

pinacols: A general term for tetrasubstituted 1,2-ethanediols. Pinacol itself is 2,3-dimethyl-2,3-butanediol $(H_3C)_2C(OH)C(OH)(CH_3)_2$.

poly: Many.

polypyrroles: See Chapter 5.

porphyrins: See Chapter 5.

propellane: A tricyclo$[m,n,o,0^{1,m+2}]$alkane, called an $[m,n,o]$propellane. A special case of paddlanes with one zero bridge.

proteins: Polypeptides of high molecular weight (above 10,000).

pseudo (Greek "false"): Prefix indicating resemblance to, especially isomerism with, e.g., pseudocumene or ψ-cumene.

pyro: Prefix designating compounds formed by heating, usually with the elimination of a simple molecule, e.g., water or CO_2.

pyrophosphoric acid: Diphosphoric acid, $(HO)_2P(O)-O-P(O)(OH)_2$.

pyrophosphorous acid: Diphosphorous acid, $(HO)_2P-O-P(OH)_2$.

pyrromethenes: Compounds containing two pyrrole rings joined by a $-CH=$ group.

quercitols: Deoxyinositols, i.e., 1,2,3,4,5-cyclohexanepentols.

quinones: Diketones derived from aromatic compounds by conversion of two CH groups into CO groups.

quinone imines (quinonimines): Compounds derived from quinones by replacement of one or more of the quinone oxygens by $HN=$.

quinone methides (quinomethides): Compounds derived from quinones by replacement of one or more of the quinone oxygens by $H_2C=$.

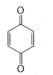

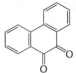

p-benzoquinone   9,10-phenanthrenequinone
                          or phenanthraquinone

retro- 1. (in carotene names): The prefix *retro-* and a pair of locants denote a shift, by one position, of all single and double bonds delineated by the pair of locants. The first locant cited is that of the carbon atom that has lost a proton, and the second that of the carbon atom that has gained a proton.

2. (in peptide names): When used with a trivially named peptide, *retro-* denotes that the amino acid sequence is the reverse of that in the naturally occurring compound.

rotaxanes: A class of molecules in which an annular component is free to rotate around a spine, but is prevented from escape by end groups on the spine. A prefix indicates the number of molecular components.

See Stoddart, J. F., et al., *J. Am. Chem. Soc.*, 114, 193, 1992.

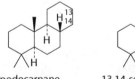

[2]rotaxane

s-: Abbreviation for symmetric(al), as in *s*-triazine (1,3,5-triazine). Also an abbreviation for *sec-*, as in *s*-butyl. Both of these usages are obsolete; the current use of *s-* is as a descriptor for pseudoasymmetric centres (see Chapter 7).

S-: Denotes sulfur as a locant. Also an important stereochemical descriptor; see Chapter 7.

Schardinger dextrins: Another name for cyclodextrins.

Schiff(s) bases: *See* azomethines.

sec-: Abbreviation of *secondary*, as in *sec*-butyl.

seco: In steroid and terpene names, *seco* denotes fission of a ring with addition of a hydrogen atom at each terminal group thus created.

podocarpane   13,14-secopodocarpane

selenane: Hantzsch-Widman systematic name for selenacyclohexane. Not a name for SeH_2, one name for which is selane.

selenenimine: $H_2Se=NH$.

selenides: Compounds R^1SeR^2, selenium analogues of ethers and sulfides. Compounds R^1SeSeR^2 are diselenides, $R^1SeSeSeR^2$ are triselenides, etc.

seleno: Denotes replacement of oxygen by selenium as in selenourea, $(H_2N)_2C=Se$. Also denotes the bridging radical $-Se-$. Usually used when the free valencies are attached to different atoms that are not otherwise connected.

selenocyanates: Compounds RSeCN. Thus, methyl selenocyanate is MeSeCN.

-selenol: Suffix denoting –SeH. Selenols are selenium analogues of alcohols and thiols.

selenones: Compounds $R^1Se(O)_2R^2$, selenium analogues of sulfones. Thus, dimethyl selenone is $Me_2Se(O)_2$.

selenoxides: Compounds $R^1Se(O)R^2$, selenium analogues of sulfoxides. Thus, dimethyl selenoxide is $Me_2Se(O)$.

selones: Compounds $R^1C(=Se)R^2$. Selenium analogues of ketones and thiones. Thus, 2-butaneselone is $H_3CC(=Se)CH_2CH_3$.

semicarbazones: Compounds $R^1R^2C=NNHCONH_2$. For example, acetone semicarbazone is $(H_3C)_2C=NNHCONH_2$.

semioxamazones: Compounds $R^1R^2C=NNHCOCONH_2$.

sesquiterpenoids: Terpenoids having a C_{15} skeleton.

sester: Numerical prefix meaning 2.5, as in sesterterpenes.

sesterterpenoids: Terpenes having a C_{25} skeleton.

silane: SiH_4. Disilane is H_3SiSiH_3, trisilane is $H_3SiSiH_2SiH_3$.

sil(a)thianes: Compounds of general formula $H_3Si-[SSiH_2]-_nSSiH_3$, named disilathiane ($n = 0$), trisilathiane ($n = 1$), etc.

silazanes: Compounds of general formula $H_3Si-[NHSiH_2]_n-NHSiH_3$, named disilazane ($n = 0$), trisilazane ($n = 1$), etc.

silicones: Polymeric or oligomeric siloxanes.

siloxanes: Compounds of general formula $H_3Si-[OSiH_2]_n-OSiH_3$, named disiloxane ($n = 0$), trisiloxane ($n = 1$), etc.

sphingoids (sphingolipids): Refers to sphingamine (D-*erythro*-2-amino-1,3-octadecanediol), its homologues, stereoisomers, and derivatives. Important biochemicals.

starburst dendrimer: *See* dendrimer.

styphnate: An ester, salt, or addition compound of styphnic acid (2,4,6-trinitro-1,3-benzenediol).

sulfanes: Compounds containing an unbranched chain of sulfur atoms may be named disulfanes, trisulfanes, etc. Thus, phenyl trisulfane is Ph–S–S–SH.

sulfenes: *S,S*-dioxides of thioaldehydes and thioketones.

sulfides: Compounds R^1SR^2. Sulfur analogues of ethers. Thus, diethyl sulfide is Et_2S. R^1S-SR^2 are disulfides, $R^1S-S-SR^2$ are trisulfides, etc. The word *sulfide* is also used to denote addition of S= to a heteroatom, as in phosphine sulfide ($H_3P=S$).

sulfines: *S*-Oxides of thiocarbonyl compounds, such as Ph(=S=O)H.

sulfones: Compounds $R^1S(O)_2R^2$. Thus, dimethyl sulfone is Me_2SO_2.

sulfonylides: Cyclic intermolecular esters of hydroxysulfonic acids. Analogues of lactides.

sulfoxides: Compounds $R^1S(O)R^2$. Thus, dimethyl sulfoxide is Me_2SO (sometimes called methyl sulfoxide). Sulfoxides having two different alkyl groups are chiral (tetrahedral S atom).

sulph-: British variant spelling of *sulf-*. IUPAC now recommends *sulf-*.

sultams: Cyclic esters of sulfonic acids. They contain the grouping $-S(O)_2N(R)-$ as part of a ring.

sultims: Tautomeric forms of sultams. They contain $-S(O)(OH)=N-$ as part of a ring.

sultines: Cyclic esters of hydroxysulfinic acids. They contain $-S(O)O-$ as part of a ring.

sultones: Cyclic esters of hydroxysulfonic acids. Analogues of lactones. They contain the grouping $-S(O)_2O-$ as part of a ring.

sydnones: A class of compounds derived from 1,2,3-oxadiazolidin-5-one, substituted in the 3-position, by loss of two hydrogen atoms, resulting in a mesoionic system (*see* mesoionic compounds). Sydnone imines are similar compounds derived from 1,2,3-oxadiazolidin-5-imine.

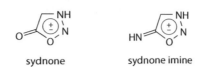

sydnone   sydnone imine

***sym-*:** Abbreviation for symmetric(al), as in *sym*-dichloroethane, $ClCH_2CH_2Cl$. Sometimes used to indicate 1,3,5-substitution in a benzene ring; e.g., *sym*-trichlorobenzene is 1,3,5-trichlorobenzene.

***t-*:** Abbreviation for tertiary, as in *tert*-butyl. Also *trans*; see Chapter 7.

tannins: Plant polyphenols.

tellurane: Hantzsch-Widman systematic name for telluracyclohexane. Not a name for TeH_2, one name for which is tellane.

tellurides: Compounds R^1TeR^2, tellurium analogues of ethers.

tellurilimine: $H_2Te=NH$.

telluro: –Te–. Used when the free valencies are attached to different atoms that are not otherwise connected.

tellurones: $R^1C(=Te)R^2$, tellurium analogues of ketones.

terpenoids: A class of organic compounds, the common structural feature of which is a carbon skeleton of repeating isoprene units.

***tert-*:** Abbreviation of tertiary as in *tert*-butyl.

thetins: Inner sulfonium salt analogues to betaines, e.g., $Me_2S^+CH_2COO^-$.

-thial: Suffix denoting –CHS at the end of an aliphatic chain. Thus, hexanethial is $H_3C(CH_2)_4CHS$.

thio: Denotes replacement of oxygen by sulfur as in thiophenol, thiourea. Also, the multiplying radical –S–. Dithio is –S–S–, trithio is –S–S–S–, etc.

thioacetals: Sulfur analogues of acetals.

thioaldehydes: Sulfur analogues of aldehydes, RCHS.

thiocarboxylic acids: Compounds RC(S)OH, RC(O)SH, and RC(S)SH, sulfur analogues of carboxylic acids.

thiocyanates: Compounds RSCN. Thus, methyl thiocyanate is MeSCN.

thioketones: Sulfur analogues of ketones.

-thiol: Suffix denoting –SH. Thiols are compounds RSH.

thiolates: Metal derivatives of thiols. Thus, sodium ethanethiolate is EtSNa.

-thione: Suffix denoting a thioketone. Thus, 2-butanethione is $H_3CC(=S)CH_2CH_3$.

thiophenol: Benzenethiol, PhSH. In order to avoid confusion, hydroxythiophene is called thiophene-ol.

thi(o)uronium salts: Quaternary derivatives of thiourea (isothiourea) with structure $[RSC(=NH)NH_2]^+ X^-$.

-thioyl: Suffix denoting an acyl radical derived from a thioic acid.

toluidides: *N*-(Methylphenyl) amides. They may be named analogously to anilides. Thus, aceto-*m*-toluidide is $H_3CCONHC_6H_4CH_3$ -3.

tosylate (tosate): An ester of *p*-toluenesulfonic acid.

tricyclo: For an explanation of names like tricyclo[5.1.0.0^{3,5}]octane, see Chapter 4 (Von Baeyer names).

triterpenoids: Terpenoids having a C_{30} skeleton.

tropones: Compounds containing the cyclohexa-2,4,6-trienone ring system.

ulosaric acids, ulosonic acids, ulosuronic acids: Acids derived from the oxidation of ketoses (see Section 5.1.3).

-ulose: Denotes a ketose; *-ulofuranose* and *-uropyranose* denote a ketose in the cyclic hemiacetal form having five- and six-membered rings, respectively (see Section 5.1.5).

***unsym-*:** Abbreviation for *unsymmetrical*, as in *unsym*-dichloroethane, H_3CCHCl_2. Sometimes used to indicate 1,2,4-substitution on a benzene ring; e.g., *unsym*-trichlorobenzene is 1,2,4-trichlorobenzene.

urethanes: Esters of carbamic acid. Urethane itself is ethyl carbamate, and hence phenylurethane is PhNHCOOEt.

uronic acids: Monocarboxylic acids derived by oxidation of the terminal CH_2OH of aldoses. Names are formed by replacing the *-ose* ending of the aldose name with *-uronic acid* (see Section 5.1.3).

uronium salts: Quaternary derivatives of urea (isourea) with structure $[ROC(=NH_2)NH_2]^+ \, X^-$.

v-: Abbreviation for vicinal, as in *v*-triazine (1,2,3-triazine).

vic-: Abbreviation for vicinal. Sometimes used to indicate 1,2,3-substitution on a benzene ring; e.g., *vic*-trichlorobenzene is 1,2,3-trichlorobenzene.

vicinal: Neighbouring.

Wittig reagents: Phosphonium ylids R_3P^+—$C^-R_2 \leftrightarrow R_3P{=}CR_2$.

xanthic acids: *O*-Esters of carbonodithioic acid, ROC(S)SH. Thus, ethylxanthic acid is EtOC(S)SH. Xanthates are salts of xanthic acids.

xylidides: *N*-(Dimethylphenyl)amides. They may be named analogously to anilides. Thus, aceto-2,4-xylidide is $CH_3CONHC_6H_3(CH_3)_2$-2,4.

-ylene: Suffix denoting a bivalent radical in which the free valencies are on different atoms.

-ylidene: Suffix denoting a bivalent radical in which the free valencies are on the same atom.

ylides: Compounds in which an anionic site is attached directly to a heteroatom carrying a positive charge; e.g., triphenylphosphonium methylide is Ph_3P^+–CH^-. Discontinued as an index term in the CAS 2006 changes. Compounds formerly indexed with a suffix *-ylide* are now indexed using the term *inner salt*.

-ylidyne: Suffix denoting a trivalent radical in which the free valencies are on the same atom.

ylium: Suffix denoting a carbonium atom; e.g., methylium is H_3C^+, acetylium is $H_3CC^+(=O)$.

zwitterionic compounds: General term for compounds containing both positive and negative charges. *See also* betaine.

7 Stereochemistry

John Buckingham

Further reading:

Eliel, E. L., and Wilen, S. H., *Stereochemistry of Organic Compounds* (Wiley Interscience, 1994).
Basic Terminology of Stereochemistry, IUPAC Recommendations 1996, www.chem.qmul.ac.uk/iupac/stereo. *Pure Appl. Chem.* 68, 2193, 1996.
Naming and Indexing of Chemical Substances for Chemical Abstracts, 2007 editon, p. 71 et. seq. (American Chemical Society, Columbus, Ohio)

Stereochemistry deals with the topography and transformations of the molecule in three dimensions, i.e., the features that go beyond the connectivity (which atoms are joined to which). It is conventional to distinguish between *configuration* (features that cannot be interconverted without bond breaking) and *conformation* (different states of the same molecule that can interconvert without bond breaking), but this distinction is not precise. There are some types of molecules (those with bond character intermediate between single and double, biaryls with medium-sized ortho-substituents, etc.) where the energy barrier to interconversion from one isomer to another is comparable to their energy content at room temperature. At sufficiently low temperatures, all conformations become configurations.

A *chiral* (handed) molecule is one capable of existence in a pair of nonsuperposable mirror-image forms. Nearly all configurations now found in the literature are *absolute configurations*, i.e., the handedness or chirality of the molecule in real space is known. This was not possible until the 1950s, so the old literature must be consulted with care. By coincidence, the arbitrary configurations assigned before the 1950s to compounds related to the standard molecules glucose and serine, and defined using the old D,L- system, were correct. (On the other hand, some terpenoid configurations that had been arbitrarily related to camphor had to be reversed.)

Chirality of a molecule (or any other object) can be more formally defined by reference to group theory. Chiral molecules belong to the lowest point groups C_n and D_n. An example of a molecule belonging to the lowest possible point group C_1 is *Cabde*. An example of a chiral molecule belonging to a higher point group is trishomocubane (D_3 symmetry). Another way of stating the symmetry requirements is that a chiral molecule cannot have a centre, plane, or alternating axis (rotation-reflection axis) of symmetry, although it may have one or more rotation axes.

D_3-Trishomocubane

The term *chiral* is also used to describe a sample of a substance. When used in this sense, it is not necessary that every molecule in the sample has the same handedness; see the definitions below for *optical purity, enantiopurity*, etc. A *racemic* sample is one containing (statistically) equal numbers of right-handed and left-handed enantiomers, and therefore showing zero optical activity at all wavelengths. A sample can also be chiral, nonracemic; i.e., it contains an excess of one enantiomer.

Chirality is most frequently studied by chiroptical methods. This term covers (1) measurement of optical rotation at a single wavelength, (2) measurement of optical rotation as a function of wavelength (optical rotatory dispersion (ORD); ORD values may be positive or negative), and (3) measurement of circular dichroism (CD) as a function of wavelength (values always positive). Definitions of terms used in these techniques are given below. A nonracemic chiral sample may have zero optical rotation at a given wavelength if that is the wavelength at which its ORD curve crosses the origin. A chiral sample always shows ORD/CD maxima, although they may be too weak to measure.

The following is a summary of the representation and description of basic stereochemistry. See also the relevant entries in Chapter 5, especially under *amino acids* and *carbohydrates*.

7.1 THE SEQUENCE RULE: *R* AND *S*

Leading references are:

> Cahn, R. S., *J. Chem. Educ.*, 41, 116, 1964.
> Cahn, R. S., et al., *Angew. Chem., Int. Ed. Engl.*, 5, 385, 1966.
> Prelog, V., et al., *Angew. Chem., Int. Ed. Engl.*, 21, 567, 1982.

The sequence rule (also known as the Cahn-Ingold-Prelog (CIP) system) is the universal system of describing absolute configurations. It provides a method of arranging atoms or groups in an order of precedence and is used to assign stereochemical descriptors, *R*-, *S*-, also *E*-, *Z*-, and others.

The molecule is viewed from opposite the group of lowest (fourth) priority. If the remaining groups in decreasing order of priority are arranged in a clockwise manner, then the configuration is *R*. If they are arranged in an anticlockwise manner, then the configuration is *S*.

In the following diagrams the order of priority of the groups is a > b > c > d. Hence, the molecule is viewed from opposite group d.

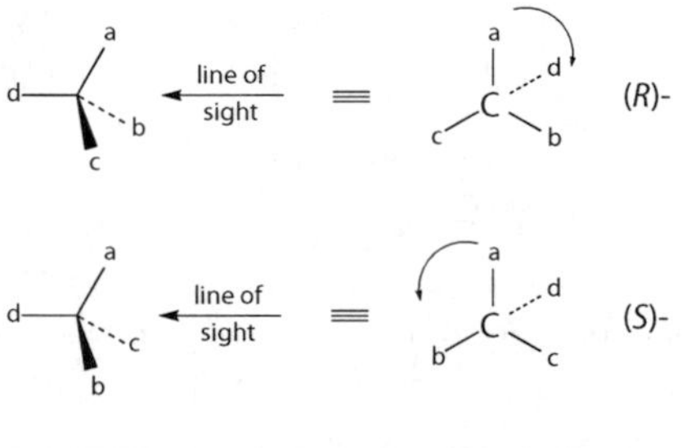

The rules as they apply to compounds with centres of chirality may be summarised as follows:

1. Atoms of higher atomic number take precedence over those of lower atomic number. Thus, $Cl > S > O > N > C > H$. Lone pairs are assigned the lowest possible priority.
2. Isotopes of higher atomic weight take precedence over those of lower atomic weight. Thus, $^3H > {}^2H > {}^1H$.
3. When the first atoms in each group are the same, then the priorities are determined by the atomic numbers of the atoms that are directly attached to these. Thus, $CH_2Cl > CH_2OH > CH_3$ because $Cl > O > H$ and $(H_3C)_3C > (H_3C)_2CH > H_3CCH_2$ because $C > H$. If no difference is observed for this second set of atoms (second sphere), then the third sphere and so on are considered in turn until there is a difference.

   When carrying out this process of outward exploration, the following principles must be adhered to: (1) all ligands in a given sphere must be explored before proceeding to the next sphere, and (2) once a precedence of one path over another has been established in one sphere, that precedence is carried over to the next sphere.

4. In groups containing a double or triple bond, for the purposes of determining priority, the multiple bond is split into two or three bonds, as follows:

Only the multiply bonded atoms themselves are duplicated and not the atoms of groups attached to them.

5. When the difference between substituents is in configuration, then in general $Z > E$ and $R > S$. However, the formal definition is that an olefinic ligand in which the substituent of higher sequence priority is on the same side of the alkene double bond as the chiral centre takes priority. This definition does not correspond with either E,Z- or *cis/trans*- (change to the rules in 1982), The subscript n (for "new") is used in cases of doubt.

Application of the 1982 rule to assignment of configuration.

The order of priority is $1 > 2 > 3 > 4$ because although 2 has Z-configuration and 1 has E-, residue 1 has the higher priority group (Cl) *cis* to the chiral centre. The compound has R_n-configuration (adapted from Eliel and Wilen).

6. In addition, a further rule was introduced in 1982 that says like precedes unlike, and this takes precedence over the rule that R- precedes S-.

Application of the like precedes unlike rule.

The configurational label at C-3 is S.

Programs are available for assigning CIP labels algorithmically, e.g., one is included in recent versions of Chemdraw.

7.1.1   LIST OF COMMON GROUPS IN CIP PRIORITY ORDER

I > Br > Cl > PR_2 > SO_3H > SO_2R > SOR > SR > SH > F > OTs > OAc> OPh > OMe > OH
> NO_2 > NMe_3^+ > NEt_2 > NMe_3 > NHCOPh > NHR > NH_2 > COOR > COOH > COPh >
$COCH_3$ > CHO > CH_2OR > CH_2OH > CN > CH_2NH_2 > Ph > C≡CH > Bu^t > cyclohexyl
> $CH(CH_3)CH_2CH_3$ > $CH=CH_2$ > $CH(CH_3)_2$ > CH_2Ph > $CH_2CH=CH_2$ > $CH_2CH(CH_3)_2$ >
CH_2CH_3 > CH_3 > D > H

R*- and *S**- are relative stereochemical descriptors. Thus, (*R**, *R**) indicates two centres of like chirality (either both *R*- or both *S*-) and (*R**, *S**) indicates two centres of unlike chirality. (*RS*) and (*SR*) are used to denote racemates (see *RS*-).

7.2   GRAPHICAL AND TEXTUAL REPRESENTATIONS OF STEREOCHEMISTRY

7.2.1   COMPOUNDS WITH ONE CHIRAL CENTRE

Where the absolute configuration is known, structures can be represented either as Fischer type diagrams or as perspective diagrams. Fischer diagrams follow the convention that the principal chain occupies the vertical position, with the head of the chain uppermost.

7.2.2   COMPOUNDS WITH TWO CHIRAL CENTRES

In addition to Fischer and perspective diagrams, physical organic chemists use Newman and sawhorse diagrams to show conformations as well as configurations of two-centre compounds.

Figure 7.1 shows 3-bromo-2-chlorobutanoic acid in Fischer-type, zigzag (closely related to flying wedge), sawhorse, and Newman representations.

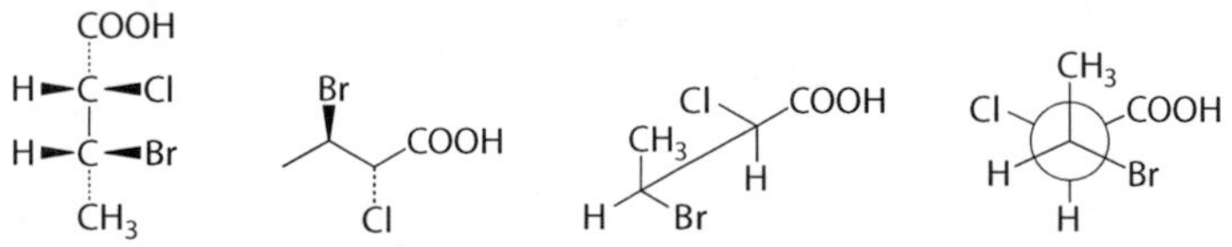

FIGURE 7.1   (2*S*,3*R*)-3-Bromo-2-chlorobutanoic acid showing some possible representations: (a) Fischer-type diagrams. (b) Zigzag. (c) Sawhorse diagram showing one of three staggered conformations. (d) Corresponding Newman projection.

In CAS presentation (9CI period), the labels *R**,*S** are used not only where the absolute configuration is unknown, but also where it is known. *R** is allocated to the centre of highest sequence priority, e.g., in the above example, position 3 (since Br > Cl). The general descriptor (*R**,*S**) for this diastereoisomer is then modified where the absolute configuration is known, and the citation refers to the optically active material. Thus. the isomer illustrated above is [*R*-(*R**,*S**)], and its racemate, when specifically referred to, is [(*R**,*S**)-(±)].

These CAS rules, which had been in use since the beginning of the 9th Collective Index period (1972), have now been thoroughly revised to give a simplified and more intuitive description. The need for a single expression to describe the total stereochemistry of a molecule has been eliminated. Stereochemical terms are now placed within the parts of a chemical name to which the stereochemical information applies. The following diagram shows the now superseded 9CI descriptors alongside the revised equivalents, which are closer to now current CAS practice.

The symbols (2*RS*,3*RS*) and (2*RS*,3*SR*) can also be used for the racemic diastereoisomers of compounds with two chiral centres though CAS does not use this system. Where the absolute configuration appears to be unknown, asterisked symbols, e.g. (2*R**, 3*R**) may be used.

Graphical representation of stereoisomers of
3-bromo-2-chlorobutanoic acid

CAS now registers and names substances with partially defined stereochemistry. Previously, partial stereochemistry was generally ignored. The presence of unknown chiral centers is indicated by the addition of the term [*partial*]- to the end of the normal stereochemical descriptor. When the reference ring or chain has incompletely defined chiral atoms/bonds, the format cites the stereochemistry using R and S terms with their nomenclature locants for all known centers. If this method is used to describe a substance for which only relative stereochemistry is known, *rel* is added to the stereochemical descriptor. Any stereochemical descriptor marked as *rel* always cites the first centre as R-.

Beilstein uses a number of additional stereochemical descriptors for specialised situations. Examples are (RS), R_a, S_a, and Ξ. For full details, see the booklet *Stereochemical Conventions in the Beilstein Handbook of Organic Chemistry*, issued by the Beilstein Institute, and Section 7.6.

7.2.3 CYCLIC STRUCTURES

The application of the above principles to simple cyclic structures is straightforward. The E,Z notation should *not* be used to define configurations of cyclic compounds such as 1,2-cyclobutanediol.

(R,S)- descriptors can be assigned to prochiral centres in more symmetrical molecules by a simple extension of the sequence rule. For example, in 1,3-cyclobutanediol the OH group at each centre has priority 1 and the H atom priority 4.

An *arbitrary* choice is made between methylene groups (2) and (3), giving $(1RS,4RS)$ chirality to the *trans* form and $(1RS,4SR)$ to the *cis* form. The result is independent of the arbitrary choice made.

An alternative and more rigorous treatment considers C-1 and C-3 as centres of pseudoasymmetry and assigns them the appropriate symbols r and s (actually r_n and s_n; see definitions below). (Note that according to this treatment, the *cis*-isomer is $1s_n,3s_n$ and the *trans*-isomer $1r_n,3r_n$; i.e., changing the configuration at one centre changes *both* descriptors.) For a full explanation, see Eliel and Wilen, p. 667.

In the case of cyclic structures with several substituents (e.g., cyclitols), the (α,β)-convention may be clearer and unambiguous. See also cyclitols in Chapter 5.

7.3 CHIRAL MOLECULES WITH NO CENTRES OF CHIRALITY

Extensions of the CIP rules deal with molecules that are chiral as a whole but contain no chiral centres.

7.3.1 ALLENES, BIARYLS, AND RELATED COMPOUNDS

A molecule such as abC=C=Cde is chiral if a ≠ b and c ≠ d (axial chirality). The additional rule is that near groups precede far groups.

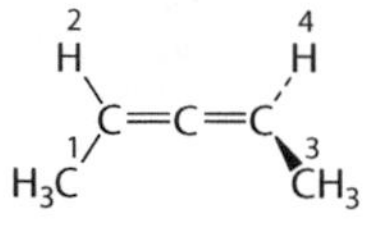

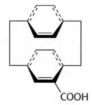

Application of the axial chirality rule to an allene: Near end of axis precedes far; chirality is *aR*.

Care is needed in some cases; e.g., an allene with four different substituents could alternatively be assigned a label using central chirality. To avoid doubt, use the descriptor $(R)_{axial}$ or *aR*.

7.3.2 MOLECULES WITH CHIRAL PLANES

The application of CIP rules to compounds showing planar chirality is complex because of ambiguities in choosing the correct plane.

The (*M,P*) system has also been used, which treats the molecule as a helix (*minus* and *plus* helicity), but is strictly redundant because *M* always ≡ *R* and *P* always ≡ *S*. For most purposes, it is better to avoid having to specify chirality whenever possible. A picture is worth a thousand words. To make it clear that planar chirality is assigned, the symbols $_pR/_pS$ (or R_{planar}/S_{planar}) can be used.

P or *pR*[2.2]Paracyclophane-
4-carboxylic acid

7.4 *E* AND *Z*

These are stereochemical descriptors used to describe the configuration about a double bond. *E*- is usually but not necessarily equivalent to *trans*-, and *Z*- to *cis*-. Priority of atoms or groups is decided in the same way as for *R* and *S* and if those of highest priority on the double bond are *trans* to each other, then the compound has *E* configuration, if *cis*, then it has *Z*.

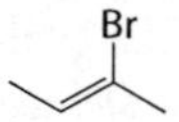

(*Z*)-2-Bromo-2-butene
equivalent to *trans*-
(priorities Br > CH₃ > H)

For many compounds with more than one double bond, CAS cites *E*- and *Z*- without locants. The *E*- and *Z*- descriptors are cited in descending order of seniority. The most senior double bond is that which has the highest-ranking (sequence rule) substituent attached. Thus, the stereochemistry of the compounds below is described as (*E,Z*)- because the phenyl group is the highest-ranked substituent attached to a doubly bonded atom.

See Blackwood, J. E., et al., *J. Chem. Doc.*, 8, 32, 1968.

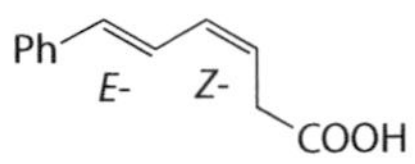

Ph
E-   *Z-*
COOH

(*E,Z*)-

7.5   THE D,L-SYSTEM

D- and L- are older configurational descriptors used to denote the configuration of chiral molecules, especially carbohydrates and α-amino acids. Fischer projections are used to assign the symbols D- and L-.

Nowadays, *R,S*- descriptors are used for all classes of molecule except for the following:

- *Carbohydrates.* Here the application of the sequence rules to the many –CH(OH)– groups is possible but tedious and confusing. Carbohydrates retain the system based on assigning the key chiral centre to the D- or L- series, as described in Chapter 5.

   (+)-Glyceraldehyde is defined as D-; the OH group attached to C(2) is on the right-hand side of the Fischer projection in which the CHO group appears at the top. Its enantiomer is defined as L- because the OH group is on the left-hand side. (The D- and L- symbols were originally assigned arbitrarily; in the 1950s it was found that (+)-glyceraldehyde has the absolute configuration represented here.)

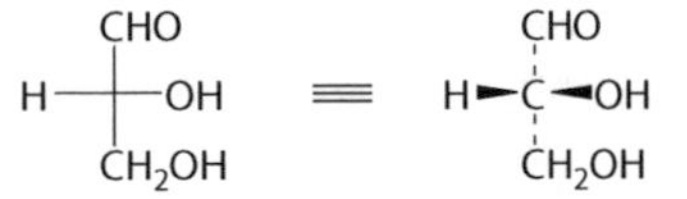

D-glyceraldehyde

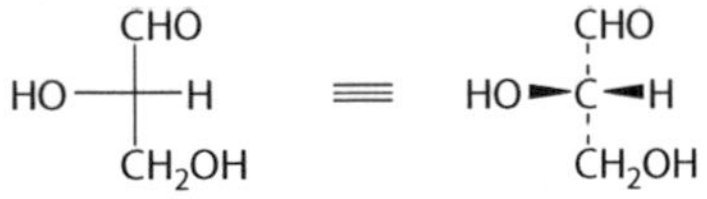

L-glyceraldehyde

For carbohydrates, in general, the position of the OH group attached to the highest-numbered carbon atom in the chain determines the assignment of D- and L-. For instance, in D-glucose the OH at position 5 is on the right-hand side of the Fischer projection.

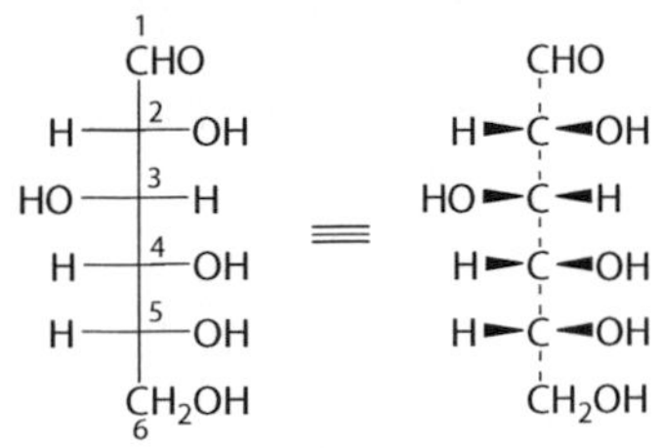

D-glucose

- *Amino acids.* These retain the D,L- system because all of the protein amino acids belong to the L- series, but not all of them are *S*- according to the sequence rule. See Chapter 5. Biochemists often use the D,L- system for synthetic compounds derived from amino acids where most organic chemists would use *R,S*-. In α-amino acids, the L-compounds are those in which the NH$_2$ group is on the left-hand side of the Fischer projection in which the COOH group is at the top. Conversely, the D-compounds are those in which the NH$_2$ group is on the right-hand side.

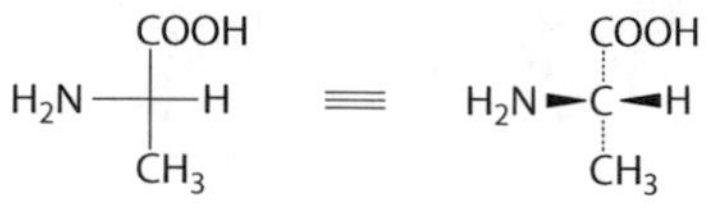

L-alanine

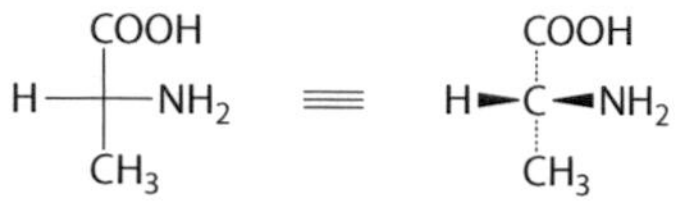

D-alanine

D- and L- do *not* relate to the sign of rotation of an optically active sample, which is designated (+)- or (–)- (formerly *d*- and *l*-).

The abbreviations D$_G$/L$_G$ and D$_S$/L$_S$ were formerly used in cases where there was potential ambiguity in assigning D/L configurations and refer to configurations relative to glucose and serine, respectively.

The D,L- system should no longer be used except for compounds that are closely and unambiguously related to either carbohydrates or amino acids. This is to avoid ambiguity. By suitably modifying the groups on, e.g., an amino acid in different ways, it is possible to arrive at compounds that can be described either as D- or L-, depending on the route used, whereas the *R,S*- system is unambiguous.

The symbol for a racemate is D,L- or (±)-.

7.6   DESCRIPTORS AND TERMS USED IN STEREOCHEMISTRY

(For designations of Greek letters, see after Z.)

a: Molar amplitude of an ORD curve, a = ([Φ]$_1$ + [Φ]$_2$)/100, where [Φ]$_1$ and [Φ]$_2$ are the molar rotations at the first and second extrema.

achiral: Not chiral, i.e., superposable on its mirror image.

achirotopic: *See* chirotopic.

allo-, altro-, arabino-: Carbohydrate-derived prefixes. See Chapter 5.

ambo-: Used after a locant to indicate a preparation containing approximately equal amounts of diastereomers at the indicated centre, e.g., (2*ambo*, 4′*R*,8′*R*)-β-tocopherol (Beilstein; not in widespread use):

anancomeric: Fixed in a single conformation by geometric constraints or by the overwhelming preponderance of one possible conformation.

anti-: (1) (Greek "opposite") Stereochemical descriptor used for bridged bicyclic compounds. In a bicyclo[*X.Y.Z*] compound (*X ≥ Y > Z*), *anti*- denotes that a substituent on the *Z* bridge points away from the *X* bridge.

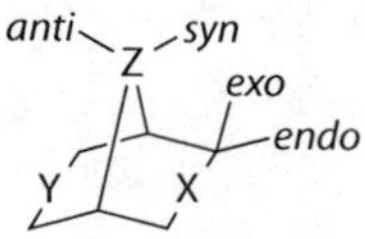

(2) Conformation of a molecule, e.g., butane, having opposite groups (distinct from *eclipsed* and *gauche*)

gauche eclipsed anti eclipsed

Conformations of butane

(3) Equivalent to trans- or *E*- when used to indicate the stereochemistry of oximes and similar C=N compounds (obsol.: use *E* or *Z*).

(4) Relative configuration of two stereogenic centres in a chain. Denotes that when drawn as a zigzag, the ligands are on opposite sides of the plane. Opposite of *syn*-.

anticlinal, antiperiplanar, synclinal: An anticlinal conformation in a molecule X-A-B-Y is when the torsion angle about the AB bond is +90° to 150° or −90° to −50° in an antiperiplanar conformation it is +150° to −150°; in a synclinal conformation it is +30° to +90° or −30° to −90°.

antimer, antipode, optical antipode: Obsolete terms for enantiomer.

asymmetric: Lacking all elements of symmetry (point group C_1). Not the same as dissymmetric, q.v.

atropisomer: An isolable stereoisomer resulting from a sufficiently high rotation barrier about a single bond. Difficult to define rigorously; a working definition is that the barrier to rotation should exceed 22.3 kcal mol^{-1}, which gives a $t_{1/2}$ for inversion of approximately 1,000 s at 300K.

axial: (1) An axial bond is one perpendicular to the plane containing or almost containing the majority of atoms in a cyclic molecule, e.g., cyclohexanes.

Position of bonds and substituents in the chair and boat conformations of cyclohexane: a = axial, e = equatorial, b = bowsprit, and f = flagpole.

(2) Axial chirality arises from the disposition of groups about an axis, e.g., in an allene; see above.

bowsprit/flagpole bonds: Bonds at the out-of-plane carbon atoms of the boat conformation of, e.g., cyclohexanes. *See* diagram under axial.

***c*-:** Abbreviation for *cis*- (obsol.). Extensively used, with elaboration, in Beilstein.

CD: Circular dichroism.

c_F, t_F, cat$_F$: Prefixes used in Beilstein to indicate *cis*- and *trans*- in a Fischer diagram (*cat* refers to the end of a chain, cat = catenoid). Not used elsewhere.

chiral carbon atom: A carbon atom in a molecule that is a centre of chirality. Better called a *chiral centre*, or even better, a *centre of chirality*, since this makes it clear that it is a portion of the molecule that is designated as chiral, not the carbon atom itself.

chirotopic: Any point in a molecule that is located in a chiral environment, not necessarily within a chiral molecule. See Eliel and Wilen, p. 53.

***cis*-:** Stereochemical descriptor denoting that two groups are on the same side of a ring or other plane. Also used to indicate the configuration of a double bond; *Z*- and *E*- are now used instead. *E*- does not always correspond to *trans*-, nor *Z*- to *cis*-. See above under *E/Z*.

cisoid: Obsolete term for *s-cis* (see below).

conformer (conformational isomer): A stable conformation of a molecule that is located at an energy minimum; e.g., ethane has three conformers.

cryptochiral: Substance that is chiral but with undetectable chiroptical properties, e.g., $(H_3C)_3CCHDOH$.

d-: Abbreviation for *dextro-* (obsol.).

D-: A configurational descriptor. Fuller description given above. D_S and D_G referred to configurations relative to serine and glucose, respectively (obsol.).

D_r-,D_s-,L_r-,L_s-: Elaborations of the D,L- notation found only in Beilstein (obsol.).

de: Diastereomeric excess. Analogous to enantiomeric excess, q.v.

dextro-: Denotes a compound that, in solution, rotates the plane of plane-polarised light to the right, as seen by the observer (obsol.). Equivalent to (+)-.

diastereo(iso)mers: Stereoisomers that are not enantiomers.

diastereotopic: Faces of a double bond that are not symmetry related. Addition of a new ligand gives different diastereomers.

dissymmetric: Old term for chiral. Distinction from asymmetric; asymmetry (e.g., molecules *Cabde*) applies only to objects of point group C_n whereas dissymmetry applies also to objects of higher point groups D_n.

dl-: Denotes a racemic mixture (*d-* + *l-*) (obsol.; avoid; use (±)-).

D,L-: Denotes a racemic mixture (D- + L-) (avoid except for carbohydrates or amino acids; use (±)- or *RS*-).

e-: Equivalent to *E-* to denote configuration at a single bond with restricted rotation (Beilstein; obsol.).

E-: Stereochemical descriptor for alkenes, cumulenes with an odd number of double bonds, and alkene analogues such as oximes. It means that the two substituents with highest CIP priority at the two ends of the bond are *trans-* to each other (German *entgegen*).

eclipsed: *See* anti-.

ee: Enantiomeric excess. The percentage excess of the enantiomer over the racemate. A pure enantiomer has 100% ee, a racemate 0%. ee = $[R - S]/[R + S] \times 100\%$.

enantiomorph: Obsolete term for *enantiomer.* Applied in the correct sense to define any mirror-image object.

endo-: Stereochemical descriptor used for bridged bicyclic systems. In a bicyclo[*X.Y.Z*] compound ($X \geq Y > Z$), *exo-* denotes that a substituent on an *X* or *Y* bridge is on the opposite side of the molecule from the *Z* bridge. For a diagram, *see* anti-.

ent-: The prefix *ent-* (a contracted form of *enantio-*) denotes configurational inversion of all the asymmetric centres whose configurations are implied in a name. It is used to designate a trivially named peptide in which the configurations of all the amino acid residues are the opposite of those in the naturally occurring compound.

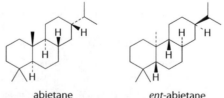

abietane   *ent*-abietane

Caution: Addition of, e.g., a *3R-OH* group to *ent*-abietane produces *ent*-3*S*-abietanol.

equatorial: A bond lying in or close to the plane containing most of the atoms in a cyclic molecule, e.g., cyclohexane. *See* diagram under axial.

erythro-: A configurational prefix. *See* carbohydrates. It is used generally to denote compounds with two chiral centres having the erythrose-like configuration (ambiguity can arise).

exo- (Greek "outside"): Stereochemical descriptor used for bridged bicyclic systems. In a bicyclo[*X.Y.Z*] compound (*X* ≥ *Y* > *Z*), *exo-* denotes that a substituent on an *X* or *Y* bridge is on the same side of the molecule as the *Z* bridge. For the diagram, *see* anti-.

fiducial group: The group that determines the assignment of a stereochemical label (conformational or configurational).

flagpole bond: *See* bowsprit and diagram under axial.

***galacto-, gluco-, glycero-, gulo-*:** Carbohydrate-derived prefixes. See Chapter 5.

***gauche*:** *See* anti-.

homochiral/heterochiral: Refers to a set of two or more molecules or fragments having the same or opposite chiralities, e.g., L-alanine/L-alanine vs. L-alanine/D-alanine.

homofacial/heterofacial: On the same or opposite side of a defined plane or face.

homotopic/heterotopic: Two or more ligands that are identical when viewed in isolation are heterotopic if replacement of each in turn by a new ligand gives a nonidentical product.

***i-*:** Abbreviation for inactive, as in *i*-tartaric acid. (obsol.).

***ido-*:** Carbohydrate-derived prefix. *See* Chapter 5 under carbohydrates.

***l-*:** (1) An abbreviated form of *levo-* or *laevo* (obsol.). (2) Stereodescriptor for diastereomers with stereocentres both *R-* or both *S-* (= "like" as opposed to *u* = "unlike"). Not widely used.

L-: A configurational descriptor. *See* D-. For L$_S$ and L$_G$, *see* D-.

***l(a)evo*:** Indicates a molecule that, in solution, rotates the plane of plane-polarised light to the left. Equivalent to (–)-.

***lyxo-, manno-*:** Carbohydrate-derived prefixes. See Chapter 5.

(*M*-), (*P*-): Stereochemical descriptors (*M* = minus, *P* = plus) introduced to describe the chirality of helical molecules. Extension of the CIP system to planar chirality gave an alternative description *aR/aS* for helical molecules such as helicenes, *aR* invariably ≡ (*M*) and *aS* ≡ (*P*), but for compounds showing planar chirality the reverse, with *pR* ≡ (*P*) and *pS* ≡ (*M*). Best avoided. See Section 7.3.2.

[M] or [Φ]: Molecular rotation, defined as [α] × MW/100. Specific rotation corrected for differences in MW. The symbol [M] and the term *molecular rotation* are now deemed incorrect, and the term *molar rotation* denoted by [Φ] is preferred.

***meso-*:** Denotes an internally compensated diastereoisomer of a chiral compound having an even number of chiral centres, e.g., *meso*-tartaric acid. Formally defined as an achiral member of a set of diastereomers that also contains chiral members.

mutarotation: Phenomenon shown by some substances, especially sugars, in which the optical activity changes with time. A correct presentation is, e.g., [α]$_D^{20}$ + 20.3 → –101.2 (2h)(c, 1.2 in H$_2$O).

op: Optical purity, defined as a percentage, op = 100[α]/[α]$_{max}$, where [α]$_{max}$ = rotation of the pure enantiomer (identical solvent, temperature, and concentration). Enantiomer excess (ee) is now preferred in careful studies because op is a physical property that may sometimes vary nonlinearly with enantiomeric composition (Horeau effect), and ee is now often measured by nonoptical methods.

ORD: Optical rotatory dispersion.

(*P*)-: *See* (*M*)-.

***pro-R, pro-S*:** These terms are used to distinguish an identical pair of atoms or groups in a prochiral compound. That which leads to an *R-* compound when considered to be preferred to the other by the sequence rule (without changing the priority with respect to the other substituents) is termed *pro-R*; the other is termed *pro-S*.

pseudoasymmetric centre, pseudoasymmetry: Term used to describe centres such as C-3 in ribitol and xylitol (see Chapter 5). C-3 is not a chiral centre and not chirotopic since it lies on a symmetry plane. It is, however, stereogenic because exchange of two of the attached ligands leads to the other *meso-* form. (The other two stereoisomers of the pentitols represent a pair of enantiomers, D- and L-arabinitol.)

pseudochiral centre, pseudochirality: Alternative terms for pseudoasymmetric centre/pseudoasymmetry. Not recommended.

quasienantiomers, quasiracemate: Terms used in place of enantiomer, racemate, where the components are similar but not identical. For example, (*R*)-2-bromobutanoic acid is quasienantiomeric with (*S*)-2-iodobutanoic acid and may form a quasiracemate with it.

R-: Stereodescriptor for chiral cenres or other stereogenic features in the CIP system. *See* above. Subscripts may be used to denote chirality as a heteroatom, e.g., R_S = chirality at a sulfur atom.

r-: Stereodescriptor applied to centres of pseudoasymmetry. In ribitol (see Chapter 5), C-3 has *s*-configuration, by application of the rule that an *R*-centre (C-4) has priority over an *S*-centre (C-2). In xylitol, C-3 has *r*-configuration.

R_a or R_{axial}/S_a or S_{axial}: Stereodescriptors for *R*- or *S*-configuration at an axis of chirality.

rac-: Prefix for racemic. Alternative to (*RS*) or (±)-. Used (especially with natural product names) to denote a racemate. In a peptide name *rac-* denotes that all the amino acids are DL. The abbreviation *racem-* is found in Beilstein.

Re/Si: Descriptors for heterotopic faces in a prochiral molecule. See Eliel and Wilen, p. 484 for a description.

rel-: Prefix indicating that a configuration is relative, not absolute. Use of the *R*,S** notation is preferred.

residual stereoisomer: The subset of the total set of stereoisomers of a compound that can be distinguished under specified conditions by a given technique. Thus, the axial and equatorial stereoisomers of chlorocyclohexane are distinguishable by NMR at room temperature or by laboratory manipulation at −160°, but not by laboratory manipulation at room temperature.

ribo-: Carbohydrate-derived prefix. See Chapter 5.

r_n/s_n (n = new): Applied to pseudoasymmetry descriptors resulting from a treatment deriving from the 1982 paper, not present in earlier CIP documentation.

R_p or R_{planar}/S_p or S_{planar}: Stereodescriptors for *R*- or *S*-configuration at a chirality plane. See Section 7.3.2.

(RS)- and (SR)-: In a one-centre compound (*RS*) means the racemate, equivalent to (±). In a compound with two or more centres of chirality, *RS* and *SR* are used to define the relative configurations of the centres in racemic diastereomers, e.g., (±)-threitol = (2*RS*,3*RS*)-1,2,3,4-butanetetrol, erythritol = (2*RS*,3*SR*)-1,2,3,4-butanetetrol. Priority is given to (*RS*)- for the lowest-numbered centre. (CAS uses *R** and *S** together with the (±)- identifier to show that a racemate is meant.)

S-: Stereodescriptor for chiral centres or other stereogenic features in the CIP system. See above.

s-: Stereodescriptor applied to centres of pseudoasymmetry; *see r-*.

S_a, S_p: *See R_a, and R_p.*

s-cis, seqcis, s-trans, seqtrans-: Obsolete forms of *Z*- and *E*-. However, *s-cis* and *s-trans* are also used to define conformations about a single bond between two double bonds, with *s-cis* = synperiplanar and *s-trans* = antiperiplanar.

Si: *See Re.*

staggered: Conformation of a molecule abcX-Ydef in which the torsion angle is 60°.

stereogenic centre: A carbon atom or other feature in a molecule that is a focus of stereoisomerism. Interchange of two ligands at a stereogenic carbon leads to inversion of configuration.

Chiral atoms are stereogenic, but not all stereogenic centres are chiral atoms. For example, in an alkene abC=Cab the double bond is a stereogenic element.

syn-: (1) Stereochemical descriptor used for bridged bicyclic systems. In a bicyclo [*X.Y.Z*] compound (*X* ≥ *Y* > *Z*), *syn*- denotes that a substituent on the Z bridge points toward the X bridge. For a diagram, *see* anti-. (2) Also used for configuration of oximes, etc. (obsol.; use *E/Z*). (3) Conformational descriptor, *see anti*-.

synclinal: *See* anticlinal.

synperiplanar: A synperiplanar conformation in a molecule X-A-B-Y is when the torsion angle about the AB bond is +30 to +90° or −30 to −90°.

***t*-:** Abbreviation for *trans*- (obsol.). Extensively used, with elaboration, in Beilstein.

***talo*-:** Carbohydrate-derived prefix. *See* Chapter 5.

t_F: *See* c_F.

***threo*-:** A configurational prefix. *See* Chapter 4 under carbohydrates. Can be used generally to denote stereoisomers of compounds having two chiral centres having the threose-like configuration. Ambiguity can occur.

***trans*-:** Stereochemical descriptor denoting that two atoms or groups are on the opposite side of a ring. Also used to indicate the configuration about a double bond. *See cis*-.

***u*-** (unlike): *See l*-.

***xylo*-:** Carbohydrate-derived prefix. *See* Chapter 4 under carbohydrates.

Z-: Opposite of *E*- for alkenes, etc. (German *zusammen*).

***z*-:** Equivalent to *Z* in denoting configuration at a single bond exhibiting restricted rotation (Beilstein; obsol.).

α-: (1) α without brackets refers to an experimentally measured rotation value, e.g., α = −19.2° (obsol.). α in square brackets refers to the specific rotation of a compound in a given solvent and at the experimental temperature, e.g., $[α]_D^{25}$ −57.4 (c, 0.25 in $CHCl_3$); it is a dimensionless number and a degree sign should *not* be used. The solvent and concentration should be stated as shown. Concentrations are given in g/100 ml.

(2) Indicates below-the-plane stereochemistry in steroids, terpenoids, etc., e.g., 5α-pregnane, and below-the-plane configuration of substituents. In such stereoparents, the α- or β-configuration at certain stereocentres may be implicit in the name of the stereoparent, while others may need to be defined. In the name 3α-chloro-5α,10α-pregnane, the three alphas perform different functions; 3α is the orientation of a substituent, 5α is inserted because the stereoparent pregnane has an undefined 5-configuration and it has to be specified, and 10α reverses the normal pregnane 10β-configuration.

(3) α,β- indicates the configuration of the glycosidic bond in glycosides (*see* Chapter 5 under carbohydrates).

(4) α,β- was formerly used to denote side chain configurations in steroids (Fieser convention). Obsolete; use *R*- and *S*-.

$α_F$, $β_F$: Used in Beilstein to denote side chain configurations in steroids (Fischer representation). Obsolete; use *R*- and *S*-.

β-: (1) Indicates above-the-plane stereochemistry in steroids, terpenoids, etc., e.g., 5β-pregnane.

(2) Indicates configuration of the glycosidic bond in glycosides. *See also* α-.

Δε: In circular dichroism, amplitude of the CD maximum; difference in molar absorption coefficients for right and left circularly polarised light. May be positive or negative.

θ: (1) Molar ellipticity in CD measurement, [θ] = [ψ] × MW/100. For small ellipticities, [θ] = 3298.2 × Δε.

(2) Symbol for bond angle.

ξ or Ξ: Lowercase xi (ξ) denotes unknown configuration at a chiral centre (alternative to α,β or *R,S*), e.g., 1β,2β,3ξ-trihydroxy-12-ursen-23-oic acid. In Beilstein, Ξ is used in place of D or L where the configuration is uncertain or undefined. In the Combined Chemical Dictionary (Section 1.2.1), the descriptor (ξ)- is also used for stereoisomers where it is uncertain which enantiomer is described, e.g., natural products isolated only by GC and characterised spectroscopically or by MS where no determination of the enantiocomposition was made.

[Φ]: *See* [M].

ψ: Specific ellipticity in CD measurement.

ω: Abbreviation for torsion angle in a conformation.

8 Graphical Representation of Organic Compounds

The effective communication of chemical structure is essential for all chemists. Over the years many different types of structure representation have been developed. Before the use of computers, chemists drew structures manually, often using a linear text notation. As more sophisticated methods for drawing have become available, the trend has been toward two-dimensional stick structures, such as the zigzag Natta projection (Figure 8.1).

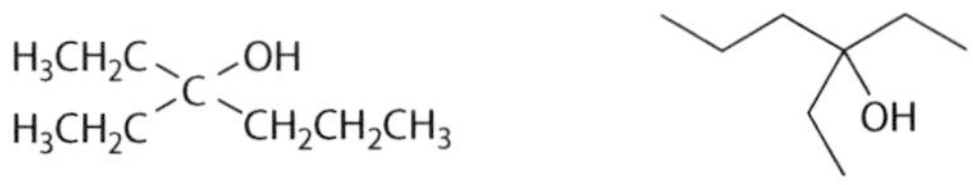

FIGURE 8.1 Linear text notation vs. Natta zigzag for 3-ethyl-3-hexanol.

There are no formal rules for the representation of chemical compounds, although a few special cases such as steroids and carbohydrates have evolved a preferred style. This chapter will outline the revised drawing conventions used in the *Combined Chemical Dictionary* (CCD) (see Section 1.2.1), which other chemists may wish to follow. (CCD diagrams have, however, been added continuously over a period of nearly thirty years. This description is of best current practice.) These rules, when followed, will result in a drawing style that is consistent and unambiguous to the reader.

The conventions adopted for CCD closely follow the International Union of Pure and Applied Chemistry (IUPAC) recommendations on graphical representation standards for chemical structure diagrams (*Pure Appl. Chem.*, 80, 227–410, 2008) and graphical representation of stereochemical configurations (*Pure Appl. Chem.*, 78, 1897–1970, 2006). Both of these publications are recommended reading for all chemists and can be downloaded via the IUPAC website.

8.1 ZIGZAG NATTA PROJECTION

For the majority of chemical structures, the Natta projection provides a clear and unambiguous representation of a compound. Generally speaking, all carbon and hydrogen atoms are implicit, with the exception of those that form part of a functional group such as a carboxylic acid (COOH) or aldehyde (CHO). The linear skeleton is drawn in the horizontal plane with numbering beginning from the right-hand side.

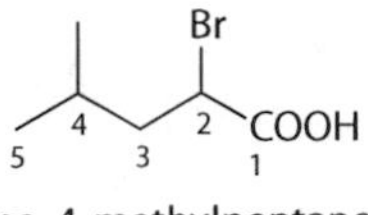

2-Bromo-4-methylpentanoic acid

In this representation the angle between bonds is 120°. Most chemical drawing packages have a chain drawing tool that will automatically draw the correct angle. For compounds containing carbon centres with four attached groups, the tetrahedral geometry is shown with the two nonhorizontal bonds separated by 60°.

159

8.1.1 Aromatic Compounds

For simple aromatic compounds the ring is orientated such that the 1 position is at the top or top right of the ring and numbered in a clockwise direction, again keeping the general horizontal layout.

8.1.2 Heterocyclic Compounds

In CCD, heterocyclic compounds are drawn with the heteroatom toward the bottom or bottom right and numbered counterclockwise. Many other information sources show the heteroatom at the top.

8.2 STEREOCHEMISTRY

Stereochemical configuration is shown with the use of solid wedge and hashed lines. There are some general rules used in CCD to avoid ambiguity:

- Wedge and dashed bonds are used as sparingly as possible to avoid confusion. The majority of tetrahedral centres require only one such bond to imply the stereochemistry of the centre.
- Bonds between adjacent stereocentres: Stereobonds between two stereocentres can be misinterpreted since it is not always clear to which chiral centre they refer. In such cases the stereobonds are drawn from the chiral atom to a nonchiral atom.

correct   correct   incorrect

- Re-entrant bonds: Similar ambiguity in stereochemical interpretation occurs when a stereobond is drawn inside the obtuse angle between two other bonds as opposed to the reflex angle.

correct   incorrect

Examples often occur in large ring systems, but it is often possible to redraw the ring to avoid a reentrant bond.

correct   *incorrect*

Using stereobonds to imply perspective: One exception to the rule above occurs when the stereo-centre is part of a bridged ring system. In this case the reentrant bonds are drawn using stereobonds since they are naturally pointing out of the plane of the paper, and the alternative results in ambiguous stereochemistry.

correct   *incorrect*

To avoid confusion, stereobonds should be drawn from the stereocentre when implying perspective whenever possible.

correct   *incorrect*

9 CAS Numbers, InChI, and Other Identifiers

See Gasteiger, J., and Engel, T., *Chemoinformatics* (Weinheim, Wiley/VCH, 2003) and Leach, A. R., and Gillet, V. J., *An Introduction to Chemoinformatics* (Dordrecht, Springer, 2007); other books are also available.

9.1 CAS REGISTRY NUMBERS

9.1.1 INTRODUCTION

Chemical Abstracts Service (CAS) developed the CAS Registry System in the early 1960s to provide a means for determining whether a chemical substance reported in the scientific literature had been indexed previously in *Chemical Abstracts*, and for retrieving the previously assigned index if it had been. Each unique chemical structure recorded in the system is assigned a permanent identifying number, the CAS registry number.

The registry number in itself has no chemical significance, but is simply a serial number assigned as a substance is entered into the registry system for the first time. The number has the format *NNNNNNN-NN-R*, where *R* is a check digit calculated by computer program from the other nine digits; by this means, errors in the transcription of registry numbers can be detected. Leading zeros are suppressed, so the first group of digits may contain fewer than seven digits.

The check digit for the registry number $N_8N_7N_6N_5N_4N_3\text{-}N_2N_1\text{-}R$ is derived from the formula below, where Q is an integer, which is discarded.

$$\frac{8N_8 + 7N_7 + 6N_6 + 5N_5 + 4N_4 + 3N_3 + 2N_2 + N_1}{10} = Q + \frac{R}{10}$$

9.1.2 SPECIFICITY

A substance is registered to the degree of structural detail given. This means that isomers, including stereoisomers, each receive their own registry number. Examples are shown below.

25167-67-3	Butene (isomer not specified
106-98-9	1-Butene
107-01-7	2-Butene (stereoisomer not specified)
624-64-6	(*E*)-2-Butene
590-18-1	(*Z*)-2-Butene
50-21-5	Lactic acid (stereochemistry unspecified)
598-82-3	(±)-Lactic acid (racemic mixture)
10326-41-7	(*S*)-Lactic acid
79-33-7	(*R*)-Lactic acid

Hydrates and salts receive their own registry numbers.

302-01-2	Hydrazine
7803-57-8	Hydrazine monohydrate
14011-37-1	Hydrazine hydrochloride
1184-66-3	Hydrazine sulfate

Labelled compounds receive their own registry numbers.

64-19-7	Acetic acid (unlabelled)
1112-02-3	Acetic-d_3 acid (D_3CCOOH)
1563-79-2	Acetic-l-^{13}C acid (H_3C^{13}COOH)

9.1.3 DUPLICATE REGISTRY NUMBERS

- CAS sometimes finds it necessary to register substances without full knowledge of their structures. Examples are trivially named natural products and trade name materials. This may lead to unintentional duplication in the registry system since the actual material may be indexed at another CA index name based on information from another literature source. Similar problems may arise when more than one structure is reported for the same chemical substance. When it is recognised that duplication has occurred and that a substance has been assigned two registry numbers, one of the numbers is retained as the preferred number, to which the other one is cross-referred.
- Certain substances are registered for non-CAS use, for example, substances registered under the provision of the U.S. Toxic Substances Control Act (TSCA), substances for the U.S. Adopted Names (USAN) Council of the U.S. Pharmacopeial Convention, and substances for the European Inventory of Existing Chemical Substances (EINECS).
- Others arise from the use of the registry system to support the preparation of index nomenclature. Thus, all parent ring systems are registered even when the parent compound has not been made. Also, all components of addition compounds, mixtures, or copolymers are registered and, occasionally, one of these components may not have been reported in the literature.

In addition to these unintended duplications, which should eventually be reconciled by CAS, there are many quasi-duplicates resulting from the liberal allocation of numbers.

9.1.4 REGISTRY NUMBERS WITH ASTERISKS

CAS, in registering substances for the preparation of CA indexes, assigns registry numbers only to substances that are described as unique chemical entities. However, through its activities in the preparation of the TSCA and EINECS inventories, CAS has assigned registry numbers to substances that are not treated as unique chemical entities in its regular CA index processing. Registry numbers assigned to substances of this type are identified by the presence of an asterisk following the number. Examples are:

Tallow (61789-97-7*)
Terphenyl, chlorinated (61788-33-8*)

These registry numbers are not found in CA Volume Indexes.

9.1.5 RACEMATES

Prior to the 14th Collective Index, registry numbers were assigned to the (+/–)-forms (racemic mixtures) of compounds with one chiral centre. From the 14th Collective Index onward these assignments have been dropped in favour of using the stereochemistry unspecified number. In cases where the (+/–)-number was earlier than the unspecified number, it replaces it as the unspecified number. Thus, DL-malic acid and malic acid (stereospecificity unspecified) now receive the same registry number and CA index name: 6915-15-7, butanedioic acid, hydroxy-. The registry number for the DL-form 617-48-1 will in the future be cross-referenced to the registry number of the nonstereospecific form 6915-15-7.

Racemates having more than one chiral center are indexed, registered, and named as having only relative stereochemistry. Thus, DL-threitol and threitol (absolute stereospecificity unspecified, but having two chiral centers with the same relative configuration) now receive the same CAS registry number and index name: 7493-90-5, 1,2,3,4-butanetetrol, ($R*,R*$)-. Again, the registry number for the DL-form will be cross-referenced to the registry number of the relative-only stereospecific form.

9.1.6 CHRONOLOGY

Originally the registry system covered substances mentioned in the chemical literature since January 1965, but in the period 1984–1986, CAS assigned registry numbers to substances indexed in the 6th (1957–1961) and 7th (1962–1966) Collective Indexes.

Because registry numbers are assigned sequentially, it is usually possible to tell from the magnitude of a number approximately when it was assigned. *Approximate* values for the highest CAS registry numbers to occur in each CAS Collective Index are shown as follows:

8CI (1967–1971)	35061-04-2
9CI (1972–1976)	61690-48-0
10CI (1977–1981)	80373-21-3
11CI (1982–1986)	106330-30-7
12CI (1987–1991)	138463-63-5
13CI (1992–1996)	183967-34-2
14CI (1997–2001)	259887-14-4
15CI (2002–2006)	915040-68-5

Thus, a substance with CAS registry number 66148-78-5 should appear for the first time in 10CI; certainly, it will not be found in 9CI. However, while the magnitude of the CAS number indicates when it was generated by CAS, a high number does not necessarily mean a compound new to science:

- It may be a compound from the old literature that has just been reported in the literature for the first time since 1967.
- It may be a number added retrospectively by CAS to compounds from various data collections. In the early years of the registry system, substances from a number of special data collections, such as the Colour Index, Merck Index, Lange's Handbook, and Pesticide Index, were added. Some of these substances may not have been reported subsequently.
- CAS has been working backwards through the literature assigning new registry numbers to substances not encountered in the previous work.
- It may be a duplicate for an existing compound.

Not all of the substances that have been registered have appeared in CA abstracts or indexes. Thus, it is quite possible to find a registry number that does not appear in any CA Substance Index.

More recently the letter *P* has been added to new registry numbers where the physical properties of the substance have been reported.

9.2 INCHI

These identifiers were developed as an IUPAC project in 2000–2004. They are the most recent technology aimed at an unambiguous text-string representation of chemical structures. (Earlier technologies included Wiswesser line notation, which is not described here, and SMILES, described below.)

InChI (pronounced "In-chee"; called IChI until 2004) stands for IUPAC International Chemical Identifier, and was developed to enable the easy linking of diverse data compilations, whether print or electronic. The name InChI™ is protected, but use and development of InChI identifiers is free access, and the source code and associated documentation can be downloaded for free from www.iupac.org/inchi. Source codes can be modified under the terms of a public licence, and IUPAC welcomes proposals for enhancements. Following beta-testing, the current version (1.02) is full release (January 2009).

The main advantages of InChI are stated as follows:

1. They are freely usable and nonproprietary.
2. They can be computed from structure information and do not have to be assigned by an organisation.
3. They can, with practice, be read to interpret the structure.

For example:

CH_3CH_2OH

ethanol

InChI = 1/C2H6O/c1-2-3/h3H,2H2,1H3

See also www.iupac.org/inchi for an extensive website on InChIs and wwmm.ch.cam.ac.uk/inchifaq for a FAQ website..

9.3   SIMPLIFIED MOLECULAR INPUT LINE ENTRY SYSTEM (SMILES)

SMILES is a line notation developed in the 1980s and since modified and extended by others, particularly Daylight Chemical Information Systems, Inc.

See Weininger, D., *J. Chem. Inf. Comput. Sci.*, 28, 31–36, 1988; 29, 97–101, 1989.

Using simple rules, a structure is represented by a string of characters unique to that structure. It can also be used to specify stereochemistry at double bonds and chiral centres. SMARTS is a further extension that allows substructure searching.

For example:

CC(=O)O	Acetic acid
c1ccccc1	Benzene
C1CCCCC1	Cyclohexane
CCN(CC)CC	Triethylamine
F/C==C\F	Z-Difluoro ethane
F/C=C/F	E-Difluoroethene

SMILES strings may be converted back to two-dimensional structures using structure diagram generation programs, of which there are several on the market.

See Helson, H. E., Structure diagram generation, in *Reviews in Computational Chemistry*, ed. K. B. Lipkowitz and D. B. Boyd (New York: Wiley-VCH, 1999), pp. 313–398.

SMILES was designed, however, such that it could be written or read without the use of a computer. Its advantage is that it is easier to interpret in this way than InChI.

10 Molecular Formulae

10.1 THE HILL SYSTEM

In most publications, including *Chemical Abstracts* and Beilstein, molecular formulae are given in Hill system order. For organic compounds, the order is C first, then H, and then the remaining element symbols alphabetically. For compounds that do not contain carbon, the element symbols are ordered alphabetically (see Hill, E. A., *J. Am. Chem. Soc.,* 22, 478–490, 1900).

Although the Hill system is now used almost exclusively, other systems have been used in the past. For example, the early formula indexes to Beilstein used the Richter system, in which the elements are cited in the order C, H, O, N, Cl, Br, I, F, S, P.

10.2 CHEMICAL ABSTRACTS CONVENTIONS

Users of *Chemical Abstracts* may occasionally have difficulty in locating certain types of compounds. For example, sodium acetate will not be found under $C_2H_3NaO_2$; it appears under $C_2H_4O_2$, which is the formula of the parent acid (acetic acid). The conventions that *Chemical Abstracts* uses include the following:

- Metal salts of acids, alcohols, and amines are indexed at the molecular formulae of the parent acids, alcohols, and amines. Thus, sodium ethoxide appears under C_2H_6O (ethanol) and not under C_2H_5NaO.
- Acid salts of amines (and other basic parents) are indexed at the molecular formulae of the amines. Thus, methanamine hydrochloride appears under CH_5N (methanamine) and not under CH_6ClN.
- Counterions of *-onium* compounds are not included in the formula heading. Thus, 1-methylpyridinium chloride appears under C_6H_8N (1-methylpyridinium) and not under C_6H_8ClN.
- Molecular addition compounds are indexed under the formulae of their components (except that entries are not made for a few common components). Thus, the 1:1 addition compound of ethanol with sulfinylbis(methane) (dimethyl sulfoxide (DMSO)) appears at C_2H_6O (ethanol) and at C_2H_6OS (sulfinylbismethane) and not at $C_4H_{12}O_2S$.

10.3 CHECKING MOLECULAR FORMULAE

When working out the molecular formula of a neutral organic compound, it is useful to remember that there must be an even number of odd-valent atoms (e.g., H, halogens, N, P). Thus, the formula $C_{27}H_{45}O$ is obviously incorrect unless it is a radical.

A more sophisticated check on the accuracy of a formula is to calculate the number of rings/ double bonds in the compound from the formula. You can then count the number of rings and double bonds and compare it with the results of the calculation.

If H = number of univalent atoms (H, halogen), N = number of trivalent atoms (N, P), and C = number of tetravalent atoms, then

$$\text{Number of rings/double bonds} = \tfrac{1}{2}(2C - H + N) + 1$$

For example, consider the following:

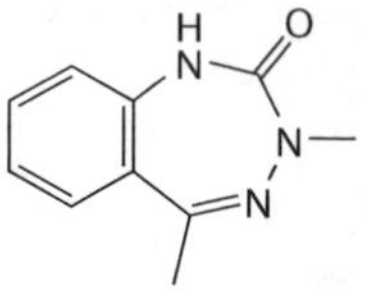

The following rapid method can be used to check the hydrogen count in a structure without using a computer, for example:

Formula $C_{10}H_{11}N_3O$.
Number of C atoms × 2 = 20.
Deduct 2 for each ring apart from the first (minus 2) and 2 for each double bond (including C=O) (minus 10), leaves 8.
Add 1 for each N, gives 11.

Note the following:

- The number of divalent atoms (O,S) does not affect the calculation. These must be checked by inspection.
- Triple bonds, including cyano, count as two doubles (subtract 4).
- Do not forget to count every ring, e.g., in a bicyclic structure.

11 Chemical Hazard Information for the Laboratory

Rupert Purchase

Two types of hazards are associated with the use of chemicals—hazards that are a direct result of the physical and reactive properties of a chemical, and health hazards resulting from the biological properties. This chapter summarises hazards that are associated with working with chemicals in a laboratory, and highlights some sources of hazard information for carrying out hazard and risk assessments.

Lack of hazard information does not mean that the consequences of handling a chemical can be disregarded. Any chemical has the capacity for harm if it is carelessly used, and for many newly synthesised materials (e.g., new synthetic reagents), hazardous properties may not be apparent or may not have been cited in the literature. The toxicity of some very reactive chemicals may not have been evaluated because of ethical considerations.

Good laboratory and manufacturing practices are encoded in national and international health and safety legislation, and place emphasis on the key attitudes to be adopted when working with chemical substances (or mixtures). Although the exact regulatory details may differ from country to country, the essential aims of national health and safety legislation relating to the handling of chemicals in laboratories (and in the workplace in general) are the same and emphasise the importance of *hazard information*:

- Identify the risks of handling hazardous substances and inform employees.
- Prevent, minimise, or control exposure.
- Ensure that control measures are correctly used and maintained, and that personal protection equipment is available.
- Monitor exposure in the workplace and comply with national occupational exposure limits.
- Provide information, training, and instruction of the risks involved.
- Keep records of risk assessments, records of the maintenance and testing of engineering controls, and occupational health records.

11.1 HAZARD AND RISK ASSESSMENT

11.1.1 DEFINITIONS

Hazard is the set of *inherent properties* of a chemical substance that make it capable of causing adverse effects in people or the environment when a particular degree of exposure occurs. *Risk* is the predicted or actual *frequency of occurrence of an adverse effect* of a chemical substance from a given exposure to humans or the environment.

Risk assessment therefore requires knowledge of both the hazard of a chemical and the purpose for which it is being used. A highly hazardous substance presents a very low risk if it is securely contained with no likely exposure. Conversely, a substance of relatively low hazard may present unacceptable risks if extensive exposure can occur. Both hazard and exposure must be considered before the risk can be adequately assessed.

11.1.2 LEGISLATION

In the UK the *Control of Substances Hazardous to Health (COSHH) Regulations 2002* oblige laboratory managers and supervisors (and employers in general) to assess the risks to health from hazardous substances used in or created by workplace activities.

The *Chemicals (Hazard Information and Packaging for Supply) (CHIP) Regulations 2009* require manufacturers and suppliers to provide users with information about hazards and health risks by labelling their products with relevant hazard information and by issuing Material Safety Data Sheets.

Other relevant legislation is the *Health and Safety at Work Act 1974*, the *Management of Health and Safety at Work Regulations 1999*, and the *Ionising Radiation Regulations 1999*.

For information on all of these, see http://www.opsi.gov.uk/stat. UK health and safety legislation is subject to amendments, updates, and harmonisation with internationally agreed health and safety directives.

11.1.3 WORKPLACE EXPOSURE LIMITS

Workplace exposure limits (WELs) were adopted in the UK in 2005 to replace maximum exposure limits (MELs) and occupational exposure standards (OESs). Workplace exposure limits—long-term exposure limits (eight-hour time-weighted average exposures) and short-term exposure limits (fifteen-minute time-weighted average exposures)—are set by the Health and Safety Executive (HSE) and published in document EH40 (http://www.hse.gov.uk/coshh/table1.pdf).

Recommendations for controlling and monitoring substances assigned WELs are part of the COSHH Regulations 2002. Exposure limits are also set by other regulatory and advisory bodies, e.g., threshold limit values (TLVs) by the American Conference of Governmental Industrial Hygienists (ACGIH) and Maximale Arbeitsplatzkonzentrationen (MAK) by German authorities. In EH40, the route of exposure is mainly by inhalation, but exposure limits are also assigned to some substances that are easily absorbed by the skin or are skin sensitizers.

11.2 PHYSICAL AND REACTIVE CHEMICAL HAZARDS

Chemicals that present a particular hazard in the laboratory as a result of their physical and reactive properties include the following categories, identified for the purposes of risk assessment and for product labelling in UK and European Union (EU) health and safety regulations:

- Flammable chemicals (Section 11.7)
- Pressurized gases
- Shock-sensitive explosive chemicals (Table 11.1)
- Water-reactive chemicals (Table 11.2)
- Pyrophoric chemicals (Table 11.3)
- Peroxide-forming chemicals (Tables 11.11 and 11.12)
- Oxidants (and reductants)
- Strong acids (and strong bases)

Additionally, the incompatibility of many of these groups of chemicals presents further hazards in experimental work, and for their safe storage and disposal.

11.3 HEALTH HAZARDS

The following groups of chemicals present health hazards for laboratory workers and others in the working environment, and are differentiated for the purposes of risk assessment and for product labelling in UK and EU health and safety regulations:

TABLE 11.1
Some Shock-Sensitive Compounds

Acetylenic compounds, especially polyacetylenes, haloacetylenes, and heavy metal salts of acetylenes (copper, silver, and mercury salts are particularly sensitive)

Acyl nitrates

Alkyl and acyl nitrites

Alkyl chlorates

Alkyl nitrates, particularly polyol nitrates such as nitrocellulose and nitroglycerine

Amine metal oxosalts: metal compounds with coordinated ammonia, hydrazine, or similar nitrogenous donors and ionic chlorate(VII), nitrate(V), manganate(VII), or other oxidizing group

Azides, including metal, nonmetal, and organic azides

Chlorate(III) salts of metals

Chlorate(VII) salts: most metal, nonmetal, amine, and organic cation chlorates(VII) can be detonated or undergo violent reaction in contact with combustible materials

Diazo compounds such as CH_2N_2

Diazonium salts, when dry

Fulminates

Hydrogen peroxide becomes increasingly treacherous as the concentration rises above 30%, forming explosive mixtures with organic materials and decomposing violently in the presence of traces of transition metals

N-Halogen compounds such as difluoroamino compounds and halogen azides

N-Nitro compounds such as N-nitromethylamine, nitrourea, nitroguanidine, and nitric amide

Oxo salts of nitrogenous bases: chlorates(VII), dichromates(VI), nitrates(V), iodates(V), chlorates(III), chlorates(V), and manganates(VII) of ammonia, amines, hydroxylamine, guanidine, etc.

Peroxides and hydroperoxides, organic

Peroxides (solid) that crystallize from or are left from evaporation of peroxidizable solvents

Peroxides, transition metal salts

Picrates, especially salts of transition and heavy metals, such as Ni, Pb, Hg, Cu, and Zn; picric acid is explosive but is less sensitive to shock or friction than its metal salts and is relatively safe as a water-wet paste

Polynitroalkyl compounds such as tetranitromethane and dinitroacetonitrile

Polynitroaromatic compounds, especially polynitro hydrocarbons, phenols, and amines

Source: Reproduced with permission from IUPAC-IPCS, *Chemical Safety Matters* (Cambridge: Cambridge University Press, 1992).

- Human carcinogens and probable human carcinogens according to the International Agency for Research on Cancer (IARC) classifications (*IARC Monographs on the Evaluation of Carcinogenic Risks to Humans: Overall Evaluations of Carcinogenicity: An Updating of IARC Monographs Volumes 1 to 42*, Suppl. 7 (Lyon: IARC, 1987); available online)
- Human teratogens and chemicals that have an effect on human reproduction
- Chemicals that are irritants to the skin, eyes, and respiratory system (data from human exposure or animal tests)
- Chemicals that are corrosive to the skin, eyes, and respiratory system (data from human exposure or animal tests)
- Skin sensitizers
- Chemicals with known target organ toxicity or toxicity due to a specific pharmacological mechanism
- Mutagenic chemicals
- Chemicals classified as very toxic or extremely toxic on the basis of acute toxicity data

TABLE 11.2
Some Water-Reactive Chemicals

Alkali metals
Alkali metal hydrides
Alkali metal amides
Metal alkyls
Grignard reagents
Halides of nonmetals, e.g., BCl_3, BF_3, PCl_3, PCl_5, $SiCl_4$, S_2Cl_2
Inorganic acid halides, e.g., $POCl_3$, $SOCl_2$, SO_2Cl_2
Anhydrous metal halides
Phosphorus(V) oxide
Calcium carbide
Organic acid halides and anhydrides of low molecular weight

Source: Reproduced with permission from IUPAC-IPCS, *Chemical Safety Matters* (Cambridge: Cambridge University Press, 1992).

TABLE 11.3
A Partial List of Pyrophoric Chemicals

Grignard reagents RMgX
Metal alkyls and aryls, e.g., RLi, RNa, R_3Al, R_2Zn
Metal carbonyls
Alkali metals, e.g., Na, K
Metal powders, e.g., Al, Co, Fe, Mg, Mn, Pd, Pt, Sn, Ti, Zn, Zr
Metal hydrides, e.g., NaH, $LiAlH_4$
Nonmetal hydrides, e.g., B_2H_6 and other boranes, PH_3, AsH_3
Nonmetal alkyls, e.g., R_3B, R_3P, R_3As
Phosphorus (white)

Source: Reproduced with permission from IUPAC-IPCS, *Chemical Safety Matters* (Cambridge: Cambridge University Press, 1992).

The toxicological criteria that are used for these classifications are described by Bender, H. F., et al., *Hazardous Chemicals: Control and Regulation in the European Market* (Weinheim: Wiley-VCH, 2007).

The health and other hazards associated with solvents are described in Section 11.7.

11.4   HANDLING AND STORAGE OF CHEMICALS

Hazard data influence the way a chemical should be handled, contained, stored, and ultimately discarded. The safe storage of chemicals requires planning and an appreciation of those chemicals that are incompatible (see Section 11.5). Chemical storage is briefly reviewed in *Chemical Safety Matters*, IUPAC-IPCS, Cambridge University Press, Cambridge, 1992, and a longer account (with a mainly North American regulatory perspective) is given in *Safe Storage of Laboratory Chemicals*, 2nd edn, ed. D.A. Pipitone, Wiley, New York, 1991.

Chemical Safety Matters also provides useful advice on the precautions to be taken when handling those chemicals that present special problems in a laboratory, e.g., substances that have a high acute toxicity or are known to be human carcinogens or can cause other chronic toxic effects. A more detailed appraisal of the problems of handling carcinogens may be found in *Safe Handling of Chemical Carcinogens, Mutagens, Teratogens and Highly Toxic Substances*, Vols. 1 and 2, ed. D.B. Walters, Ann Arbor Science, Michigan, 1980, and in Castegnaro, M. et al., *Chemical Carcinogens: Some Guidelines for Handling and Disposal in the Laboratory*, Springer, Berlin, 1986.

Awareness of very reactive chemicals is essential. Advice on handling highly flammable and/or potentially explosive reagents is provided in the IUPAC-IPCS book *Chemical Safety Matters*, and the properties of many common but hazardous laboratory chemicals are succinctly summarised in the 'yellow pages' section of *Hazards in the Chemical Laboratory*, 5th edn., ed. S.G. Luxon, Royal Society of Chemistry, Cambridge, 1992. One particular explosive hazard, peroxide-forming chemicals, is described in more detail in Section 11.8.

11.4.1 GASES

Handling gases poses special problems for laboratory personnel, from the correct way to store, transport, and use compressed gas cylinders to the dangers from water being sucked back into the cylinders of hydrolysable gases. *Chemical Safety Matters* provides sound practical advice on using gases. *Hazards in the Chemical Laboratory* contains summaries of the hazardous and toxic properties of commonly used laboratory gases. See also Yaws, C. L., *Matheson Gas Data Book*, 7th ed. (Matheson Tri-Gas, NJ: McGraw-Hill, 2001); *Effects of Exposure to Toxic Gases—First Aid and Medical Treatment,* 3rd ed., ed. F. Scornavacca et al. (Secausus, NJ: Matheson Gas Products, 1988). The use of liquefied gases presents additional hazards, e.g., the use and disposal of liquid nitrogen, which can be contaminated with liquid oxygen.

11.5 HAZARDOUS REACTION MIXTURES

The potential for chemicals to interact in a violent and uncontrolled manner should be foremost in the mind of everyone concerned with the planning and execution of chemical operations. Not only can syntheses and purifications go disastrously wrong if the elementary principles of chemistry are overlooked, but the inadequate storage of incompatible chemicals has led to many a gutted and blackened factory, warehouse and laboratory.

Luckily for the laboratory chemist, many of these mishaps of yesteryear have been collated, most notably (and authoritatively) by Leslie Bretherick. *Bretherick's Handbook of Reactive Chemical Hazards*, which by 2006 had reached its 7th edition, details the predictable and the unexpected from the literature of reactive chemical hazards. In a review, published in *Hazards in the Chemical Laboratory*, 5th edn, ed. S.G. Luxon, Royal Society of Chemistry, Cambridge, 1992, Bretherick has also summarised some frequently encountered incompatible chemicals that present either a reactive hazard or a toxic hazard if combined. These two lists are reprinted here as Tables 11.4 and 11.5 by kind permission of the Royal Society of Chemistry. In addition, potentially explosive combinations of some commonly-encountered laboratory reagents are shown in Table 11.6 (reproduced with permission from *Chemical Safety Matters*, IUPAC-IPCS, Cambridge University Press, Cambridge, 1992).

11.6 DISPOSAL OF CHEMICALS

Careful disposal is required in three commonly encountered situations in laboratories:

- The containment of accidental spillages of chemicals
- The disposal of residues from syntheses in which organometallic reagents were used (toxic, pyrophoric, water reactive, and flammable hazards)
- The disposal of column chromatographic materials and any absorbed residues (toxic, particulate, and flammable hazards)

TABLE 11.4
A Partial List of Incompatible Chemicals—Reactive Hazards

Substances in the left-hand column should be stored and handled so that they cannot possibly accidentally contact corresponding substances in the right-hand column under uncontrolled conditions, when violent reactions may occur.

Acetic acid	Chromic acid, nitric acid, peroxides, and permanganates
Acetic anhydride	Hydroxyl-containing compounds, ethylene glycol, perchloric acid
Acetone	Concentrated nitric and sulfuric acid mixtures, hydrogen peroxide
Acetylene	Chlorine, bromine, copper, silver, fluorine, and mercury
Alkali and alkaline-earth metals, such as sodium, potassium, lithium, magnesium, calcium	Carbon dioxide, carbon tetrachloride, and other chlorinated hydrocarbons (also prohibit water, foam, and dry chemicals on fires involving these metals—dry sand should be available)
Aluminium powder	Halogenated or oxygenated solvents
Ammonia, anhydrous	Mercury, chlorine, calcium hypochlorite, iodine, bromine, and hydrogen fluoride
Ammonium nitrate	Acids, metals powder, flammable liquids, chlorates, nitrites, sulphur, finely divided organics or combustibles
Aniline	Nitric acid, hydrogen peroxide
Bromine	Ammonia, acetylene, butadiene, butane and other petroleum gases, sodium carbide, turpentine, benzene, and finely divided metals
Calcium oxide	Water
Carbon activated	Calcium hypochlorite, other oxidants
Chlorates	Ammonium salts, acids, metal powders, phosphorus, sulfur, finely divided organics or combustibles
Chromic acid and chromium trioxide	Acetic acid, naphthalene, camphor, glycerol, turpentine, alcohol, and other flammable liquids
Chlorine	Ammonia, acetylene, butadiene, butane, other petroleum gases, hydrogen, sodium carbide, turpentine, benzene, and finely divided metals
Chlorine dioxide	Ammonia, methane, phosphine, and hydrogen sulfide
Copper	Acetylene, hydrogen peroxide
Fluorine	Isolate from everything
Hydrazine	Hydrogen peroxide, nitric acid, any other oxidant, heavy metal salts
Hydrocarbons (benzene, butane, propane, gasoline, turpentine, etc.)	Fluorine, chlorine, bromine, chromic acid, concentrated nitric acid, peroxides
Hydrogen cyanide	Nitric acid, alkalis
Hydrogen fluoride	Ammonia, aqueous or anhydrous
Hydrogen peroxide	Copper, chromium, iron, most metals or their salts, any flammable liquid, combustible materials, aniline, nitromethane
Hydrogen sulfide	Fuming nitric acid, oxidising gases
Iodine	Acetylene, ammonia (anhydrous or aqueous)
Mercury	Acetylene, fulminic acid,[a] ammonia
Nitric acid (concentrated)	Acetic acid, acetone, alcohol, aniline, chromic acid, hydrogen cyanide, hydrogen sulfide, flammable liquids, flammable gases, nitratable substances, fats, grease
Nitromethane, lower nitroalkanes	Inorganic bases, amine, halogens, 13X molecular sieve
Oxalic acid	Silver, mercury, urea
Oxygen	Oils, grease, hydrogen, flammable liquids, solids, or gases
Perchloric acid	Acetic anhydride, bismuth and its alloys, alcohol, paper, wood, grease, oils, dehydrating agents
Peroxides, organic	Acids (organic or mineral, avoid friction, store cold)

TABLE 11.4 (continued)
A Partial List of Incompatible Chemicals—Reactive Hazards

Phosphinates	Any oxidant
Phosphorous (white)	Air, oxygen
Potassium chlorate	Acids (see also chlorates)
Potassium perchlorate	Acids (see also perchloric acid)
Potassium permanganate	Glycerol, ethylene glycol, benzaldehyde, sulfuric acid
Silver	Acetylene, oxalic acid, tartaric acid, fulminic acid,[a] ammonium compounds
Sodium	See alkali metals (above)
Sodium nitrite	Ammonium nitrate and other ammonium salts
Sodium peroxide	Any oxidisable substrate, such as ethanol, methanol, glacial acetic acid, acetic anhydride, benzaldehyde, carbon disulfide, glycerol, glycerol, ethylene glycol, ethyl acetate, methyl acetate, and furfural
Sulfuric acid	Chlorates, perchlorates, permanganates
Thiocyanates	Metal nitrates, nitrites, oxidants
Trifluoromethanesulfonic acid	Perchlorate salts

Source: Reproduced with permission from L. Bretherick, *Hazards in the Chemical Laboratory*, ed. S.G. Luxon (Cambridge: Royal Society of Chemistry, 1992).

[a] Produced in nitric acid–ethanol mixtures.

TABLE 11.5
A Partial List of Incompatible Chemicals—Toxic Hazards

Substances in the left-hand column should be stored and handled so that they cannot possibly accidentally contact corresponding substances in the centre column, because toxic materials (right-hand column) would be produced.

Arsenical materials	Any reducing agent[a]	Arsine
Azides	Acids	Hydrogen azide
Cyanides	Acids	Hydrogen cyanide
Hypochlorites	Acids	Chlorine or hypochlorous acid
Nitrates	Sulfuric acid	Nitrogen dioxide
Nitric acid	Copper, brass, any heavy metals	Nitrogen dioxide (nitrous fumes)
Nitrites	Acids	Nitrous fumes
Phosphorus	Caustic alkalis or reducing agents	Phosphine
Selenides	Reducing agents	Hydrogen selenide
Sulfides	Acids	Hydrogen sulfide
Tellurides	Reducing agents	Hydrogen telluride

Source: Reproduced with permission from L. Bretherick, *Hazards in the Chemical Laboratory*, ed. S.G. Luxon (Cambridge: Royal Society of Chemistry, 1992).

[a] Arsine has been produced by putting an arsenical alloy into a wet galvanized bucket.

TABLE 11.6
Potentially Explosive Combinations of Some Common Reagents

Acetone with chloroform in the presence of base

Acetylene with copper, silver, mercury, or their salts

Ammonia (including aqueous solutions) with Cl_2, Br_2, or I_2

Carbon disulfide with sodium azide

Chlorine with an alcohol

Chloroform or carbon tetrachloride with powdered Al or Mg

Decolorizing carbon with an oxidizing agent

Diethyl ether with chlorine (including a chlorine atmosphere)

Dimethyl sulfoxide with an acyl halide, $SOCl_2$, or $POCl_3$ or with CrO_3

Ethanol with calcium chlorate or silver nitrate

Nitric acid with acetic anhydride or acetic acid

Picric acid with a heavy metal salt, such as of Pb, Hg, or Ag

Silver oxide with ammonia with ethanol

Sodium with a chlorinated hydrocarbon

Sodium chlorate with an amine

Source: Reproduced with permission from IUPAC-IPCS, *Chemical Safety Matters* (Cambridge: Cambridge University Press, 1992).

An account of the safe disposal of laboratory chemicals is given in Pitt, M. J., et al., *Handbook of Laboratory Waste Disposal* (Chichester: Ellis Horwood, 1985). Detailed experimental procedures have been published on how to convert particularly reactive and toxic substances into less harmful products before their disposal; see, for example, *Hazardous Laboratory Chemicals Disposal Guide*, 3rd ed., ed. M.-A. Armour (Boca Raton, FL: CRC Press, 2003). *Destruction of Hazardous Chemicals in the Laboratory,* 2nd ed., ed. G. Lunn et al. (New York: Wiley, 1994) contains methods for the degradation and disposal of the following chemicals:

Acid halides and anhydrides

Aflatoxins

Alkali and alkaline-earth metals

Alkali-metal alkoxides

Antineoplastic alkylating agents

Aromatic amines

Azides

Azo and azoxy compounds and tetrazenes

Biological stains

Boron trifluoride and inorganic fluorides

Butyllithium

Calcium carbide

Carbamic acid esters

Chloromethylsilanes and silicon tetrachloride

N-Chlorosuccinimide

Chlorosulfonic acid

Cr(VI)

Cisplatin

Citrinin

Complex metal hydrides

Cyanides and cyanogen bromide

Cycloserine

Dichloromethotrexate, vincristine, and vinblastin

Diisopropyl fluorophosphate

Dimethyl sulfate and related compounds

Doxorubicin and daunorubicin

Drugs containing hydrazine and triazene groups

Ethidium bromide

Haloethers

Halogenated compounds

Halogens

Heavy metals

Hexamethylphosphoramide

Hydrazines

Hypochlorites

Mercury

Methotrexate

2-Methylaziridine

l-Methyl-4-phenyl-l,2,3,6-tetrahydro-
   pyridine (MPTP)

Mitomycin C

4-Nitrophenol

N-Nitrosamines and *N*-nitrosamides

Nitrosourea drugs

Ochratoxin A

Organic nitriles

OsO_4

Patulin

Peracids

Peroxides and hydroperoxides

Phosgene

Phosphorus and P_4O_{10}

Picric acid

Polycyclic aromatic and heterocyclic
   hydrocarbons

$KMnO_4$

β-Propiolactone

Protease inhibitors

$NaNH_2$

Sterigmatocystin

Sulfonyl fluoride enzyme inhibitors

6-Thioguanine and 6-mercaptopurine

Uranyl compounds

Methods for the conversion of the major classes of chemical carcinogens into nonmutagenic residues are also described by Castegnaro, M., et al., *Chemical Carcinogens: Some Guidelines for Handling and Disposal in the Laboratory* (Berlin: Springer, 1986).

Disposal methods for some of the more common classes of organic compounds may be found in *Chemical Safety Matters* (hydrocarbons; halogenated hydrocarbons; alcohols and phenols; ethers, thiols, and organosulfur compounds; carboxylic acids and derivatives; aldehydes; ketones; amines; nitro and nitroso compounds; and peroxides).

11.7   SOLVENTS

Solvents are *fire and health hazards*, and caution is necessary when using these substances in a laboratory environment. The flammable properties and *flammability classifications* of many solvents impose restrictions on their handling and storage. Particular concerns are vapour leaks of solvents as sources of ignition, and the inappropriate storage of Winchester bottles containing solvents (especially if exposed to sunlight, which can result in peroxidation) in laboratories. The peroxidation of solvents during storage as a reactive hazard is described in more detail in Section 11.8. Both acute and chronic low-level exposures contribute to the recognised health hazards of solvents.

11.7.1   FLAMMABILITY CLASSIFICATIONS

Flammability classifications of solvents (and other chemicals) are based on flash point (fl.p.) measurements. Flash point is the lowest temperature at which a liquid has sufficient vapour pressure to form an ignitable mixture with air near the surface of the liquid. The following criteria currently apply (CHIP Regulations 2009):

Extremely flammable: liquids with fl.p. < 0°C and Bp ≤ 35°C
Highly flammable: fl.p. ≥ 0°C and < 21°C
Flammable: fl.p. ≥ 21°C and < 55°C

Substances with fl.p. > 55°C should be regarded as combustible if brought to a high temperature.

By 2015 the United Nations Globally Harmonized System of Classification and Labelling of Chemicals (GHS) will replace these categories. The GHS system divides flammable liquids into four new categories:

Category 1: fl.p. < 23°C and initial Bp ≤ 35°C
Category 2: fl.p. < 23°C and initial Bp > 35°C
Category 3: fl.p. ≥ 23°C and ≤ 60°C
Category 4: fl.p. > 60°C and ≤ 93°C

Flammable substances used and stored in the laboratory are also subject to further risk assessment and control in UK law under the the Health and Safety at Work Act 1974, the Management of Health and Safety at Work Regulations 1999, the COSHH Regulations 2002, the Dangerous Substances and Explosive Atmospheres Regulations 2002 (DSEAR), and the Regulatory Reform (Fire Safety) Order 2005.

Flammability classifications for a selection of solvents (and some other substances) are given in Table 11.7. The chemicals are listed in order of increasing boiling point to the nearest 1°C. Solvents in Table 11.7 that are also peroxidation hazards may be identified from data in Tables 11.11 and 11.12.

11.7.2 HEALTH HAZARDS

Apart from the acute toxic effects of high concentrations of the more volatile solvents, there are health hazards from the long-term (chronic) exposure to low levels of solvents. *Reproductive effects* that are associated with chronic exposure to some solvents used in laboratories are shown in Table 11.8. Evidence from animal studies suggests there are reproductive hazards from handling other solvents. For example:

- 2-Ethoxyethanol and 2-butanone are teratogenic (in animal models).
- Dichloromethane, styrene, 1,1,1-trichloroethane, tetrachloroethylene, and xylene isomers have foetotoxic properties (in animal models).

The IARC classifications for the *carcinogenic risk* from exposure to some laboratory solvents (and other selected reagents) are summarised in Table 11.9. *Other toxic effects* for classes of solvents categorised by functional group are given in Table 11.10.

Solvents that are currently assigned a workplace exposure limit (eight-hour long-term exposure limit) that is less than or equal to 100 ppm are marked in Table 11.7 with an arrowhead (▶) (data from EH40/2005).

11.8 PEROXIDE-FORMING CHEMICALS

Peroxide-forming solvents and reagents should be dated at the time they are first opened, and should be either discarded or tested for peroxides within a fixed period of time after their first use. Peroxides can be detected with NaI/AcOH, though dialkyl peroxides may need treatment with concentrated HCl or 50% H_2SO_4 before detection with iodide is possible. A commercially available test paper, which contains a peroxidase, can detect hydroperoxides and dialkyl peroxides, as well as oxidizing anions, in organic and aqueous solvents.

The types of structures that have been identified as likely to produce peroxides are listed in Table 11.11, and some common peroxidisable chemicals are given in Table 11.12.

Hydroperoxides, but not dialkyl peroxides, can be removed from peroxide-forming solvents by passage through basic activated alumina, by treatment with a self-indicating activated molecular sieve (type 4A) under nitrogen, or by treatment with Fe^{2+}/H^+, CuCl, or other reductants.

The following references provide further information:

Detection and removal of peroxides from solvents: *Organic Solvents: Physical Properties and Methods of Purification,* 4th ed., ed. J. A. Riddick et al. (Chichester: Wiley, 1986).
Deperoxidation of ethers with molecular sieves: Burfield, D. R., *J. Org. Chem.,* 47, 3821–3824, 1982.
Determination of organic peroxides: Mair, R. D., et al., in *Treatise on Analytical Chemistry,* ed. I. M. Kolthoff et al., Vol. 14, Part II (New York: Interscience, 1971), p. 295.

TABLE 11.7
Fire Hazards of Some Common Laboratory Solvents and Other Substances

Bp (°C)	Mp (°C)	Name[a]	Flash Point (°C)[b]	Flammability Classification[c]
30–60		Petrol[d]		Extremely flammable
30	−161	2-Methylbutane	<−51	Extremely flammable
32	−99	Methyl formate	<−19	Extremely flammable
35	−116	► Diethyl ether	−45	Extremely flammable
36	−129	Pentane	−49	Extremely flammable
38	−98	Dimethyl sulfide	−34	Highly flammable
40	−97	► Dichloromethane		Concentrated 12–19% in air, flammable
46	−112	► Carbon disulfide	−30	Extremely flammable
46	−14	1,1,1-Trichloro-2,2,2-trifluoroethane		Nonflammable
47	−111	1,2-Dibromo-1,1,2,2-tetrafluoroethane		Nonflammable
50	−94	Cyclopentane	−37	Extremely flammable
54	−109	► 2-Methoxy-2-methylpropane	−28	Highly flammable
56	−94	Acetone	−17	Highly flammable
56	−98	Methyl acetate	−9	Highly flammable
61	−63	► Chloroform		Nonflammable
65	−108	► Tetrahydrofuran	−14	Highly flammable
65	−98	Methanol	10	Highly flammable
69	−87	Diisopropyl ether	−28	Highly flammable
69	−94	► Hexane	−23	Highly flammable
72	−15	Trifluoroacetic acid		Nonflammable
74	−32	► 1,1,1-Trichloroethane		Nonflammable
75	−95	1,3-Dioxolane	2 (oc)	Highly flammable
77	−84	Ethyl acetate	−4	Highly flammable
77	−21	► Carbon tetrachloride		Nonflammable
78	−117	Ethanol	12	Highly flammable
78	−123	1-Chlorobutane	−12	Highly flammable
80	−86	2-Butanone	−1	Highly flammable
80	6	► Benzene	−11	Highly flammable
81	6	► Cyclohexane	−20	Highly flammable
82	−45	► Acetonitrile	6 (oc)	Highly flammable
82	−90	2-Propanol	12	Highly flammable
83	26	2-Methyl-2-propanol	11	Highly flammable
84	−35	► 1,2-Dichloroethane	13	Highly flammable
85	−58	1,2-Dimethoxyethane	1	Highly flammable
87	−85	► Trichloroethylene		Nonflammable
88	−45	Tetrahydropyran	−20	Highly flammable
97	−127	1-Propanol	15	Highly flammable
98	−92	Heptane	−4	Highly flammable
99	−108	2,2,4-Trimethylpentane	−12	Highly flammable
100	−115	► 2-Butanol	24	Highly flammable
100	0	Water		Nonflammable
101	11	► 1,4-Dioxane	11	Highly flammable
101	−127	Methylcyclohexane	−4	Highly flammable
101	−29	► Nitromethane	35	Flammable

(continued on next page)

TABLE 11.7 (continued)
Fire Hazards of Some Common Laboratory Solvents and Other Substances

Bp (°C)	Mp (°C)	Name[a]	Flash Point (°C)[b]	Flammability Classification[c]
101	8	► Formic acid	69	
102	−42	3-Pentanone	13	Highly flammable
103	15	Trimethyl orthoformate	15	Highly flammable
104	−6	Bromotrichloromethane		Nonflammable
108	−108	2-Methyl-1-propanol	28	Flammable
111	−95	► Toluene	4	Highly flammable
114	−36	► 1,1,2-Trichloroethane		Nonflammable
116	−42	► Pyridine	20	Flammable
117	−80	► 4-Methyl-2-pentanone	17	Highly flammable
118	−90	1-Butanol	29	Flammable
118	17	Acetic acid	39	Flammable
121	−19	► Tetrachloroethylene		Nonflammable
125	−86	► 2-Methoxyethanol	43	Flammable
126	−77	Butyl acetate	22	Flammable
126	−57	Octane	13	Highly flammable
132	−117	3-Methyl-1-butanol	43	Flammable
132	10	► 1,2-Dibromoethane		Nonflammable
132	−45	► Chlorobenzene	24	Flammable
135	−70	► 2-Ethoxyethanol	44	Flammable
136	−94	► Ethylbenzene	15	Highly flammable
138	14	► 1,4-Dimethylbenzene	25	Flammable
139	−47	► 1,3-Dimethylbenzene	25	Flammable
142	−79	Isopentyl acetate	25	Flammable
142	−98	Dibutyl ether	25	Flammable
144	−25	► 1,2-Dimethylbenzene	17	Highly flammable
146	30	Triethyl orthoformate	30	Flammable
150	−51	Nonane	30	Flammable
153	−61	► Dimethylformamide	55	Flammable
155	−38	Methoxybenzene	52 (oc)	Flammable
155	−45	► Cyclohexanone	44	Flammable
156	−31	Bromobenzene	51	Flammable
161	−68	Diglyme	67	Flammable
166	−20	► N,N-Dimethylacetamide	67 (oc)	Flammable
172	−75	► 2-Butoxyethanol	61	Flammable
175	−42	2,4,6-Trimethylpyridine	57	Flammable
180	−17	► 1,2-Dichlorobenzene	66	Flammable
185	−31	trans-Decahydronaphthalene	54	Flammable
189	18	Dimethyl sulfoxide	95 (oc)	
191	−13	Benzonitrile	72	
195	−17	1-Octanol	81	
196	−46	Trimethyl phosphate	107	
196	−43	cis-Decahydronaphthalene	54	Flammable
197	−13	► 1,2-Ethanediol	111	
202	20	Acetophenone	77	

TABLE 11.7 (continued)
Fire Hazards of Some Common Laboratory Solvents and Other Substances

Bp (°C)	Mp (°C)	Name[a]	Flash Point (°C)[b]	Flammability Classification[c]
202	−2	Hexachloro-2-propanone		Nonflammable
202	−24	► 1-Methyl-2-pyrrolidinone	96 (oc)	
205	−15	Benzyl alcohol	93	
207	<−50	1,3-Butanediol	109	
207	−35	1,2,3,4-Tetrahydronaphthalene	71	
210	3	► Formamide	>77	
211	6	► Nitrobenzene	88	
214	17	► 1,2,4-Trichlorobenzene	105	
215	−12	Dodecane	74	
216	−45	1,2-Bis(2-methoxyethoxy)ethane	111	
222	82	Acetamide	>104	
235	7	Hexamethylphosphoric triamide	>55	
240	−55	4-Methyl-1,3-dioxolan-2-one	135	
255	72	Biphenyl	113	
279	96	Acenaphthene	>66	
285	27	Tetrahydrothiophene 1,1-dioxide	177	
290	18	Glycerol	160	
328	−6	Tetraethylene glycol	174 (oc)	

Note: Carbon-, sulfur-, nitrogen-, and phosphorus-containing solvents will evolve oxides of their constituent elements, including CO, on combustion, and these gases are toxic and probably irritants if a fire involving such materials is encountered. Some chlorinated solvents can form phosgene (carbonyl chloride) in fires.

[a] ►indicates a substance currently assigned a workplace exposure limit (eight-hour long-term exposure limit) that is less than or equal to 100 ppm (data from EH40/2005 as consolidated with amendments October 2007).

[b] Flash point measurements from the closed-cup method are quoted unless only data from the open-cup (oc) method are available. Data from Stephenson, R. M., *Flash Points of Organic and Organometallic Compounds* (New York: Elsevier, 1987); Bond, J., *Sources of Ignition* (Oxford: Butterworth, 1991).

[c] Substances having flash points above 55°C are considered nonflammable, but may ignite if brought to a high temperature.

[d] Mixture of hydrocarbons, typically 73% *n*-pentane, 23% branched pentanes, 3% cyclopentane. Higher boiling petrols have correspondingly decreasing flammability hazards.

TABLE 11.8
Reproductive Effects of Some Solvents

Reproductive Effects	Solvent(s)
Menstrual disorders	Toluene, styrene, benzene
Abortion or infertility	Formaldehyde, benzene
Testicular atrophy	2-Ethoxyethanol
Decreased foetal growth, low birth weight	Toluene, formaldehyde, vinyl chloride

Source: Reproduced with permission from *Occupational Toxicology*, 2nd ed., ed. C. Winder et al. (Boca Raton, FL: CRC Press, 2004).

TABLE 11.9
IARC Classifications[a] for Some Laboratory Solvents

Solvent	IARC Group
Benzene	Group 1
Carbon tetrachloride	Group 2B
Chloroform	Group 2B
Cyclohexanone	Group 3
1,2-Dichloroethane	Group 2B
Dichloromethane	Group 2B
Dimethylformamide	Group 3
1,4-Dioxane	Group 2B
Mineral oils (untreated)	Group 1
Tetrachloroethylene	Group 2A
Toluene	Group 3
1,1,1-Trichloroethane	Group 3
1,1,2-Trichloroethane	Group 3
Trichloroethylene	Group 2A
Xylene	Group 3

Source: Reproduced with permission from *Occupational Toxicology*, 2nd ed., ed. C. Winder et al. (Boca Raton, FL: CRC Press, 2004).

[a] IARC classifications: Group 1, agents that are carcinogenic to humans; Group 2A, agents that are probably carcinogenic to humans; Group 2B: agents that are possibly carcinogenic to humans; Group 3: agents that are not classifiable; Group 4: agents that are probably not carcinogenic to humans. From: *IARC Monographs on the Evaluation of Carcinogenic Risks to Humans: Overall Evaluations of Carcinogenicity: An Updating of IARC Monographs Volumes 1 to 42*, Suppl. 7 (Lyon: IARC, 1987); available online.

11.9 FURTHER LITERATURE SOURCES

11.9.1 Risk and Hazard Assessment (General)

Toxic Hazard Assessment of Chemicals, ed. M. L. Richardson (London: Royal Society of Chemistry, 1986). Definitions of risk and hazard.

King's Safety in the Process Industries, 2nd ed., ed. R. W. King et al. (London: Arnold, 1998).

Handbook of Occupational Safety and Health, 2nd ed., ed. L. J. DiBerardinis (New York: Wiley, 1999).

Risk Assessment of Chemicals, 2nd ed., ed. C. J. Van Leeuwen et al. (Dordrecht: Springer, 2007).

11.9.2 Physical Properties Related to Hazard

Riddick, J. A., et al., *Organic Solvents: Physical Properties and Methods of Purification*, 4th ed. (New York: Wiley-Interscience, 1986).

Stephenson, R. M., *Flash Points of Organic and Organometallic Compounds* (New York: Elsevier, 1987).

Bond, J., *Sources of Ignition* (Oxford: Butterworth, 1991) (flash points, explosive limits, and autoignition temperatures).

TABLE 11.10
Toxic Effects of Groups of Solvents

| | | Effects | |
| | | | |
Solvent Group	Examples	Acute	Chronic
Aliphatic hydrocarbons	Petrol, kerosene, diesel, *n*-hexane	Nausea, pulmonary irritation, ventricular arrhythmia	Weight loss, anaemia, proteinuria, haematuria, bone marrow hypoplasia
Aromatic hydrocarbons	Toluene, xylene, benzene	Nausea ventricular arrhythmia, respiratory	Headache, anorexia, lassitude
Halogentaed hydrocarbons	Carbon tetrachloride, dichloromethane, trichloroethane, trichloroethylene, tetrachloroethylene	Irritant, liver, kidney, heart	Fatigue, anorexia, liver, kidney, cancer[a]
Ketones	Acetone, methyl ethyl ketone, methyl *n*-butyl ketone	Irritant, respiratory depression	
Alcohols	Methanol, ethanol, isopropanol	Irritant, gastrointestinal	Liver, immune function
Esters	Methyl formate, methyl acetate, amyl acetate	Irritant, liver, palpitations	
Glycols	Ethylene glycol, diethylene glycol, propylene glycol	Kidney	Kidney
Ethers	Diethyl ether, isopropyl ether	Irritant, nausea	
Glycols ethers	Ethylene glycol monomethyl ether, ethylene glycol, monoethyl ether, propylene glycol monomethyl ether	Irritant, nausea, anaemia, liver, kidney, reproductive system	

Source: Reproduced with permission from *Occupational Toxicology*, 2nd ed., ed. C. Winder et al. (Boca Raton, FL: CRC Press, 2004).

[a]   In experimental animals, nongenotoxic.

Lide, D. R., *Handbook of Organic Solvents* (Boca Raton, FL: CRC Press, 1995).

Verschueren, K., *Handbook of Environmental Data on Organic Chemicals*, 4th ed. (Chichester: Wiley, 2001).

Yaws, C. L., *Matheson Gas Data Book*, 7th ed. (New York: McGraw-Hill, 2001).

Kirk-Othmer's Encyclopedia of Chemical Technology, 5th ed. (New York: Wiley, 2004–2007).

11.9.3 OCCUPATIONAL EXPOSURE LIMITS

Occupational Exposure Limits for Airborne Toxic Substances, 3rd ed. (Geneva: ILO, 1991) (data from sixteen countries).

EH40/2005 Workplace Exposure Limits (Norwich: HSE Books, 2005; available online with updates http://www.hse.gov.uk/coshh/table1.pdf).

2009 TLVs® and BEIs®, American Conference of Governmental Industrial Hygienists, Ohio, 2009.

List of MAK and BAT Values 2005 (Weinheim: Deutsche Forschungsgemeinschaft, Wiley-VCH, 2005).

11.9.4 REACTIVE HAZARDS

Jackson, H. L., et al., *J. Chem. Ed.*, 47, A175, 1970 (peroxidizable compounds).

Hazards in the Chemical Laboratory, 5th ed., ed. S. G. Luxon (Cambridge: Royal Society of Chemistry, 1992).

IUPAC-IPCS, *Chemical Safety Matters* (Cambridge: Cambridge University Press, 1992).

Kelly, R. J., *Chem. Health Saf.*, 3, 28–36, 1996 (peroxidizable organic compounds).

TABLE 11.11
Types of Chemicals That May Form Peroxides

Organic Structures

Ethers and acetals with α-hydrogen atoms

Olefins with allylic hydrogen atoms

Chloroolefins and fluoroolefins

Vinyl halides, esters, and ethers

Dienes

Vinylacetylenes with α-hydrogen atoms

Alkylacetylenes with α-hydrogen atoms

Alkylarenes that contain tertiary hydrogen atoms

Alkanes and cycloalkanes that contain tertiary hydrogen atoms

Acrylates and methacrylates

Secondary alcohols

Ketones that contain α-hydrogen atoms

Aldehydes

Ureas, amides, and lactams that have a H atom linked to a C attached to a N

Inorganic Substances

Alkali metals, especially potassium, rubidium, and caesium

Metal amides

Organometallic compounds with a metal atom bonded to carbon

Metal alkoxides

Source: Reproduced with permission from IUPAC-IPCS, *Chemical Safety Matters* (Cambridge: Cambridge University Press, 1992).

Clark, D. E., *Chem. Health Saf.*, 8(5), 12–22, 2001 (peroxidizable organic compounds).

Pohanish, R. P., et al., *Wiley Guide to Chemical Incompatibilities*, 2nd ed. (New York: Wiley, 2003).

Bretherick's Handbook of Reactive Chemical Hazards, 7th ed., ed. P. G. Urben (Oxford: Elsevier, 2007).

11.9.5 Toxicology

General

IARC, *IARC Monographs on the Evaluation of the Carcinogenic Risk of Chemicals to Humans* (Lyon: IARC, 1971–).

Clinical and Experimental Toxicology of Cyanides, ed. B. Ballantyne et al. (Bristol: Wright, 1987).

Effects of Exposure to Toxic Gases—First Aid and Medical Treatment, 3rd ed., ed. F. Scornavacca et al. (Secaucus, NJ: Matheson Gas Products, 1988).

Dangerous Properties of Industrial Materials Report, 1980–1996 (toxicological and ecotoxicological data on chemicals produced on a large scale).

Grandjean, P., *Skin Penetration: Hazardous Chemicals at Work* (London: Taylor & Francis, 1990) (three hundred chemicals that are toxic by skin absorption).

Patty's Industrial Hygiene and Toxicology, 5th ed. (Hoboken, NJ: Wiley, 2001).

TABLE 11.12
Common Peroxide-Forming Chemicals

Severe peroxide hazard on storage with exposure to air. *Discard within 3 months.*

Diisopropyl ether	Sodium amide (sodamide)
Divinylacetylene[a]	Vinylidene chloride (1,1-dichloroethylene)[a]
Potassium metal	Potassium amide

Peroxide hazard on concentration: Do not distil or evaporate without first testing for the presence of peroxides. *Discard or test for peroxides after 6 months.*

Acetaldehyde diethyl acetal (1,1-diethoxyethane)	Ethylene glycol dimethyl ether (glyme)
Cumene (isopropylbenzene)	Ethylene glycol ether acetates
Cyclohexene	Ethylene glycol monoethers (cellosolves)
Cyclopentene	Furan
Decalin (decahydronaphthalene)	Methylacetylene
Diacetylene (1,2-butadiyne)	Methylcyclopentane
Dicyclopentadiene	Methyl isobutyl ketone
Diethyl ether (ether)	Tetrahydrofuran
Diethylene glycol dimethyl ether (diglyme)	Tetralin (tetrahydronaphthalene)
Dioxan/dioxolan (dioxane)	Vinyl ethers[a]

Hazard or rapid polymerization initiated by internally formed peroxides.[a]

(A) Normal liquids. *Discard or test for peroxides after 6 months.*[b]

Chloroprene (2-chloro-1,3-butadiene)[c]	Vinyl acetate
Styrene	Vinylpyridine

(B) Normal gases. *Discard after 12 months.*[d]

Butadiene[c]	Vinylacetylene[c]
Tetrafluoroethylene[c]	Vinyl chloride

Source: Reproduced with permission from IUPAC-IPCS, *Chemical Safety Matters* (Cambridge: Cambridge University Press, 1992).

[a] Monomers may polymerize and should be stored with a polymerization inhibitor from which the monomer can be separated by distillation just before use.

[b] Although common acrylic monomers such as acrylonitrile, acrylic acid, ethyl acrylate, and methyl methacrylate can form peroxides, they have not been reported to develop hazardous levels in normal use and storage.

[c] The hazard from peroxide formation in these compounds is substantially greater when they are stored in the liquid phase.

[d] Although air cannot enter a gas cylinder in which gases are stored under pressure, these gases are sometimes transferred from the original cylinder to another in the laboratory, and it is difficult to be sure that there is no residual air in the receiving cylinder. An inhibitor should be put into any secondary cylinder before transfer. The supplier can suggest an appropriate inhibitor to be used. The hazard posed by these gases is much greater if there is a liquid phase in the secondary container. Even inhibited gases that have been put into a secondary container under conditions that create a liquid phase should be discarded within 12 months.

Occupational Toxicology, 2nd ed., ed. C. Winder et al. (Boca Raton, FL: CRC Press, 2004).

Proctor and Hughes' Chemical Hazards of the Workplace, 5th ed., ed. G. J. Hathaway et al. (Hoboken, NJ: Wiley, 2004).

Comprehensive Toxicology, ed. I. G. Sipes et al. (New York: Elsevier, 1996).

Lewis, R. J., Sr., *Sax's Dangerous Properties of Industrial Materials*, 11th ed. (Hoboken, NJ: Wiley, 2004).

REPRODUCTIVE TOXICOLOGY

Lewis, R. J., *Reproductively Active Chemicals: A Reference Guide* (New York: Van Nostrand-Reinhold, 1991).

Kolb, V. M., Ed., *Teratogens*, 2nd ed. (Amsterdam: Elsevier, 1993).

Shepard, T. H., *Catalog of Teratogenic Agents*, 9th ed. (Baltimore: The John Hopkins University Press, 1998).

SOLVENT TOXICOLOGY

Solvents in Common Use: Health Risks to Workers (London: Royal Society of Chemistry, 1988).

Chemical Safety Data Sheets: Solvents, Vol. 1 (Cambridge: Royal Society of Chemistry, 1989).

Ethel Browning's Toxicity and Metabolism of Industrial Solvents, 2nd ed., ed. R. Snyder, Vols. 1–3 (Amsterdam: Elsevier, 1987–1992).

Henning, H., ed., *Solvent Safety Sheets: A Compendium for the Working Chemist* (Cambridge: Royal Society of Chemistry, 1993).

Long-Term Neurotoxic Effects of Paint Solvents (London: Royal Society of Chemistry, 1993) (neurotoxicity).

Toxicology of Solvents, ed. M. McParland et al. (Shrewsbury, Shropshire, UK: RAPRA Technology Ltd., 2002) (toxicity and treatment of solvent exposure for all the commonly used laboratory solvents).

METAL TOXICOLOGY

Barnes, J. M., et al., *Organometallic Chemistry Reviews*, 3, 137, 1968 (toxicology of organo-metallic compounds).

Venugopal, B., et al., *Metal Toxicity in Mammals*, Vols. 1–2 (New York: Plenum Press, 1977–1978).

Biological Monitoring of Toxic Metals, ed. T. W. Clarkson (New York: Plenum Press, 1988).

Handbook on Toxicity of Inorganic Compounds, ed. H. G. Seiler (New York: M. Dekker, 1988).

Metal Neurotoxicity, ed. S. C. Bondy (Boca Raton, FL: CRC Press, 1988).

Harmful Chemical Substances: Elements in Groups I–IV of the Periodic Table and Their Inorganic Compounds, ed. V. A. Filov et al., Vol. 1 (New York: Ellis Horwood, 1993).

Hostýnek, J. J., et al., *CRC Crit. Rev. Toxicol.*, 23, 171, 1993 (skin effects of metals).

Metal Toxicology, ed. R. A. Goyer (San Diego: Academic Press, 1995).

Toxicology of Metals, ed. L. W. Chang (Boca Raton, FL: CRC Press, 1996).

Handbook on the Toxicology of Metals, 3rd ed., ed. G. F. Nordberg et al. (Amsterdam: Elsevier, 2007).

11.9.6 MATERIAL SAFETY DATA SHEETS

International Chemical Safety Cards, Commission of the European Communities, Luxembourg (produced for the International Programme on Chemical Safety); available online.

Compendium of Safety Data Sheets for Research and Industrial Chemicals, ed. L. H. Keith, Parts I–VI (Deerfield Park, FL: VCH, 1985–1987).

The Sigma-Aldrich Library of Chemical Safety Data, 2nd ed., ed. R. E. Lenga (Milwaukee, WI: Sigma-Aldrich Corp., 1988).

Chemical Safety Sheets (Dordrecht: Kluwer Academic, 1991) (includes a section on the prediction of chemical handling properties from physical data).

11.9.7 LABORATORY SAFETY

Journal of Chemical Health & Safety. Official publication of the American Chemical Society Division of Chemical Health and Safety. Published by Elsevier B.V., Amsterdam.

Laboratory Hazards Bulletin. Published monthly by the Royal Society of Chemistry, Cambridge.

Laboratory Safety: Theory and Practice, ed. A. A. Fuscaldo (New York: Academic Press, 1980).

Degradation of Chemical Carcinogens: An Annotated Bibliography, ed. M. W. Slein et al. (New York: Van Nostrand Reinhold, 1980).

Furniss, B. S., et al., *Vogel's Textbook of Practical Organic Chemistry*, 5th ed. (Harlow, Essex: Longman Scientific & Technical, 1989), pp. 35–51 (hazards in organic chemistry laboratories).

Lunn, G., et al., *Destruction of Hazardous Chemicals in the Laboratory* (New York: Wiley, 1990).

Improving Safety in the Chemical Laboratory: A Practical Guide, 2nd ed., ed. J. A. Young (New York: Wiley, 1991).

Safe Storage of Laboratory Chemicals, 2nd ed., ed. D. A. Pipitone (New York: Wiley, 1991).

IUPAC-IPCS, *Chemical Safety Matters* (Cambridge: Cambridge University Press, 1992) (useful laboratory safety advice. including storage and disposal of waste chemicals).

Hazards in the Chemical Laboratory, 5th ed., ed. S. G. Luxon (Cambridge: Royal Society of Chemistry, 1992).

Palluzi, R. P., *Pilot Plant and Laboratory Safety* (New York: McGraw Hill, 1994).

Stricoff, R. S., and Walters, D. B., *Handbook of Laboratory Health and Safety*, 2nd ed. (New York: J. Wiley, 1995).

Prudent Practices in the Laboratory (Washington, D.C.: National Academic Press, 1995).

Errington, R. J., *Advanced Practical Inorganic and Metalorganic Chemistry* (London: Blackie Academic, 1997) (techniques for the safe handling of organometallic reagents).

Furr, A. K., *CRC Handbook of Laboratory Safety*, 5th ed. (Boca Raton, FL: CRC Press, 2000).

Handbook of Chemical Health and Safety, ed. R. J. Alaimo (New York: American Chemical Society/Oxford University Press, 2001).

Wiener, J. J. M., and Grice, C. A., "Practical Segregation of Incompatible Reagents in the Organic Chemistry Laboratory," *Org. Process Res. Dev.*, 13(6), 1395–1400, 2009.

11.9.8 HEALTH AND SAFETY LEGISLATION

Croner's Laboratory Manager, Croner Publications, 1997–, (revised quarterly). Provides updated information on changes to health and safety legislation affecting the management of laboratories.

Selwyn, N. M., *The Law of Health and Safety at Work 2008/2009*, 17th ed. (Kingston upon Thames: Croner, 2009). *Tolley's Health and Safety at Work Handbook 2009*, 21st ed. (London: LexisNexis, 2009).

11.9.9 ELECTRONIC SOURCES FOR HAZARD INFORMATION

The web is a vast resource for hazard information and advice on safe practices in the chemical laboratory. Many UK and U.S. university chemistry departments have posted their safety policies and guidance for laboratory workers on the web and added links to other health and safety websites. The websites of the following organisations are also useful sources of hazard information:

Organisation	Internet Address and Description of Content
Agency for Toxic Substances and Disease Registry	http://www.atsdr.cdc.gov/ Health effects information concerning chemicals, chemicals released from hazardous waste disposal sites, physician case studies
American Conference of Governmental Industrial Hygienists	www.acgih.org Sources of information on TLVs, biological exposure indices, chemicals under study, and revisions to TLVs
Health and Safety Executive (HSE)	http://www.hse.gov.uk/coshh/index.htm COSHH home page
International Agency for Research On Cancer	www.iarc.fr/
International Programme on Chemical Safety	http://www.inchem.org/
National Institute for Occupational Health and Safety	www.cdc.gov/niosh Research studies, health hazard evaluations, extensive links to occupational safety and health resources on the Internet
National Library of Medicine	www.nlm.nih.gov Databases include PubMed and TOXLINE
National Toxicology Program	http://ntp.niehs.nih.gov/ Extensive information on chemicals, reactivity, long-term and short-term effects
NIOSH Pocket Guide to Chemical Hazards	http://www.cdc.gov/niosh/npg/ Also gives a link to the Registry of Toxic Effects of Chemical Substances (RTECS) database
Royal Society of Chemistry Environment Health & Safety Committee Notes	http://www.rsc.org/ *COSHH in Laboratories*; *Fire Safety in Chemical Laboratories*

12 Spectroscopy

The regions of the electromagnetic spectrum are shown in Table 12.1. The following sections deal with infrared (IR) spectroscopy, ultraviolet (UV) spectroscopy, and nuclear magnetic resonance (NMR)

TABLE 12.1
The Electromagnetic Spectrum

Region	Range
Vacuum ultraviolet	100–180 nm
Ultraviolet	180–400 nm
Visible	400–750 nm
Near infrared	0.75–2.5 μm
Infrared	2.5–15 μm
Far infrared	15–300 μm

12.1 INFRARED SPECTROSCOPY

12.1.1 WINDOW MATERIALS, MULLING OILS, AND SOLVENTS

Note: IR absorption can depend on whether mull or solvent is used

12.1.1.1 Window Materials

The transmission ranges of various window materials are listed in Table 12.2.

TABLE 12.2
Window Materials

Material	Transmission Range (cm^{-1})
NaCl	40 000–590
KBr	40 000–400
AgCl	25 000–435
CaF_2	67 000–1100
CsBr	10 000–270
ZnS	10 000–680

12.1.1.2 Mulling Oils

Nujol® (a high-molecular-weight hydrocarbon) can be used from 650 cm^{-1} to the far infrared. It gives IR absorptions around 2900 (vs), 1460, and 1350 cm^{-1}. Fluorolube® (a high-molecular-weight fluorinated hydrocarbon) is useful for the range 4000 to 1370 cm^{-1}. Hexachlorobutadiene can also be used.

12.1.1.3   Solvents

The following solvents are commonly used to record IR spectra. They *cannot* be used in the regions shown (cm⁻¹).

- Carbon disulfide
  1 mm cell: 2340–2100, 1640–1385, 875–845
  0.1 mm cell: 2200–2140, 1595–1460

- Carbon tetrachloride
  1 mm cell: 1610–1500, 1270–1200, 1020–960, <860
  0.1 mm cell: 820–720

- Chloroform
  1 mm cell: 3090–2980, 2440–2380, 1555–1410, 1290–1155, 940–910, <860
  0.1 mm cell: 3020–3000, 1240–1200, <805

12.1.2   Characteristic Infrared Absorption Bands

The characteristic IR absorption bands of various types of compounds are listed in Table 12.3, in two complementary formats.

TABLE 12.3
Characteristic IR Absorption Bands

Type of Compound	Bond	Type of Vibration	Frequency (cm⁻¹)
(a) Presented alphabetically by type of compound			
Alcohols	C–O	Stretching	1300–1050
(Not H-bonded)	C–H	Stretching	3650–3600
(H-bonded)	O–H	Stretching	3600–3200
Aldehydes	C–H	Stretching	2900–2700
	C=O	Stretching	1740–1690
Alkanes	C–H	Stretching	3000–2800
Alkenes	C=C	Stretching	1680–1600
	C–H	Bending	995–675
	C–H	Stretching	3100–3000
Alkyl bromides	C–Br	Stretching	680–500
chlorides	C–Cl	Stretching	850–600
fluorides	C–F	Stretching	1400–1000
iodides	C–I	Stretching	500–200
Alkynes	C–H	Stretching	3350–3300
	C≡C	Stretching	2250–2100
Amides	C=O	Stretching	1715–1630
Amines	N–H	Bending	1650–1550
	C–H	Stretching	1350–1000
	N–H	Stretching	3500–3100

TABLE 12.3 (continued)
Characteristic IR Absorption Bands

Type of Compound	Bond	Type of Vibration	Frequency (cm^{-1})
Aromatics	C–H	Bending	900–680
	C=C	Stretching	1625–1570
			1525–1475
	C–H	Stretching	3150–3000
Carboxylic acids	O–H	Stretching	3400–2400
	C=O	Stretching	1750–1690
	C–O	Stretching	1300–1080
Esters	C–O	Stretching	1300–1080
	C=O	Stretching	1780–1730
Ethers	C–O	Stretching	1300–1080
Imines/oximes	C=N	Stretching	1690–1640
Ketones	C=O	Stretching	1730–1650
Nitriles	C≡N	Stretching	2260–2240
Nitro	N–O	Stretching	1550–1500
Phosphorus compounds	P=O	Stretching	1300–960
	P–O	Stretching	1260–855
	P–H	Bending	1090–910
Thiols	S–H	Stretching	2600–2500

(b) Presented in order of decreasing frequency

Type of Compound	Bond	Type of Vibration	Frequency (cm^{-1})
Alcohols	O–H	Stretching	3650–3600
Alcohols	O–H	Stretching	3600–3200
Amines	N–H	Stretching	3500–3100
Carboxylic acids	O–H	Stretching	3400–2400
Alkynes	C–H	Stretching	3350–3300
Aromatics	C–H	Stretching	3150–3000
Alkenes	C–H	Stretching	3100–3000
Alkanes	C–H	Stretching	3000–2800
Aldehydes	C–H	Stretching	2900–2700
Thiols	S–H	Stretching	2600–2500
Nitriles	C≡N	Stretching	2260–2240
Alkynes	C≡C	Stretching	2250–2100
Esters	C=O	Stretching	1750–1730
Carboxylic acids	C=O	Stretching	1750–1690
Aldehydes	C=O	Stretching	1740–1690
Ketones	C=O	Stretching	1730–1650*
Amides	C=O	Stretching	1715–1630
Imines/oximes	C=N	Stretching	1690–1640
Alkenes	C=C	Stretching	1680–1600

(continued on next page)

TABLE 12.3 (continued)
Characteristic IR Absorption Bands

Type of Compound	Bond	Type of Vibration	Frequency (cm^{-1})
Amines	N–H	Bending	1650–1550
Alkyl fluorides	C–F	Stretching	1400–1000
Amines	C–N	Stretching	1350–1000
Carboxylic acids	C–O	Stretching	1300–1080
Esters	C–O	Stretching	1300–1080
Ethers	C–O	Stretching	1300–1080
Alcohols	C–O	Stretching	1300–1050
Phosphorus compounds	P=O	Stretching	1300–960
Phosphorus compounds	P–O	Stretching	1260–855
Phosphorus compounds	P–H	Bending	1090–910
Alkenes	C–H	Bending	975–675
Aromatics	C–H	Bending	900–680
Alkyl chlorides	C–Cl	Stretching	850–600
Alkyl bromides	C–Br	Stretching	680–500
Alkyl iodides	C–I	Stretching	500–200

* cyclobutanone and cyclopentanone absorb up to 1780 cm^{-1}.

12.2 ULTRAVIOLET SPECTROSCOPY

12.2.1 ULTRAVIOLET CUTOFF LIMITS FOR SOLVENTS

These cutoff limits, which are listed in Table 12.4, are the wavelengths at which the absorbance approaches 1.0 in a 10 mm cell.

TABLE 12.4
UV Cutoff Limits for Solvents

Solvent	Wavelength (nm)
Acetonitrile	190
Water	205
Methanol	210
Cyclohexane	210
Hexane	210
Ethanol (95%)	210
1,4-Dioxane	215
Diethyl ether	215
Tetrahydrofuran	220
Dichloromethane	235
Chloroform	245
Carbon tetrachloride	265
Benzene	280
Toluene	285
Acetone	330

12.2.2 Characteristic Ultraviolet/Visible Absorption Bands

The characteristic UV/VIS absorption bands for some representative chromophores are listed in Table 12.5.

TABLE 12.5
UV/VIS Absorption Bands for Representative Chromophores

Chromophore		λ_{max} (ε_{max})
Aldehydes	$-CHO$	180–210 (10 000), 280–300 (15)
Amides	$-CONH_2$	175–180 (7000), 210–220 (60)
Amines	$-NH_2$	190–200 (3000)
Azides	$-N_3$	287 (20)
Azo compounds	$-N=N-$	330–400 (10)
Bromides	$-Br$	200–210 (300)
Carboxylic acids	$-COOH$	195–210 (50)
Chlorides	$-Cl$	170–175 (300)
Disulfides	$-S-S-$	194 (5500), 250–255 (400)
Esters	$-COOR$	195–210 (50)
Ethers	$-O-$	180–185 (2000)
Imines	$>C=N-$	190 (5000)
Iodides	$-I$	255–260 (400)
Ketones	$>C=O$	180–195 (1000), 270–290 (20)
Nitriles	$-C\equiv N$	160–165 (5)
Nitro compounds	$-NO_2$	200–210 (10 000), 275 (20)
Nitroso compounds	$-N=O$	300 (100), 600–665 (20)
Oximes	$=N-OH$	190–195 (5000)
Sulfides	$-S-$	194 (4600), 210–215 (1500)
Sulfones	$-SO_2-$	180
Sulfoxides	$-S(O)-$	210–230 (1500)
Thiols	$-SH$	190–200 (1500)

Unsaturated Systems

Alkenes	$-C=C-$	162–175 (15 000), 190–195 (10 000)
Alkynes	$-C\equiv C-$	175–180 (10 000), 195 (2000), 223 (150)
Allenes	$C=C=C$	170–185 (5000), 225–230 (600)
Ketenes	$C=C=O$	225–230 (600), 375–380 (20)[a]

Conjugated Systems (see Section 12.2.3 for Woodward-Fieser Rules)

$-(C=C)_2-$ (acyclic)	210–230 (21 000)
$-(C=C)_3-$	260 (35 000)
$-(C=C)_4-$	300 (52 000)
$-(C=C)_5-$	330 (118 000)
$-(C=C)_2-$ (cyclic)	230–260 (3000–8000)
$-C=C-C\equiv C-$	219–230 (7500)
$-C=C-C=N-$	220 (23 000)
$-C=C-C=O$	210–250 (10 000–20 000), 300–350 (30)
$-C=C-NO_2$	229–235 (9500)

(continued on next page)

TABLE 12.5 (continued)
UV/VIS Absorption Bands for Representative
Chromophores

Chromophore	λ_{max} (ε_{max})
$-C{\equiv}C-C{=}O$	214 (4500), 308 (20)
$-C{=}C-COOH$	206 (13 500), 242 (250)
$-C{\equiv}C-COOH$	210 (6000)
$-C{=}C-C{\equiv}N$	215 (680)
$-C(O)C(O)-$	195 (25), 280–285 (20), 420–460 (10)
Aromatic Systems	
Benzene	184 (46 700), 204 (6900), 255 (170)
Biphenyl	246 (20 000)
Naphthalene	222 (112 000), 275 (5600), 312 (175)
Anthracene	252 (199 000), 375 (7900)
Pyridine	174 (80 000), 195 (6000), 257 (1700)
Quinoline	227 (37 000), 270 (3600), 314 (2750)
Isoquinoline	218 (80 000), 266 (4000), 317 (3500)

12.2.3   UV/VIS Absorption of Dienes and Polyenes

The Woodward-Fieser rules can be used to estimate the UV/VIS absorption as follows:

Parent Diene System

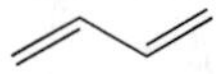	Acyclic	215 nm
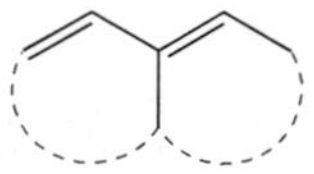	Heteroannular	214 nm
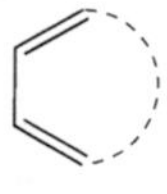	Homoannular	253 nm

Increments

For each additional conjugated double bond		+30 nm
For each exocyclic double bond	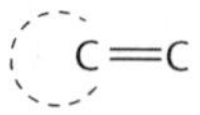 C=C	+5 nm
For each substituent		
C substituent		+5 nm
OAc		0 nm
OR (R = alkyl)		+6 nm
SR (R = alkyl)		+30 nm
Cl, Br		+5 nm
NR$_2$ (R = alkyl)		+60 nm
Solvent Correction		0 nm

Examples

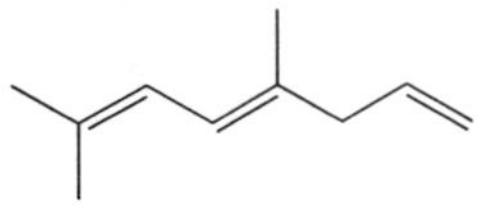

Acyclic   215 nm
Four alkyl substituents   20 nm
                                                                             235 nm

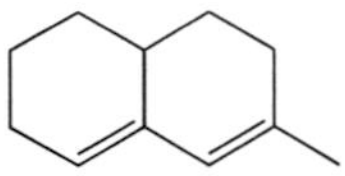

Heteroannular   214 nm
Four alkyl substituents   20 nm
Exocyclic double bond   5 nm
                                                                             239 nm

12.2.4 UV/VIS Absorption of α,β-Unsaturated Carbonyl Compounds

The Woodward-Fieser rules can be used to estimate the UV/VIS absorption as follows:

Parent System

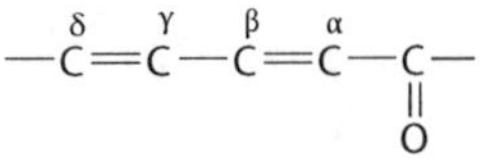

$$\overset{\delta}{-C}=\overset{\gamma}{C}-\overset{\beta}{C}=\overset{\alpha}{C}-\underset{\underset{O}{\|}}{C}-$$

Acyclic α,β-unsaturated ketone   215 nm
α,β-Unsaturated aldehyde   207 nm
α,β-Unsaturated carboxylic acid or ester   193 nm
Six-membered cyclic α,β-unsaturated ketone   215 nm
Five-membered cyclic α,β-unsaturated ketone   202 nm

Increments
For each additional conjugated double bond   +30 nm

For each exocyclic double bond $C=C$ +5 nm

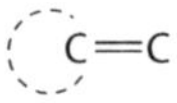

For each homoannular diene system 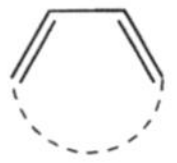   +39 nm

For each substituent at the π-electron system (nm)

	α	β	γ	δ and Beyond
C substituent	10	12	18	18
OH	35	30		50
OAc	6	6	6	6
OR (R = alkyl)	35	30	17	31
SR (R = alkyl)		85		
Cl	12	12		
Br	25	30		
NR$_2$ (R = alkyl)		95		

Solvent Corrections

Water	+8 nm
Ethanol, methanol	0 nm
Chloroform	−1 nm
Dioxane	−5 nm
Diethyl ether	−7 nm
Hexane, cyclohexane	−11 nm

Examples

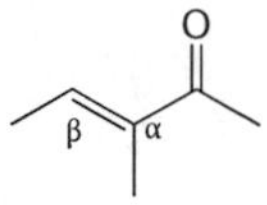

Acyclic ketone	215 nm
α-Alkyl group	10 nm
β-Alkyl group	12 nm
	237 nm

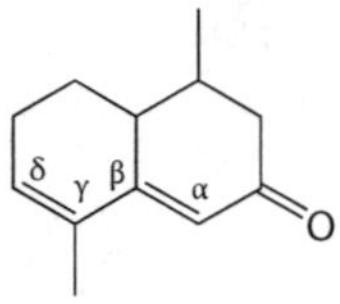

Six-membered cyclic ketone	215 nm
Additional conjugated bond	+30 nm
Exocyclic bond	+5 nm
β-Alkyl group	+12 nm
γ-Alkyl group	+18 nm
δ-Alkyl group	+18 nm
	298 nm

12.3 NUCLEAR MAGNETIC RESONANCE SPECTROSCOPY

Ross Denton

Nuclear magnetic resonance (NMR) spectroscopy is the most powerful spectroscopic method for structural elucidation of organic molecules and is routinely used by organic chemists. Summarised below are common NMR active nuclei; chemical shift data for NMR solvents, common impurities, and functional groups; coupling constants; and details of common NMR experiments used to determine the connectivity and stereochemistry of small organic molecules.

12.3.1 COMMON NUCLEI USED IN NMR

These are listed in Table 12.6, along with details on NMR frequency and isotopic abundance.

12.3.2 CHEMICAL SHIFT DATA

Table 12.7 contains a summary of chemical shift data for residual protons in commonly used NMR solvents. Table 12.8 contains chemical shift data for solvents and other common impurities. The ranges of the ^{1}H, ^{13}C, ^{19}F, and ^{31}P NMR chemical shifts of various functional groups are shown in Figures 12.1 to 12.4, respectively and in a different format in Tables 12.9 to 12.12.

TABLE 12.6
Common Nuclei Used in NMR

Nucleus	Spin	NMR Frequency (Hz) at 11.74 T	Isotopic Abundance (%)
^{1}H	1/2	500.000	99.98
^{2}H	1	76.753	0.01
^{11}B	3/2	160.419	80.42
^{13}C	1/2	125.721	1.11
^{14}N	1	36.118	99.63
^{15}N	(−)1/2	50.664	0.37
^{17}O	(−)5/2	67.784	0.037
^{19}F	1/2	470.385	100
^{31}P	1/2	202.404	100

TABLE 12.7
Chemical Shift Data for Residual Protons in Common NMR Solvents

Solvent	δ (ppm) of Residual Protons	δ ^{13}C (ppm)
Acetic acid-d$_4$	2.0, 11.5[a]	21, 177
Acetone-d$_6$	2.0	30, 205
Acetonitrile-d$_3$	2.0	0.3, 117
Benzene-d$_6$	7.2	128
Carbon disulfide	—	1931
Carbon tetrachloride	—	97
Chloroform-d	7.2	77
Deuterium oxide	4.8[a]	—
Dimethyl-d$_6$ sulfoxide	2.5	43
1,4-Dioxane	3.7	67
Methanol-d$_4$	3.4, 4.8[a]	49
Hexachloroacetone	—	124, 126
Pyridine-d$_5$	7.2, 7.6, 8.5	124-150
Toluene-d$_8$	2.4, 7.3	21, 125–138
Trifluoroacetic acid-d	13.0	115, 163

[a] Value may vary considerably depending on the solute.

TABLE 12.8
Chemical Shift Data for Common Solvents and Impurities in CDCl$_3$

Compound	^{1}H NMR δ (ppm)	^{13}C NMR δ (ppm)
Acetic acid	2.10 (s), 11.4 (s)	177.0, 20.8
Acetone	2.17 (s)	207.1, 30.9
Acetonitrile	2.10 (s)	116.4, 1.9
Benzene	7.34 (s)	128.4
1,2-Dichloroethane	3.73 (s)	43.5
Dichloromethane	5.30 (s)	53.5
Diethylene glycol dimethyl ether (diglyme)	3.65 (m), 3.57 (m)	71.9, 70.5, 59.0
Diethyl ether	3.47 (q), 1.21 (t)	65.9, 15.2
N,N-Dimethylacetamide	3.02 (s), 2.94 (s), 2.09 (s)	171.1, 38.1, 35.3, 21.5
N,N-Dimethylformamide	8.02 (s), 2.96 (s), 2.88 (s)	162.6, 36.5, 31.5
Dimethylsulfoxide	2.62 (s)	40.8
1,4-Dioxane	3.71 (s)	67.1
Ethanol	3.72 (q), 1.32 (s), 1.25 (t)	58.3, 18.4
Ethyl acetate	4.12 (q), 2.05 (s), 1.26 (t)	171.4, 60.5, 21.0, 14.2
Ethylene glycol	3.76 (s)	63.8
Grease	1.26 (m), 0.86 (broad s)	29.8
n-Hexane	1.26 (m), 0.88 (t)	31.6, 22.7, 14.1
Methanol	3.49 (s), 1.09 (s)	50.4
Nitromethane	4.33 (s)	62.5
2-Propanol	4.04 (sep), 1.22 (d)	64.5, 25.1
Pyridine	8.62 (m), 7.68 (m), 7.29 (m)	149.0, 136.0, 123.8
Tetrahydrofuran	3.76 (m), 1.85 (m)	68.0, 25.6
Toluene	2.36 (s), 7.17 (m), 7.25 (m)	137.9, 129.1, 128.3, 125.3, 21.5
Triethylamine	2.53 (q), 1.03 (t)	46.3, 11.6
o-Xylene	7.07 (m), 2.22 (s)	136.8, 130.3, 126.5, 18.8

Note: Multiplicities are designated using the following abbreviations: s = singlet, d = doublet, t = triplet, q = quartet, sep = septet.

See Gottlieb, H. E., et al., *J. Org. Chem.*, 62, 7512–7515, 1997.

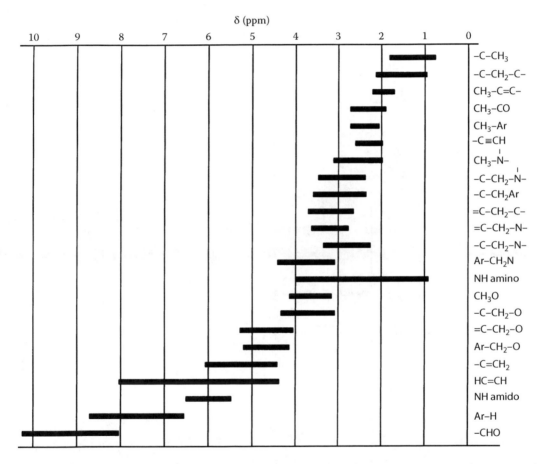

FIGURE 12.1 Ranges of ¹H NMR chemical shifts for various groups (Ar = aromatic ring) relative to δ (TMS) = 0.

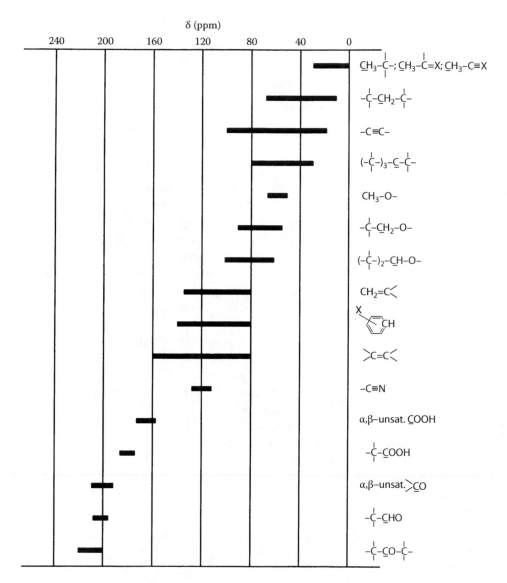

FIGURE 12.2 Ranges of ^{13}C NMR chemical shifts for various groups (X = any group) relative to δ(TMS) = 0.

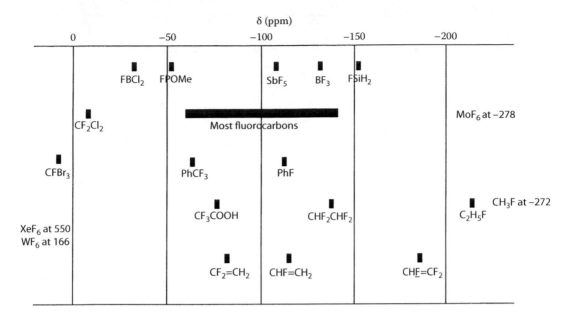

FIGURE 12.3   Ranges of ^{19}F NMR chemical shifts relative to δ ($CFCl_3$) = 0. (Reproduced with permission from W. Kemp, *NMR in Chemistry*, published by Macmillan Press Ltd., 1986.)

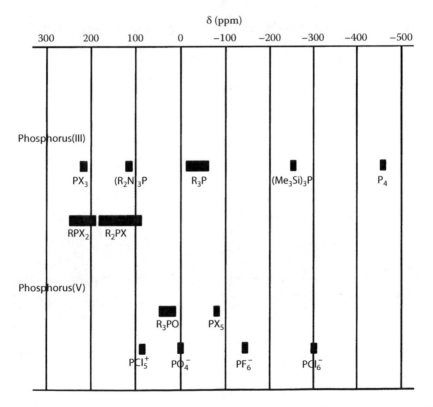

FIGURE 12.4   Ranges of ^{31}P NMR chemical shifts relative to δ (H_3PO_4(aq.)) = 0. (Reproduced with permission from W. Kemp, *NMR in Chemistry*, published by Macmillan Press Ltd., 1986.)

TABLE 12.9
^1H and ^{13}C Chemical Shifts for a Methyl Group in Various Situations

	^1H (δ ppm)	^{13}C (δ ppm)		^1H (δ ppm)	^{13}C (δ ppm)
$H_3C-\overset{\mid}{\underset{\mid}{C}}-$	0.7–1.3	8–24	$H_3C-N\overset{/}{\underset{\backslash}{}}$	2.1–2.5	30–45
$H_3C-\overset{\mid}{C}=C\overset{/}{\underset{\backslash}{}}$	1.7–2.0	15–27[a]	H_3C-O-	3.3–3.5	56–59
$H_3C-\overset{O}{\overset{\|}{C}}-$	2.0–2.1	26–31	$H_3C-O-\overset{O}{\overset{\|}{C}}-$	3.6–3.9	51–52
$H_3C-\overset{O}{\overset{\|}{C}}-O-$	2.0–2.1	20–22			

[a] Dependent on stereochemistry.

TABLE 12.10
Aromatic Substituent Effects in NMR

	^1H (ppm)				^{13}C (ppm)		
Parent	7.27				128		
			Increments				
Substituent	*ortho*-H	*meta*-H	*para*-H	C-1 (*ipso*)	*ortho*-C	*meta*-C	*para*-C
–CH₃	–0.2	–0.1	–0.2	9	0	0	–2
C=C	0.2	0.2	0.2	9	0	0	–2
–F	–0.3	0	–0.2	35	–14	1	–5
–Cl	0	0	–0.1	6	0	1	–2
–Br	0.2	–0.1	–0.05	5	3	2	–2
–I	0.35	–0.2	0	–32	10	3	–1
–OH	–0.45	–0.1	–0.2	27	–13	1	–7
–OCH₃	–0.2	–0.2	–0.2	30	–15	1	–8
–OCOCH₃	–0.2	0	–0.1	23	–6	1	–2
–SR	0.1	–0.1	–0.2	4	1	1	–3
–SO₃H	0.4	–0.1	0.1	16	0	0	4
–NH₂, –NMe₂	–0.8	–0.15	–0.4	20	–15	1	–10
–NO₂	1.0	0.2	0.4	20	–5	1	6
–CHO	0.65	0.2	0.4	9	1	1	6
–CO.R	0.6	0.3	0.3	9	0	0	5
–CO₂H	0.8	0.15	0.2	2	2	0	5
–CN	0.3	0.3	0.3	–15	4	1	4

Note: Aromatic compounds also have distinctive UV absorptions.

TABLE 12.11
Variation in ^{13}C Chemical Shifts with Chain Length and Ring Size

Chain Length	^{13}C (δ ppm)					Ring Size	^{13}C (δ ppm)
CH_4	-2.3					3	-2.9
$CH_3.CH_3$	5.7	5.7				4	22.5
$CH_3.CH_2.CH_3$	15	16	15			5	25.7
$CH_3.CH_2.CH_2.CH_3$	13	25	25	13		6	27.0
$CH_3.CH_2.CH_2.CH_2.CH_3$	14	23	33	23	14	7	28.9
$CH_3.CH_2.CH_2.CH_2$ ...	14	23	33	29.5	...	8	27.5

Note: These values change in the presence of substituents and chain branching.

norbornane   *trans*-decalin   *cis*-decalin

TABLE 12.12
^{13}C Chemical Shifts for Various Alkenes (δ ppm)

12.3.3 Coupling Constants

The sign and magnitude of H–H coupling constants and C–H coupling constants are summarized in Tables 12.13 and 12.14, respectively.

TABLE 12.13
Summary of H–H Coupling Constants

	J_{H-H} (Hz)	Sign
^2J	0–30	–
^3J	0–18	+
^{3+n}J	0–7	+ or –

TABLE 12.14
Summary of C–H Coupling Constants

	J_{C-H} (Hz)	Sign
^1J	125–250	+
^2J	–10 to +20	+ or –
^3J	1–10	+
^{3+n}J	<1	+ or –

See the following references for more information:

Williams, D. H., and Fleming, I., *Spectroscopic Methods in Organic Chemistry* (New York: McGraw-Hill, 1989).

Harwood, L. M., and Claridge, T. D. W., *Introduction to Organic Spectroscopy* (Oxford: Oxford University Press, 1997).

Friebolin, H., *Basic One- and Two-Dimensional NMR Spectroscopy* (Weinheim Wiley-VCH, 2005).

12.3.3.1 Geminal H–H Coupling ($^2J_{H-H}$)

The magnitude of geminal coupling constants $^2J_{H-H}$ depends on the hybridisation of the carbon atom, the H–C–H bond angle, and electronegative substituents. In general, the observed coupling constant becomes more positive as the H–C–H bond angle increases (see Table 12.15; Williams and Fleming, Harwood and Claridge, and Friebolin, as above).

TABLE 12.15
Common $^2J_{H-H}$ Coupling Constants (R = Alkyl Group)

	$^2J_{H-H}$ (Hz)		$^2J_{H-H}$ (Hz)
	–4.5	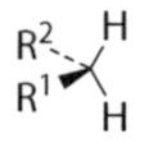	–12.5
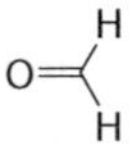	+41	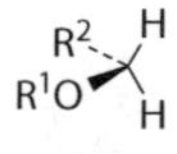	10.5
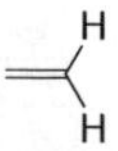	+3 to –3	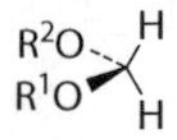	–6.0

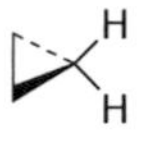

12.3.3.2 Vicinal H–H Coupling ($^3J_{H-H}$)

The average $^3J_{H-H}$ value for a "freely" rotating carbon-carbon bond is approximately 7–8 Hz. Vicinal coupling constants are reduced (ca. less than 1 Hz) by electronegative substituents and reduced as the length of the carbon-carbon bond increases (see Williams and Fleming, Harwood and Claridge, and Friebolin, as above). Vicinal coupling constants also vary as a function of the dihedral angle according to the Karplus equation $^3J_{H-H} = 4.22 - 0.5\cos\theta + 4.5\cos2\theta$ (where θ is the dihedral angle) (Karplus, M., *J. Am. Chem. Soc.*, 85, 2870–2871, 1963). Figure 12.5 illustrates this relationship, while Table 12.16 contains common $^3J_{H-H}$ values.

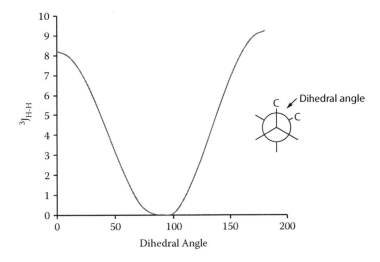

FIGURE 12.5   Variation of $^3J_{H-H}$ as a function of the dihedral angle.

TABLE 12.16
Common $^3J_{H-H}$ Coupling Constants

	$^3J_{H-H}$ (Hz)		$^3J_{H-H}$ (Hz)		$^3J_{H-H}$ (Hz)
Freely rotating	8	Cyclohexane axial-axial	10–12		8–10
	8–9	Cyclohexane axial-equatorial	2–5		14–16
	10–12	Cyclohexane equatorial-equatorial	0–5		9
	9–13	Cyclobutane	*trans* 5–9 *cis* 6–10		5
	4–8	Cyclopropane	*trans* 3–6 *cis* 6–10		3
	4–10		7.5		1

12.3.3.3   Long-Range Coupling Constants ($^{3+n}J_{H-H}$)

Couplings through more than three bonds are typically less than 1 Hz. An exception occurs when the bonds are fixed in a "W" conformation. Common $^{3}J_{H-H}$ coupling constants are listed in Table 12.17 (Williams and Fleming, Harwood and Claridge, and Friebolin, as above).

TABLE 12.17
Common J_{H-H} Coupling Constants

12.3.4   MODERN NMR TECHNIQUES FOR STRUCTURAL ELUCIDATION OF SMALL MOLECULES

Modern NMR experiments are used extensively for structure elucidation. A summary of the most important one- and two-dimensional methods for small molecules is given below. The experiments, which can be fully automated and used routinely in academic and industrial laboratories, are subdivided into homo- and heteronuclear one-dimensional methods and homo- and heteronuclear two-dimensional methods (see Friebolin, as above; Sanders, J. K. M., and Hunter, B. K., *Modern NMR Spectroscopy: A Guide for Chemists* (Oxford: Oxford University Press, 1993)).

12.3.4.1   1D Methods

12.3.4.1.1   APT (Attached Proton Test)

An experiment for assigning multiplicities to signals in decoupled ^{13}C spectra. The experiment shows all carbon signals (as opposed to DEPT) with CH and CH_3 appearing positive, while quaternary carbons and CH_2s appear as negative peaks.

12.3.4.1.2   DEPT (Distortionless Enhancement of Polarisation Transfer)

An experiment for assigning multiplicities to signals in decoupled ^{13}C spectra. It is more sensitive than the APT; however, it must be run with three different final pulse angles (45, 90, and 135) and compared to the original decoupled ^{13}C spectrum. DEPT 45 shows CH, CH_2, and CH_3 as positive; DEPT 90 shows CH as positive; DEPT 135 shows CH and CH_3 as positive and CH_2 negative.

*12.3.4.1.3   1D INADEQUATE (Incredible Natural Abundance
              Double Quantum Transfer Experiment)*

An experiment for obtaining $^{1}J_{C-C}$ values. The names are characteristic of the carbon-carbon bond order. For example, $^{1}J_{C-C} = 35$–45 for a C–C single bond while $^{1}J_{C-C} = 65$ for a double bond. The main decoupled signals are removed and the satellite peaks appear as positive and negative signals. The experiment requires ^{13}C-enriched or very concentrated samples.

12.3.4.2   2D Methods

*12.3.4.2.1 ^1H–^1H COSY (**C**orrelated **S**pectroscopy)*

An experiment that correlates spin-coupled protons. The spectrum contains a "diagonal," which contains the 1D spectrum. The correlated protons appear as cross-peaks off the diagonal; therefore, a pair of coupled protons, whose signals appear on the diagonal, and their associated cross-peaks form the corners of a square. A very useful experiment when overlapping signals and non-first-order effects complicate the 1D ^1H spectrum.

*12.3.4.2.2 ^1H–^1H TCOSY (**T**otal **C**orrelated **S**pectroscopy, also known*
*as HOHAHA (**Ho**monuclear **Ha**rtman **Ha**hn))*

An experiment that correlates spin-coupled protons. It differs from ^1H–^1H COSY in that correlations are seen between all protons in the spin system and not just those directly coupled. Correlations appear as cross-peaks.

*12.3.4.2.3 ^{13}C–^{13}C INADEQUATE (**I**ncredible **N**atural **A**bundance*
***D**ouble **Q**uantum **T**ransfer **E**xperiment)*

An experiment that correlates spin-coupled carbons. A very insensitive experiment that can be made practical if the sample can be ^{13}C enriched. At natural abundance extremely concentrated samples and long acquisition times are required; however, direct carbon-carbon connectivity can be obtained.

*12.3.4.2.4 ^1H–^1H NOESY (**N**uclear **O**verhauser **E**ffect **S**pectroscopy)*

An experiment that correlates protons that are close in space. The experiment can be performed in a 1D fashion (NOE or nOe) if individual resonances are preselected. Usually used for molecules with high molecular weights (>1,500). The diagonal contains the 1D spectrum; protons near to each other in space are correlated as cross-peaks that appear off the diagonal.

*12.3.4.2.5 ^1H–^1H ROESY (**R**otating **O**verhauser **E**ffect **S**pectroscopy)*

An experiment that correlates protons that are close in space. The experiment can be performed in a 1D fashion (NOE) if individual resonances are preselected. Usually used for molecules with low molecular weights (<800). The diagonal contains the 1D spectrum; protons near to each other in space are correlated as cross-peaks that appear off the diagonal.

*12.3.4.2.6 ^1H–^{13}C HMQC (**H**eteronuclear **M**ultiple **Q**uantum **C**oherence)*

An experiment that correlates spin-coupled protons and carbons. This experiment is selective for one-bond couplings and therefore provides direct carbon-hydrogen connectivity. The spectrum does not contain a diagonal; proton and carbon signals are correlated via cross-peaks.

*12.3.4.2.7 ^1H–^{13}C HMBC (**H**eteronuclear **M**ultiple **B**ond **C**oherence)*

An experiment that correlates spin-coupled protons and carbons. This experiment is selective for two- to four-bond couplings and therefore provides long-range carbon-hydrogen connectivity. The spectrum does not contain a diagonal; proton and carbon signals are correlated via cross-peaks.

13 Mass Spectrometry

James McCullagh

13.1 INTRODUCTION

A fundamental aspect of mass spectrometry is the formation of positive or negative ions and the subsequent gas phase measurement of their mass to charge ratio (*m/z*). A ubiquitous method of ion formation and analysis does not exist for all compounds, and hence a range of mass spectrometer systems has been developed with different ion sources, sensitivity, resolution, mass range, mass accuracy, and fundamental suitability for different compounds. This chapter provides information relevant to organic chemists preparing samples for mass spectrometry analysis or analysing their results. Since the first edition of *The Organic Chemist's Desk Reference* significant growth in mass spectrometer systems, performance, and their applications has taken place, and this section has been extended and updated to reflect these developments.

13.2 IONISATION TECHNIQUES AND MASS SPECTROMETER SYSTEMS

A number of different ionisation methods are used in mass spectrometry to form analyte gas phase ions. These are generated through the transfer of an electron to or from an uncharged analyte, protonation, de-protonation, cationisation, anionisation, or the transfer of charge from the solid to the gas phase. Table 13.1 lists a number of the more common ionisation methods used in organic mass spectrometry, and Table 13.2 provides comparative attributes, including appropriate ionisation techniques, for several common mass spectrometer systems.

TABLE 13.1
Common Ionisation Methods

Ionisation Sources	Sample Type	Typical Analytes	Ions Formed	Ion Sensitivity	Advantages	Disadvantages
Electrospray ionisation (ESI)	Nonvolatile liquids and solids in solution	Wide range of polar and nonvolatile compounds sufficiently basic to accept a proton (positive mode) or sufficiently acidic to lose a proton (negative mode)	$(M + nH)^{n+}$ $(M - nH)^{n-}$ $(M + cation)^+$ $(M + NH_4)^+$	~High femtomole	Amenable to a broad range of compounds, very little fragmentation, useful for LC/MS with nonvolatile compounds	Not amenable to nonprotonatable/de-protonable species such as hydrocarbons
Electron impact (EI)	Gasses, volatile liquids, and solids	Hydrocarbons Aromatics	M^+, M^-	~Low picomole	Fragmentation is characteristic for a given compound providing a uniquely identifiable mass spectrum	High energy, leads to multiple cleavages and rearrangements, complex mass spectra to interpret
Chemical ionisation (CI)	Gasses, volatile liquids, and solids	Small compounds (<1,000 Da) containing a heteroatom, for example, halogenated aromatics, sugars, and organic acids	$(M + H)^+$ $(M - H)^-$	~Low picomole	Soft ionisation technique; can form pseudomolecular ions with little fragmentation	Still leads to fragmentation and rearrangements
Matrix-assisted laser desorption (MALDI)	Volatile and nonvolatile solids	Synthetic and biopolymers and a wide range of polar and nonvolatile compounds; good for large molecules	$(M + H)^+$ $(M - H)^-$ $(M + cation)^+$ M^+	~Femtomole	Very little fragmentation, predominantly singly charged species formed; low sample volumes required	Analysis <500 Da prohibited due to prevalence of matrix ions
Fast atom bombardment (FAB)	Nonvolatile solids in solution	Carbohydrates, organometallics, peptides, nonvolatiles	$(M + H)^+$ $(M - H)^-$	~Picomole	Mild ionisation up to ~5,000 Da	Mass range limited; ESI has now largely replaced FAB due to greater sensitivity and ease of use
APCI	Soluble, polar, and ionic compounds	Small, soluble nonvolatile polar and ionic compounds	$(M + H)^+$ $(M - H)^-$ $(M + cation)^+$	~High femtomole	Very efficient ionisation at atmospheric pressure; very little fragmentation	Limited to molecular weights up to ~1,500 Da
Field desorption (FD)	Nonpolar compounds	High molecular mass, nonpolar compounds; good examples: larger organometallics	M^+, M^-, MH^+	~Micromole	Only molecular ions are formed, no fragmentation	Limited mass range and sensitivity, difficult to use, slow throughput, no automation; largely superseded by ESI and MALDI
Field ionisation (FI)	Any polar or nonpolar compound of low mass	Small molecules (<500 Da)	M^+	~Micromole	Only molecular ions are formed, no fragmentation, easier to use than FD	Limited mass range; requires an experienced operator

Source: Data compiled from Siuzdak, 2006; Watson and Sparkman, 2007.

TABLE 13.2
Typical Mass Spectrometers Used for the Analysis of Organic Compounds

Mass Analyser	Compatible Ion Sources	Accuracy (ppm)	Resolution (FWHM)	Mass Range (Da)	Typical Analysis
Time of flight	ESI, MALDI, APCI, EI, CI, FI	2–10	10,000–40,000	Unlimited	LC/MS, nanoelectrospray, proteomics, small molecules and metabolites
Magnetic sector	EI, ESI, FAB	3–10	30,000	10,000	Isotope ratio mass spectrometry and accelerator mass spectrometry
Quadrupole	ESI, EI, CI,	100	4,000[a]	4,000	Low-resolution LC/MS and GC/MS; triple quadrupole configuration provides MS/MS capability
Ion trap	ESI, EI, CI, MALDI	100	4,000[a]	4,000	LC-MS/MS, useful for accumulating ion when ion signal is weak
Fourier transform Ion cyclotron resonance	ESI, APCI, MALDI, EI,CI	0.1–5	>1,500,000	~250,000	Very high resolution, high-accuracy m/z analysis; LC/MS, nanoLC/MS, and MALDI

Source: Data compiled from Siuzdak, 2006.
[a] Large non-standard quadrupoles are available commercially.

13.3   INTERPRETING MASS SPECTRA AND MOLECULAR MASS

Interpretation of mass spectra depends on the type of mass spectrometer and ionisation technique used. Hard ionisation methods such as EI produce molecular ion fragmentation, which can be used to identify diagnostic fragmentation patterns and functional groups. Softer ionisation techniques such as ESI and MALDI provide pseudomolecular ion formation, and rules in accordance with spectral information can be used to identify corresponding molecular structure and elemental composition. Table 13.3 lists some of the types of information that can be provided by mass spectrometry, and Table 13.4 gives definitions of molecular masses that are highly relevant in mass spectrometry.

The molecular weight of a species has a significant effect on the number of possible molecular formulae associated with a certain mass accuracy, and Figure 13.1 demonstrates examples of this relationship for a range of mass measurement accuracies covered by current mass spectrometer systems.

TABLE 13.3
Interpreting Mass Spectra: Types of Mass Spectrometry Experiment for Organic Chemists

Mass Spectrometry Experiment	Information Provided by Experiment
Accurate mass measurement	Accurate mass measurement of a pseudomolecular ion such as $[M+nH]^{n+}$ found in a mass spectrum can be used to determine possible molecular formulae. Accuracy of 0.5 ppm is achievable using FT-ICR-MS, and typically TOF instruments can achieve 2 ppm with appropriate calibration.
Fragmentation pattern interpretation	EI mass spectra provide fragmentary ions that can be used as a fingerprint to identify species. This is suitable for small molecules (<1,000 Da), and most mass spectrometers were used for this until the development of softer ionisation techniques in the 1970s and 1980s.
High-resolution mass spectra	Resolution up to 40,000 (FWHM) is achievable using TOF MS, and FT-ICR-MS can provide resolution over 1,000,000. This is suitable for determining monoisotopic exact mass up to four decimal places.
Nitrogen rule	Nitrogen is the only element that does not have both odd or even valence and nominal mass. Valence (+3) is odd while nominal mass (14Da) is even. Any molecule that contains an odd number of nitrogen atoms will have an odd nominal mass. This can be used to limit the number of potential molecular formulae.
Low-resolution mass spectra	Suitable for determining the nominal mass of a molecular ion.
Isotopic abundance	Elements with distinctive isotope ratios (Cl, Br, and transition metals, for example) will provide a distinctive isotopic cluster in the mass spectrum of a compound. This can be used to identify the presence of elements within unknown compounds.
Isotope peaks and number of carbon atoms	For a compound containing carbon atoms the peaks representing ^{13}C [M + 1] will register an intensity 1.1× total number of C atoms.
MS/MS	Purposeful fragmentation of molecular ion peaks can be used to provide structural information. This technique has been exploited using ESI ionisation in conjunction with LC/MS for the identification of peptide and proteins.
Quantitation	ESI and MALDI ion intensities represent the ease with which an analyte will protonate or de-protonate, and hence generally cannot be used to compare concentrations between different compounds. However, for molecules with similar functional groups, ion intensity and concentration are often closely correlated. When internal and external calibration can be made, quantitation using ion intensities is possible.
IMS	Ion mobility mass spectrometry separates ions by their cross-sectional area as well as mass. This provides the opportunity to study conformational changes to a molecule's structure.

TABLE 13.4
Definition of Molecular Masses Relevant in Mass Spectrometry

Molecular Masses	Definitions	Example: $C_{25}H_{15}N_5O_{26}$	Calculated Mass
Average mass	Calculated using the average of the mass of each element weighted for its natural isotopic abundance	C: $25 \times 12.011 = 300.275$ H: $15 \times 1.0079 = 15.1185$ N: $5 \times 14.0067 = 70.0335$ O: $26 \times 15.999 = 415.974$	801.401
Nominal mass	Calculated using the mass of the most abundant isotope of each element	C: $25 \times 12 = 300$ H: $15 \times 1 = 15$ N: $5 \times 14 = 70$ O: $26 \times 16 = 416$	801
Monoisotopic mass	Calculated using the mass of the most abundant isotope of each element	C: $25 \times 12.000 = 300.000$ H: $15 \times 1.0078 = 15.1170$ N: $5 \times 14.0031 = 70.0155$ O: $26 \times 15.994 = 415.844$	800.9765
Exact mass	Calculated using the exact mass of a single isotope of each element in the molecule	C: $25 \times 12.000 = 300.000$ H: $15 \times 1.0078 = 15.1170$ N: $5 \times 14.0031 = 70.0155$ O: $26 \times 15.994 = 415.844$	800.9765
Accurate mass	Experimentally determined mass of an ion usually used to determine the molecular formula	Measured at 2 ppm mass accuracy	800.9740–800.9770

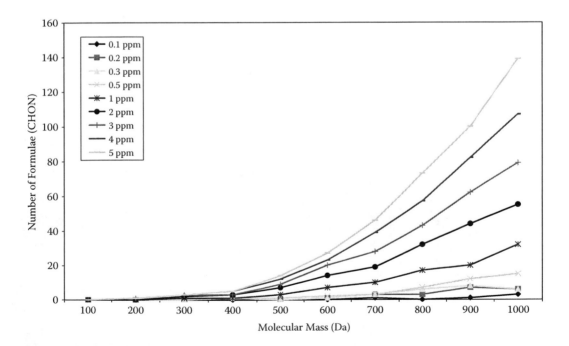

FIGURE 13.1 Shows the relationship between the number of molecular formulae and molecular mass for a range of mass measurement accuracies.

13.4 SAMPLE INTRODUCTION AND SOLVENT SYSTEMS FOR ELECTROSPRAY MASS SPECTROMETRY

Table 13.5 lists some common methods of introducing analytes for electrospray mass spectrometry, and Table 13.6 lists compatible electrospray solvent systems for organic compounds.

TABLE 13.5
Common Sample Introduction Methods using Electrospray Ionisation

MS Sample Inlet	Typical Flow Rates/ Quantity Used (µl/min)	Suitable Compounds
Direct infusion (ESI)	3–10	Nonvolatile solutions where sample is not limited
Nanoelectrospray	0.01–0.1	Single analysis of nonvolatile solutions where sample is limited
Nanomate direct infusion	0.05–0.5	Multiple analysis of nonvolatile solutions where sample is limited
LC/MS	200–1,000	Separation of mixtures in solution
Capillary LC/MS	1–100	Nonvolatile solids and liquids
nanoLC/MS	0.2–100	Nonvolatile solids and liquids

TABLE 13.6
Solvent Compatibility with Electrospray Ionisation

Common Solvents and Modifiers for ESI-MS	Suitability	Comments
Water	√	Water and organic solvent mixture is the default electrospray solvent system
Methanol	√	
Acetonitrile	√	
Dichloromethane	√	If mixed with methanol
Tetrahydrofuran	√	For air or protic sensitive samples use freshly distilled nitromethane
Nitromethane	√	
Ethanol, propanol, butanol	√	
Acetone	√	
Pyridine	√	
Acetic acid	√	
Volatile salts, e.g., ammonium acetate	√	
Volatile buffers, e.g., ammonium bicarbonate	√	
Trifluoroacetic acid (TFA)	Suitable in small quantities	Suppresses ion signal, particularly in negative ion mode; can be difficult to flush from the instrument, causing problems with negative ionisation.
DMSO	Suitable in small quantities	High viscosity and interaction with PEEK tubing
DMF	Suitable in small quantities	Difficult to maintain a stable ion signal
Benzene	X	
Toluene	X	
Carbon tetrachloride	X	
Hexane	X	
Involatile salts	X	
Involatile buffers e.g., potassium chloride	X	
Detergents	X	
Sodium Dodecyl Sulfate (SDS)	X	
EDTA	X	

13.5   COMMON ADDUCTS AND CONTAMINANTS IN MASS SPECTRA

Tables 13.7 and 13.8 provide examples of common adduct and contaminant ions found in positive and negative ionisation modes.

TABLE 13.7
Common Positive and Negative Molecular Ion Adducts

Positive Ion Mode	Negative Ion Mode
$[M + 23]^+$ (Na^+)	$[M+45]^-$ (Formate)
$[M + 32]^+$ (MeOH)	$[M+59]^-$ (Acetate)
$[M + 39]^+$ (K^+)	$[M+58]^-$ (NaCl)
$[M + 41]^+$ (CH_3CN^+)	$[M+78]^-$ (DMSO)
$[M + 59]^+$ ($CH_3CN + NH_4$)$^+$	$[M+113]^-$ (TFA)
	$[M+35.5]^-$ (chloride)

Source: Data compiled from Keller et al., 2008.

TABLE 13.8
Common Contaminants

m/z	Ion	Compound
33	$[M + H]^+$	Methanol
42	$[M + H]^+$	Acetonitrile
59	$[M + NH_4]^+$	Acetonitrile
64	$[M + Na]^+$	Acetonitrile
65	$[2M + H]^+$	Methanol
77	$[M + H]^+$	Polypropylene glycol
79	$[M + H]^+$	DMSO
83	$[2M + H]^+$	Acetonitrile
85	$[M + H]^+$	d_6-DMSO
88	$[M + H]^+$	Acetonitrile/formic acid
101	$[M + Na]^+$	DMSO
102	$[M + H]^+$	Triethylamine (TEA)
104/106	$[M + Cu]^+$	Acetonitrile
105	$[2M + Na]^+$	Acetonitrile
120	$[M + Na + CH_3CN]^+$	DMSO
122	$[M + H]^+$	Tris buffer
123	$[M + H]^+$	Dimethylaminopyridine
130	$[M + H]^+$	Diisopropylethylamine
144	$[M + H]^+$	Tripropylamine (TPA)
145/147	$[2M + Cu]^+$	Acetonitrile
146	$[3M + Na]^+$	Acetonitrile
150	$[M + H]^+$	Phenyldiethylamine
153	$[M + H]^+$	1,8-Diazabicyclo[5.4.0]undec-7-ene
157	$[2M + H]^+$	DMSO
169	$[2M + H]^+$	d_6-DMSO
179	$[2M + Na]^+$	DMSO
183	$[M + H]^+$	Diphenylketone
186	$[M + H]^+$	Tributylamine
225	$[M + H]^+$	Dicyclohexyl urea (DCU)
239/241	$[(M.HCl)2 - Cl]^+$	Triethamine
242	M^+	Tetrabutylammonium
243	M^+	Trityl cation
257	$[3M + H]^+$	DMSO
273	M^+	Monomethoxytrityl
279	$[M + H]^+$	Dibutyl phthalate (plasticiser)
301	$[M + Na]^+$	Dibutyl phthalate (plasticiser)
317	$[M + K]^+$	Dibutyl phthalate (plasticiser)
338	$[M + H]^+$	Erucamide
391	$[M + H]^+$	Diisooctyl phthalate (plasticiser)
413	$[M + Na]^+$	Diisooctyl phthalate (plasticiser)
429	$[M + K]^+$	Diisooctyl phthalate (plasticiser)
449	$[2M + H]^+$	Dicyclohexyl urea (DCU)
454	$[M + Na + CH_3CN]^+$	Diisooctyl phthalate (plasticiser)
798	$[2M + NH_4]^+$	Diisooctyl phthalate (plasticiser)
803	$[2M + Na]^+$	Diisooctyl phthalate (plasticiser)

Source: Data compiled from author's experience and Keller, B. O., Sui, J., Young, A. B., and Whittal, R. M., "Interferences and Contaminants Encountered in Modern Mass Spectrometry," *Anal. Chim. Acta*, 627, 71–81, 2008.

13.6   MALDI MATRICES

Table 13.9 provides details of suitable matrices for a range of common MALDI analytes and appropriate solvent systems.

TABLE 13.9
Common Matrices for MALDI

Common Sample Substrates	Common MALDI Matrices	Structure	m/z [M + H]+	Suitable Solvent
Peptides Polymers Intact bacteria	CHCA (α-cyano-4-hydroxy cinnamic acid)		189.04	Methanol Tetrahydrofuran Acetone
Proteins Peptides Polymers	Sinapinic acid (3,5-dimethoxy-4-hydroxycinnamic acid)		224.07	Methanol Tetrahydrofuran Acetone Ethanol/water
Polar and nonpolar synthetic polymers Oligonucleotides Proteins	HABA (2-(4-Hydroxyphenylazo) benzoic acid)		244.08	Tetrahydrofuran Acetonitrile/methanol
Resins Unsaturated aromatic polyesters	Dithranol (1,8-Dihydroxy-9(10H)-anthracenone)		226.06	Tetrahydrofuran Carbontetrachloride HFIP
Peptides Carbohydrates Glycolipids Glycopeptides Polymers	DHB (2,5-dihydroxybenzoic acid)		154.03	Methanol Acetonitrile Water
Polymethyl methacrylates	IAA (β-indole acrylic acid)		187.06	Acetone
Oligonucleotides Nucleic acids Carbohydrates Peptides	THAP (2,4,6-Trihydroxyacetophenone)		186.16	Acetonitrile Ethanol Water

13.7   FRAGMENTATION IONS AND NEUTRAL LOSSES

Hard ionisation techniques commonly fragment molecular ions, leading to the loss of neutral species and the formation of fragmentation ions. Some common species lost in mass spectra, and possible chemical inferences that can be drawn from this information, are shown in Table 13.10. In contrast, examples of common fragment ions that are formed are listed in Table 13.11.

TABLE 13.10
Some Common Fragments Lost in Mass Spectra

Ions	Groups	Possible Inference	Ions	Groups	Possible Inference
$M-1$	H	Labile H, aldehydes	$M-34$	H_2S	Thiol
$M-2$	H_2		$M-35, 37$	Cl	Labile chloride
$M-15$	CH_3		$M-41$	C_3H_5	Propyl ester
$M-16$	O	Nitro compound, sulfoxide	$M-42$	CH_2CO	Methyl ketone, aryl acetate
$M-16$	NH_2	Sulfonamide, carboxamide	$M-42$	C_3H_6	Butyl or isobutyl ketone, aryl propyl ether
$M-17$	OH	Acid, oxime	$M-43$	C_3H_7	Propyl ketone, $ArCH_2CH_2CH_3$
$M-17$	NH_3		$M-43$	CH_2CO	Methyl ketone
$M-18$	H_2O	Alcohol, aldehyde, ketone	$M-44$	CO_2	Ester, anhydride
$M-19$	F	Fluoride	$M-44$	C_3H_8	
$M-20$	HF	Fluoride	$M-45$	COOH	Carboxylic acid
			$M-45$	OC_2H_5	Ethyl ester
$M-26$	C_2H_2	Aromatic hydrocarbon	$M-46$	C_2H_5OH	Ethyl ester
$M-26$	CN	Aliphatic nitrile	$M-46$	NO_2	Aromatic nitro compound
$M-27$	HCN	Nitrile, nitrogen heterocycle	$M-48$	SO	Aromatic sulfoxide
$M-28$	CO	Quinone, phenol			
$M-28$	C_2H_4	Aromatic ethyl ether, propyl ketone	$M-55$	C_4H_7	Butyl ester
$M-29$	CHO	Ketone	$M-56$	C_4H_8	ArR (R = butyl, 2-methyl-propyl, pentyl, 3-methyl-butyl, pentyl ketone)
$M-29$	C_2H_5	Ethyl ketone, $ArCH_2CH_2CH_3$, ethyl ester	$M-57$	C_4H_9	Butyl ketone
$M-30$	C_2H_6		$M-57$	C_2H_5CO	Ethyl ketone
$M-30$	CH_2O	Aryl methyl ether	$M-58$	C_4H_{10}	
$M-30$	NO	Aromatic nitro compound	$M-60$	CH_3COOH	Acetate
$M-31$	OCH_3	Methyl ester	$M-79, 81$	Br	Bromide
$M-32$	CH_3OH	Methyl ester	$M-127$	I	Iodide
$M-32$	S	Sulfide, aromatic thiol			
$M-33$	$H_2O + CH_3$				
$M-33$	HS	Thiol			

Source: Data compiled from Wieser, 2006.

TABLE 13.11
Common Fragment Ions in Mass Spectra

m/e	Ion	Possible Inference
15	CH_3^+	
18	H_2O^+	
26	$C_2H_2^+$	
27	$C_2H_3^+$	
28	CO^+	Carbonyl compound
28	$C_2H_4^+$	Ethyl compound
28	N_2^+	Azo compound
29	CHO^+	Aldehyde
29	$C_2H_5^+$	Ethyl compound
30	$H_2C=NH_2^+$	Primary amine
31	$H_2O=OH^+$	Primary alcohol
35, 37	Cl^+	Chloro compound
36, 38	HCl^+	Chloro compound
39	$C_3H_3^+$	
40	$C_3H_4^+$	
41	$C_3H_5^+$	
42	$C_2H_2O^+$	Acetate
42	$C_3H_6^+$	
43	H_3CCO^+	H_3CCOX
43	$C_3H_7^+$	C_3H_7X
44	$C_2H_6N^+$	Aliphatic amine
44	$O=C=NH_2^+$	Primary amine
44	CO_2^+	
44	$C_3H_8^+$	
44	$H_2C=CH(OH)^+$	Aldehyde
45	$H_2C=OCH_3^+$	Ether, alcohol
45	$H_3CCH=OH^+$	Ether, alcohol
47	$H_2C=SH^+$	Aliphatic thiol
49, 51	H_2CCl^+	Chloromethyl compound
50	$C_4H_2^+$	Aromatic compound
51	$C_4H_3^+$	C_6H_5X
55	$C_4H_7^+$	Unsaturated hydrocarbon
56	$C_4H_8^+$	
57	$C_4H_9^+$	C_6H_9X
57	$H_3CCH_2CO^+$	Ethyl ketone, propionate ester
58	$H_2C=C(OH)CH_3^+$	Methyl ketone, dialkyl ketone
58	$Me_2N=CH_2^+$	Aliphatic amine
59	$COOMe^+$	Methyl ester
59	$H_2C=C(OH)NH_2^+$	Primary amide
59	$H_2C=OC_2H_5^+$	Ether
59	$C_2H_5CH=OH^+$	$C_2H_5CH(OH)X$
60	$H_2C=C(OH)OH^+$	Carboxylic acid
61	$H_3CCO(OH_2)^+$	Acetate ester
61	$H_8CH_2CH_2^+$	Aliphatic thiol
66	$H_2S_2^+$	Dialkyl disulfide
68	$N\equiv CCH_2CH_2CH_2^+$	RX (R = pyrrolyl)

TABLE 13.11 (continued)
Common Fragment Ions in Mass Spectra

m/e	Ion	Possible Inference
69	CF_3^+	
69	$C_5H_9^+$	
70	$C_5H_{10}^+$	
71	$C_5H_{11}^+$	$C_5H_{11}X$
71	$C_3H_7CO^+$	Propyl ketone, butyrate ester
72	$H_2C=C(OH)C_2H_5^+$	Ethyl alkyl ketone
72	$C_3H_7CH=NH_2^+$	Amine
73	$C_4H_9O^+$	
73	$COOEt^+$	Ethyl ester
73	Me_3Si^+	Me_3SiX
74	$H_2C=C(OH)OCH_3^+$	Methyl ester
75	$Me_2Si=OH^+$	Me_3SiOX
75	$C_2H_5CO(OH_2)^+$	Propionate ester
76	$C_6H_4^+$	C_6H_5X, XC_6H_4Y
77	$C_6H_5^+$	C_6H_5X
78	$C_6H_6^+$	C_6H_5+
78	$C_5H_4N^+$	RX (X = pyridinyl)
79	$C_6H_7^+$	C_6H_5X
79, 81	Br^+	Bromo compound
80, 82	HBr^+	Bromo compound
80	$C_5H_6N^+$	RCH_2X (R = pyrrolyl)
81	$C_5H_5O^+$	RCH_2X (R = pyranyl)
83, 85, 87	$HCCl_2^+$	$HCCl_3$
85	$C_6H_{13}^+$	$C_6H_{13}X$
85	$C_4H_9CO^+$	C_4H_9COX
85	$C_5H_9O^+$	RX (X = 2-pyranyl)
85	$C_4H_5O_2^+$	RX (R = 5-oxo-2-furanyl)
86	$C_4H_9CH=NH_2^+$	Amine
86	$H_2C=C(=OH)C_3H_7^+$	Propyl alkyl ketone
87	$H_2C=CHC(=OH)$ OMe^+	XCH_2CH_2COOMe
91	$C_7H_7^+$	$C_6H_5CH_2X$, $H_3CC_6H_4X$
91, 93	$C_4H_8Cl^+$	RCl (R = n-alkyl ≥ hexyl)
92	$C_7H_8^+$	$C_6H_5CH_2R$ (R = alkyl)
92	$C_6H_6N^+$	RCH_2X (R = pyridinyl)
93, 95	$BrCH_2^+$	$BrCH_2X$
94	$C_6H_6O^+$	C_6H_5OR (R = alkyl)
94	$C_5H_4NO^+$	RCOX (R = pyrrolyl)
95	$C_5H_3O_2^+$	RCOX (R = pyranyl)
97	$C_5H_5S^+$	RCH_2X (R = thienyl)
105	$C_6H_5CO^+$	C_6H_5COX
105	$C_8H_9^+$	$H_3CC_6H_4CH_2X$
107	$C_7H_7O^+$	$HOC_6H_4CH_2X$
107, 109	$C_2H_4Br^+$	
111	$C_5H_3OS^+$	RCOX (R = thienyl)

(continued on next page)

TABLE 13.11 (continued)
Common Fragment Ions in Mass Spectra

m/e	Ion	Possible Inference
121	$C_8H_9O^+$	$MeOC_6H_4CH_2X$
123	$C_6H_5COOH_2^+$	Alkyl benzoate
127	I^+	
128	HHI^+	
135, 137	$C_4H_8Br^+$	RBr (R = n-alkyl ≥ hexyl)
141	CH_2I^+	

13.8   NATURAL ABUNDANCE AND ISOTOPIC MASSES OF SELECTED ISOTOPES AND NUCLEAR PARTICLES

The mass difference a single electron makes is observable using high-accuracy mass spectrometry. Table 13.12 lists the atomic weight of a proton, neutron, and electron. Table 13.13 lists selected isotopes along with their atomic number, atomic weight, monoisotopic mass, and relative abundance.

TABLE 13.12
Atomic Weight of Nuclear Particles

Symbol	Name	Weight (amu)
H^+	Proton	1.0073
n	Neutron	1.0087
e	Electron	0.0006

TABLE 13.13
Natural Abundance and Isotopic Masses of Selected Isotopes

Element	Isotope	Atomic No. (Z)	Atomic Weight of Element (Ar)	Monoisotopic Mass $^{12}C=12.000$	Natural Abundance (%)
Hydrogen	^1H	1	1.00794(7)	1.0078250	99.9885(70)
Deuterium	^2H	1		2.0141018	0.0115(70)
Tritium	^3H	1		3.0160293	0.000137(3)
Helium	^3He	2	4.002602(2)	3.0160293	0.00137(3)
	^4He	2		4.0026032	99.999863(3)
Lithium	^6Li	3	6.941(2)	6.0151223	7.59(4)
	^7Li	3		7.0160040	92.41(4)
Beryllium	^9Be	4	9.01212(3)	9.0121821	100
Boron	^{10}B	5	10.811(7)	10.012937	19.9(7)
	^{11}B	5		11.009305	80.1(7)
Carbon	^{12}C	6	12.0107(8)	12.000000	98.93(8)
	^{13}C	6		13.003354	1.07(8)
	^{14}C	6		14.003241	1×10^{-14}
Nitrogen	^{14}N	7	14.0067(2)	14.003074	99.632(7)
	^{15}N	7		15.000108	0.368(7)
Oxygen	^{16}O	8	15.9994(3)	15.994914	99.757(16)
	^{17}O	8		16.999131	0.038(1)
	^{18}O	8		17.999160	0.205(14)
Fluorine	^{19}F	9	18.9984032(5)	18.998403	100
Neon	^{20}Ne	10	20.1797(6)	19.992440	90.48(3)
	^{21}Ne	10		20.993846	0.27(1)
	^{22}Ne	10		21.991385	9.25(3)
Sodium	^{23}Na	11	22.989770(2)	22.989770	100
Magnesium	^{24}Mg	12	24.3050(6)	23.985041	78.99(4)
	^{25}Mg	12		24.985837	10.00(1)
	^{26}Mg	12		25.982593	11.01(3)
Aluminium	^{27}Al	13	26.981538(2)	26.981358	100
Silicon	^{28}Si	14	28.0855(3)	27.976926	92.2297(7)
	^{29}Si	14		28.976494	4.6832(5)
	^{30}Si	14		29.973770	3.0872(5)
Phosphorus	^{31}P	15	30.973761(2)	30.973761	100
Sulfur	^{32}S	16	32.065(5)	31.972070	94.93(31)
	^{33}S	16		32.971458	0.76(2)
	^{34}S	16		33.967866	4.29(28)
	^{36}S	16		35.967080	0.02(1)
Chlorine	^{35}Cl	17	35.453(2)	34.968852	75.78(4)
	^{37}Cl	17		36.965902	24.22(4)
Bromine	^{79}Br	35	79.904(1)	78.918 337	50.69(7)
	^{81}Br	35		80.916 291	49.31(7)
Iodine	^{127}I	53	126.904 47(3)	126.904 468(4)	100

Source: Data compiled from Wieser, M. E., "Atomic Weights of the Elements 2005," IUPAC Technical Report, *Pure Appl. Chem.*, 78, 2051–2066, 2006.

Note: The number in parentheses indicates the uncertainty in the last digit of the atomic weight. Monoisotopic mass (relative atomic mass) refers here to the mass of a specific nuclide (isotope). Atomic weight from a specified source is the ratio of the average mass per atom of the element to 1/12 of the mass of an atom of 12C.

13.9   GLOSSARY OF ABBREVIATIONS AND TERMS COMMONLY USED IN MASS SPECTROMETRY

Amu	Atomic mass unit
APCI	Atmospheric pressure chemical ionisation
CI	Chemical ionisation
Da	Dalton
EI	Electron impact ionisation
ESI	Electrospray ionisation
FAB	Fast atom bombardment
FD	Field desorption
FI	Field ionisation
FT-ICR-MS	Fourier transform ion cyclotron resonance mass spectrometry
FWHM	Full width at half maximum
GC-C-IRMS	Gas chromatography combustion isotope ratio mass spectrometry
GC-MS	Gas chromatography mass spectrometry
ICP-MS	Inductively coupled plasma mass spectrometry
ICR	Ion cyclotron resonance
IMS	Ion mobility mass spectrometry
IRMPD	Infrared multiphoton dissociation
IRMS	Isotope ratio mass spectrometry
LC-MS	Liquid chromatography mass spectrometry
LDMS	Laser desorption mass spectrometry
LOD	Limit of detection
LOQ	Limit of quantification
M^+	Singly charged ion
$[M + H]^+$	Protonated pseudomolecular ion
$[M - H]^-$	De-protonated pseudomolecular ion
MALDI	Matrix-assisted laser desorption ionisation
MS/MS	Mass spectrometry–mass spectrometry (tandem MS)
m/z	Mass to charge ratio of an ion
QTOF	Quadrupole time of flight mass spectrometry
SIM	Selected ion monitoring
SIMS	Secondary ion mass spectrometry
SRM	Selected reaction monitoring
TIMS	Thermal ionisation mass spectrometry
TOF	Time of flight mass spectrometry

REFERENCES

Keller, B.O., Sui, J., Young, A.B., Whittal, R.M. 2008. Interferences and contaminants encountered in modern mass spectrometry. *Analytica Chimica Acta* 627: 71–81.

Siuzdak, G. 2006. *The Expanding Role of Mass Spectrometry in Biotechnology*. 2nd edition. San Diego: MCC Press.

Watson, T.J. and Sparkman, D.O. 2007. *Introduction to Mass Spectrometry*. 4th edition. Chichester: Wiley.

Wieser, M.E. 2006. Atomic Weights of the Elements 2005 (IUPAC Technical Report). *Pure Appl. Chem.* 78: 2051–66.

14 Crystallography

Maureen Julian

14.1 INTRODUCTION

Crystallography is the study of molecular and crystalline structures and their properties. The unit cell is the building block of the crystal. Once the unit cell has been measured and the fractional coordinates are known, then bond distances and angles can be calculated. By varying the temperature of the crystal, the coefficients of thermal expansion can be calculated from the change in the lattice parameters. By varying the pressure, the bulk modulus can also be calculated. Crystals exhibit symmetry such as rotation axes and glides and can be classified into 32 point groups and 230 space groups. The *International Tables for Crystallography* are the standard guide for the literature in crystallography. Volume A is devoted to the space group symmetries. Associated with every direct lattice is a reciprocal lattice. The planes of the direct lattice correspond to the points of the reciprocal lattice. Mathematical applications of the reciprocal lattice give straightforward calculations of the Bragg *d*-spacings and the interfacial angles of the crystal. X-rays were discovered in 1895, and x-ray diffraction is the main technique for studying molecular and crystal structures. The scattering and interference due to the individual atoms located within the unit cell contribute to the variation in intensity of the individual diffracted reflections. The structure factors are proportional to the coefficients in the Fourier series that are used to calculate an electron density map.

14.2 DEFINITIONS

Ångström (Å): A unit of length used in x-ray crystallography and spectroscopy, $1\text{Å} = 10^{-10}$ m = 0.1 nm = 10^{-8} cm.

Asymmetric unit: Smallest part of the unit cell that, when operated on by the symmetry operations, produces the whole unit cell.

Basis vectors: Linearly independent vectors **a**, **b**, and **c** that generate the lattice.

Bragg's law: $n\lambda = 2\,d_{hkl}\sin\theta_{hkl}$, where n is an integer, which is the order of the diffracted beam, λ is the wavelength of the incoming beam, d_{hkl} is the *d*-spacing, and θ_{hkl} is the Bragg angle for the *(hkl)* planes.

Bravais lattice: Classification of fourteen three-dimensional lattices based on primitive and nonprimitive unit cells. Named after Auguste Bravais, who first used them.

Bulk modulus, K: The reciprocal of the volumetric compressibility.

Crystal: A solid composed of atoms arranged in a periodic array.

Crystal systems: A classification of point groups as triclinic, monoclinic, orthorhombic, trigonal, tetragonal, hexagonal, or cubic as determined by symmetries.

Crystallographic direction: Vector between two lattice points where the direction is indicated by [*u v w*], where *u*, *v*, and *w* do not contain a common integer. The integers *u*, *v*, and *w* are called the indices of the crystallographic direction and specify an infinite set of parallel vectors.

Fourier series: Representation of a continuous periodic function expressed as a sum of a series of sine or cosine terms. It is useful for the calculation of electron density.

Fractional coordinates: Coordinates of the atoms written as fractions of the basis vectors.

Friedel's law: In diffraction patterns, the intensity of the *hkl* reflection is equal to the intensity of the $\bar{h}\,\bar{k}\,\bar{l}$ reflection. Therefore, all x-ray diffraction spectra have an inversion point.

Glide: Operation that is a product of a mirror and a translation that is a fraction of the lattice vector in the plane of the mirror. There are axial glides, double glides, diagonal glides, and diamond glides.

Interfacial crystal angle: The angle between the two normals to the crystal planes or crystal faces.

Lattice: (1) An array of points in a crystal with identical neighbourhoods. (2) An array defined by vector $\mathbf{t} = u\mathbf{a} + v\mathbf{b} + w\mathbf{c}$, where u, v, w are integers and $\mathbf{a}$, $\mathbf{b}$, $\mathbf{c}$ are basis vectors.

Lattice parameters: The scalar values a, b, c, α, β, and γ. Also called lattice constants.

Miller indices, *hkl*: Three relatively prime integers, *hkl*, that are reciprocals of the fractional intercepts that the crystallographic plane makes with the crystallographic axes. The **crystallographic plane** (*hkl*) is described by its Miller indices.

Point group: A group whose symmetry operations leave at least one point unmoved.

Reciprocal lattice: Array defined by vectors $\mathbf{H}(hkl) = h\mathbf{a}^* + k\mathbf{b}^* + l\mathbf{c}^*$, where $\mathbf{a}^*$, $\mathbf{b}^*$, $\mathbf{c}^*$ are basis vectors for the reciprocal lattice and h, k, l, are integers between $-\infty$ and $+\infty$.

Reciprocal lattice basis vectors: Given the basis vectors $\mathbf{a}$, $\mathbf{b}$, $\mathbf{c}$ in direct space, the reciprocal lattice basis vectors $\mathbf{a}^*$, $\mathbf{b}^*$, $\mathbf{c}^*$ are defined by the equation

$$\begin{pmatrix} \mathbf{a}^*\!\cdot\!\mathbf{a} & \mathbf{a}^*\!\cdot\!\mathbf{b} & \mathbf{a}^*\!\cdot\!\mathbf{c} \\ \mathbf{b}^*\!\cdot\!\mathbf{a} & \mathbf{b}^*\!\cdot\!\mathbf{b} & \mathbf{b}^*\!\cdot\!\mathbf{c} \\ \mathbf{c}^*\!\cdot\!\mathbf{a} & \mathbf{c}^*\!\cdot\!\mathbf{b} & \mathbf{c}^*\!\cdot\!\mathbf{c} \end{pmatrix} = \begin{pmatrix} 1 & 0 & 0 \\ 0 & 1 & 0 \\ 0 & 0 & 1 \end{pmatrix}$$

Space group: Symmetry group of a regularly repeating infinite pattern. Each group has an infinite set of translations. There are 230 space groups.

Unit cell: Parallelepiped defined by basis vectors $\mathbf{a}$, $\mathbf{b}$, and $\mathbf{c}$. Unit cell fills space under translation.

14.3 CRYSTALLOGRAPHIC POINT GROUPS

The periodicity of a lattice limits the number of compatible rotation operations to onefold, twofold, threefold, fourfold, and sixfold. This, in turn, limits the number of point groups to thirty-two. Point groups are used to describe individual molecules. Table 14.1 shows the thirty-two point groups in both the Hermann-Mauguin notation and the Schoenflies notation divided into seven crystal systems: triclinic, monoclinic, orthorhombic, tetragonal, trigonal, hexagonal, and cubic.

TABLE 14.1
Crystal Systems and Their Point Groups

Crystal System	Point Groups (Hermann-Mauguin)	Point Groups (Schoenflies)
Triclinic	1, $\bar{1}$	C_1, C_i
Monoclinic	2, m, $2/m$	C_2, C_s, C_{2h}
Orthorhombic	222, $mm2$, mmm	D_2, C_{2v}, D_{2h}
Tetragonal	4, $\bar{4}$, $4/m$, 422, $4mm$, $\bar{4}2m$, $4/mmm$	C_4, S_4, C_{4h}, D_4, C_{4v}, D_{2d}, D_{4h}
Trigonal	3, $\bar{3}$, 32, $3m$, $\bar{3}m$	C_3, C_{3i}, D_3, C_{3v}, D_{3d}
Hexagonal	6, $\bar{6}$, $6/m$, 622, $6mm$, $\bar{6}m2$, $6/mmm$	C_6, C_{3h}, C_{6h}, D_6, C_{6v}, D_{3h}, D_{6h}
Cubic	23, $m\bar{3}$, 432, $\bar{4}3m$, $m\bar{3}m$	T, T_h, O, T_d, O_h

Source: From Julian, M. M., *Foundations of Crystallography with Computer Applications* (Boca Raton, FL: CRC Press, 2008), p. 114.

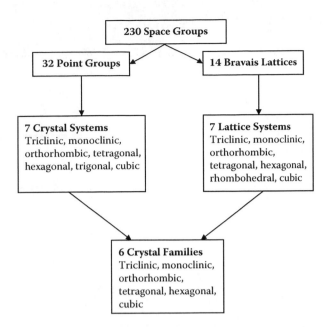

FIGURE 14.1 Classification of space groups. (From Julian, M. M., *Foundations of Crystallography with Computer Applications* (Boca Raton, FL: CRC Press, 2008), p. 174.

14.4   SPACE GROUPS

The usage of the terms *triclinic*, *monoclinic*, *orthorhombic*, *tetragonal*, and *cubic* is consistent for crystal systems, Bravais lattices, and crystal families. Unfortunately, the word *hexagonal* takes on three different meanings, depending on whether it is applied to crystal systems, Bravais lattices, or crystal families. The word *hexagonal* is found throughout the crystallographic literature and caution must be used in interpreting it (Figure 14.1).

14.5   RECIPROCAL LATTICE

Use of the reciprocal lattice unites and simplifies crystallographic calculations. The motivation for the reciprocal lattice is that the x-ray pattern can be interpreted as the reciprocal lattice with the x-ray diffraction intensities superimposed on it. See Section 14.2 for the definition of the reciprocal lattice vectors a^*, b^*, and c^* in terms of the direct basis vectors a, b, and c. Table 14.2 shows the parallel between the properties of the direct lattice and the reciprocal lattice, and Table 14.3 relates the direct and reciprocal lattices.

14.6   EXAMPLES OF ORGANIC CRYSTALS

Examples are shown in Table 14.4.

14.7   CIF DATA FORMAT

The Crystallographic Interchange File (CIF) format is used for distributing crystallographic information. It is an open-access system of distribution of information where no charge is made to the reader. See *Acta Crystallographica Section E: Structure Reports Online*, http://journals.iucr.org/e/. This journal contains structural information including the CIF file.

TABLE 14.2
Properties of a Direct Lattice in Parallel with Those of its Reciprocal Lattice

Direct Lattice

Direct lattice vector:

$$\mathbf{t}(uvw) = u\mathbf{a} + v\mathbf{b} + w\mathbf{c}$$

where $\mathbf{a}$, $\mathbf{b}$, $\mathbf{c}$ are basis vectors for the direct lattice, and u, v, w are integers between $-\infty$ and $+\infty$ (including zero)

$\mathbf{G}$, the metric matrix, for the direct lattice is

$$\mathbf{G} = \begin{pmatrix} \mathbf{a}\cdot\mathbf{a} & \mathbf{a}\cdot\mathbf{b} & \mathbf{a}\cdot\mathbf{c} \\ \mathbf{b}\cdot\mathbf{a} & \mathbf{b}\cdot\mathbf{b} & \mathbf{b}\cdot\mathbf{c} \\ \mathbf{c}\cdot\mathbf{a} & \mathbf{c}\cdot\mathbf{b} & \mathbf{c}\cdot\mathbf{c} \end{pmatrix}$$

Volume, V, of a unit cell in direct space is

$$V = \sqrt{\det(\mathbf{G})}$$

where $\det(\mathbf{G})$ is the determinant of $\mathbf{G}$

The dot product of two vectors in direct space is

$$\mathbf{t}(u_1\, v_1\, w_1)\cdot\mathbf{t}(u_2\, v_2\, w_2) =$$

$$(u_1\ v_1\ w_1)\, \mathbf{G} \begin{pmatrix} u_2 \\ v_2 \\ w_2 \end{pmatrix}$$

The magnitude squared of a vector in direct space is

$$t^2(u\ v\ w) = (u\ v\ w)\, \mathbf{G} \begin{pmatrix} u \\ v \\ w \end{pmatrix}$$

The $\cos\theta$ of the angle between two vectors in direct space is

$$\cos\theta = \frac{(u_1 v_1 w_1)\, \mathbf{G} \begin{pmatrix} u_2 \\ v_2 \\ w_2 \end{pmatrix}}{t_1 t_2}$$

where t_1 and t_2 are the magnitudes of the vectors $\mathbf{t}(u_1\, v_1\, w_1)$ and $\mathbf{t}(u_2\, v_2\, w_2)$, respectively

Reciprocal Lattice

Reciprocal lattice vector:

$$\mathbf{H}(hkl) = h\mathbf{a}^* + k\mathbf{b}^* + l\mathbf{c}^*$$

where $\mathbf{a}^*$, $\mathbf{b}^*$, $\mathbf{c}^*$ are basis vectors for the reciprocal lattice, and h, k, l are integers between $-\infty$ and $+\infty$ (including zero)

$\mathbf{G}^*$, the metric matrix, for the reciprocal lattice is

$$\mathbf{G}^* = \begin{pmatrix} \mathbf{a}^*\cdot\mathbf{a}^* & \mathbf{a}^*\cdot\mathbf{b}^* & \mathbf{a}^*\cdot\mathbf{c}^* \\ \mathbf{b}^*\cdot\mathbf{a}^* & \mathbf{b}^*\cdot\mathbf{b}^* & \mathbf{b}^*\cdot\mathbf{c}^* \\ \mathbf{c}^*\cdot\mathbf{a}^* & \mathbf{c}^*\cdot\mathbf{b}^* & \mathbf{c}^*\cdot\mathbf{c}^* \end{pmatrix}$$

Volume, V^*, of a unit cell in reciprocal space is

$$V^* = \sqrt{\det(\mathbf{G}^*)}$$

where $\det(\mathbf{G}^*)$ is the determinant of $\mathbf{G}^*$

The dot product of two vectors in reciprocal space isΣ

$$\mathbf{H}(h_1\, k_1\, l_1)\cdot\mathbf{H}(h_2\, k_2\, l_2) =$$

$$(h_1\ k_1\ l_1)\, \mathbf{G}^* \begin{pmatrix} h_2 \\ k_2 \\ l_2 \end{pmatrix}$$

The magnitude squared of a vector in reciprocal space is

$$H^2(h\ k\ l) = (h\ k\ l)\, \mathbf{G}^* \begin{pmatrix} h \\ k \\ l \end{pmatrix}$$

The $\cos\theta$ of the angle between two vectors in reciprocal space is

$$\cos\theta^* = \frac{(h_1\ k_1 l_1)\, \mathbf{G}^* \begin{pmatrix} h_2 \\ k_2 \\ l_2 \end{pmatrix}}{H_1 H_2}$$

where H_1 and H_2 are the magnitudes of the vectors $\mathbf{H}(h_1\, k_1\, l_1)$ and $\mathbf{H}(h_2\, k_2\, l_2)$, respectively

Source: From Julian, M. M., *Foundations of Crystallography with Computer Applications* (Boca Raton, FL: CRC Press, 2008), p. 215.

TABLE 14.3
Relationship between the Direct and Reciprocal Lattices

$$\mathbf{a} = \frac{\mathbf{b}^* \times \mathbf{c}^*}{V^*} \qquad \mathbf{a}^* = \frac{\mathbf{b} \times \mathbf{c}}{V}$$

$$\mathbf{b} = \frac{\mathbf{c}^* \times \mathbf{a}^*}{V^*} \qquad \mathbf{b}^* = \frac{\mathbf{c} \times \mathbf{a}}{V}$$

$$\mathbf{c} = \frac{\mathbf{a}^* \times \mathbf{b}^*}{V^*} \qquad \mathbf{c}^* = \frac{\mathbf{a} \times \mathbf{b}}{V}$$

TABLE 14.4
Examples of Crystallographic Data for a Few Organic Compounds

Name	Crystal System	Point Group	Space Group	a, Å	b, Å	c, Å	α, °	β, °	γ, °
Anthracene,[a] $C_{14}H_{10}$	Monoclinic	$2/m$	$P2_1/a$	8.559	6.014	11.171	90	124.58	90
Urea,[a] $CO(NH_2)_2$	Tetragonal	$\bar{4}2m$	$P\bar{4}2_1m$	5.576	5.576	4.692	90	90	90
Caffeine,[a] $C_8H_{10}N_4O_3$	Monoclinic	$2/m$	$P2_1/a$	14.8	16.7	3.97	90	95.81	90
Benzene,[a] C_6H_6	Orthorhombic	mmm	$Pbca$	7.460	9.66	7.034	90	90	90
Hexamethylbenzene,[b] $C_{12}H_{18}$	Triclinic	$\bar{1}$	$P\bar{1}$	5.2360	6.1845	7.9520	103.816	98.460	100.057
Muscle fatty acid binding protein[c]	Orthorhombic	222	$P2_12_12_1$	35.4	56.7	72.7	90	90	90

[a] ICDD, *Powder Diffraction File,* ed. W. F. McClune (Newton Square, PA: International Centre for Diffraction Data, 2000).
[b] CIF from library of crystal files in Centre for Innovation & Enterprise, *CrystalMaker Software Limited* (Oxford: Oxford University, 2006). See example in Section 14.7.
[c] Giacovazzo, C., Monaco, H. L., Artioli, G., Viterbo, D., Ferraris, G., Gilli, G., Zanotti, G., and Catti, M., *Fundamentals of Crystallography*, 2nd ed., ed. C. Giacovazzo (Oxford: Oxford University Press, 2002), p. 697.

A CIF file is given below[2] for hexamethylbenzene. Information includes chemical formula, formula weight, lattice constants, volume of unit cell, information from the *International Tables for Crystallography*, fractional coordinates of the individual atoms, and thermal parameters.[3]

```
_chemical_formula_sum      'C12 H18'
_chemical_formula_weight  162.274
_cell_length_a   5.2360
_cell_length_b   6.1845
_cell_length_c   7.9520
_cell_angle_alpha   103.816
_cell_angle_beta   98.460
_cell_angle_gamma  100.057
_cell_volume   241.4
_symmetry_int_tables_number   2
_symmetry_space_group_name_H-M      'P -1'
_symmetry_space_group_name_Hall     '-P_1'
loop_
```

```
_atom_type_symbol
_atom_type_oxidation_number
_atom_type_radius_bond
C       ?       1.200
H       ?       1.200
loop_
_atom_site_label
_atom_site_type_symbol
_atom_site_fract_x
_atom_site_fract_y
_atom_site_fract_z
_atom_site_occupancy
_atom_site_symmetry_multiplicity
_atom_site_Wyckoff_symbol
_atom_site_attached_hydrogens
_atom_site_calc_flag
_atom_site_thermal_displace_type
_atom_site_u_iso_or_equiv
C1   C -0.5659 -0.6165 0.3192 ? 2 i ? d Uiso 0.00670
C2   C -0.6790 -0.4306 0.3870 ? 2 i ? d Uiso 0.01400
C3   C -0.6131 -0.3167 0.5689 ? 2 i ? d Uiso 0.02160
C11  C -0.6485 -0.7475 0.1238 ? 2 i ? d Uiso 0.00870
C21  C -0.8704 -0.3491 0.2613 ? 2 i ? d Uiso 0.01830
C31  C -0.7526 -0.1236 0.6369 ? 2 i ? d Uiso 0.02960
H11A H -0.5128 -0.6816 0.0588 ? 2 i ? d Uiso 0.03800
H11B H -0.8232 -0.6994 0.0685 ? 2 i ? d Uiso 0.08940
H11C H -0.6745 -0.9230 0.1142 ? 2 i ? d Uiso 0.06450
H21A H -0.8658 -0.1752 0.3195 ? 2 i ? d Uiso 0.10270
H21B H -1.0648 -0.4342 0.2551 ? 2 i ? d Uiso 0.05150
H21C H -0.8067 -0.3714 0.1419 ? 2 i ? d Uiso 0.06000
H31A H -0.9516 -0.1777 0.5787 ? 2 i ? d Uiso 0.06080
H31B H -0.6463 0.0283 0.6208 ? 2 i ? d Uiso 0.03480
H31C H -0.7178 -0.0831 0.7800 ? 2 i ? d Uiso 0.03320
```

14.8   BRAGG'S LAW AND THE X-RAY SPECTRUM

In Bragg's law, $n\lambda = 2\,d_{hkl} \sin \theta_{hkl}$, where n is an integer, which is the order of the diffracted beam, λ is the wavelength of the incoming beam, d_{hkl} is the d-spacing, and θ_{hkl} is the Bragg angle for the (hkl) planes. The d-spacing is a property of the crystal, the Bragg's angle θ_{hkl} is an experimental observation, and the wavelength, λ, depends on the material in the x-ray tube. When high-speed electrons from the cathode crash into the anode, characteristic discrete x-rays are emitted. Two examples of the x-rays emitted are K_β and K_α, where $K_\beta > K_\alpha$. The wavelength of these x-rays depends on the atomic number, Z, of the material making up the anode. Table 14.5 shows the characteristic radiation for several elements with their atomic number. Different experiments may require different anodes in the x-ray tube.

14.9   CRYSTAL SPECIMEN PREPARATION FOR X-RAY ANALYSIS

There are two general crystal preparations for x-ray analysis. The first is for x-ray powder analysis and the second is for single-crystal analysis. These procedures complement one another. For x-ray

TABLE 14.5
Characteristic Radiation for Several Elements Commonly Used as Anodes

Atomic Number, Z	Element	K_α, Å	K_β, Å
24	Cr	2.29	2.08
25	Mn	2.10	1.91
26	Fe	1.94	1.76
27	Co	1.79	1.62
28	Ni	1.66	1.50
29	Cu	1.54	1.39

Source: Julian, M. M., *Foundations of Crystallography with Computer Applications* (Boca Raton, FL: CRC Press, 2008), p. 266.

powder analysis the sample consists of many, maybe thousands, of tiny crystals oriented randomly. The principal use of x-ray powders is for identification. For single-crystal analysis the idea is to grow a single perfect crystal. The latter group can be further divided into protein crystallography, or the study of biological macromolecules, and all other crystals.

14.9.1 PREPARATION OF X-RAY POWDERS

Over 250,000 x-ray diffraction patterns have been compiled in a library by the Joint Committee on Powder Diffraction Standards (JCPDS). Figure 14.2 shows the Powder Diffraction File (PDF) for hexamethylbenzene. The crystallographic information includes a literature reference, cell parameters, space group, volume of unit cell, density, intensity pattern, and identification of the diffraction

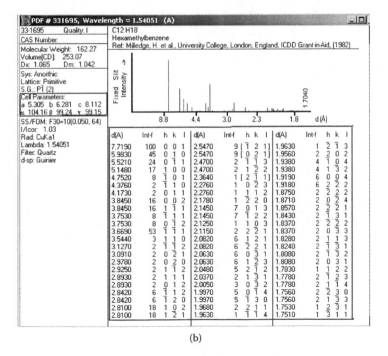

(b)

FIGURE 14.2 Powder Diffraction File (PDF) for hexamethylbenzene, PDF 33-1695.

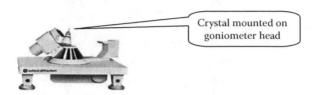

Crystal mounted on goniometer head

FIGURE 14.3   Goniometer head holding a crystal. (Oxford Diffraction Ltd.)

peaks. Note there is a difference, within experimental error of the parameters, between Figure 14.2 and Table 14.4.

Crystalline material is ground into equiaxial, randomly oriented grains of about 50 μm. Appropriate sieves can be used. The thin layer of crystals is spread onto a glass microscope slide or a holder specially designed for the particular x-ray diffraction setup. If there is preferred rather than random orientation of the grains, the diffraction pattern will be distorted.

14.9.2   PREPARATIONS OF SINGLE CRYSTALS

Single-crystal analysis is generally more difficult than powder analysis, but the results are more informative.

14.9.2.1   Protein Crystal Preparation

The growth of protein crystals is a difficult, complex, and often frustrating procedure. The protein crystal is precipitated from a supersaturated solution of the macromolecule in which the protein is partitioned between the solid phase and the solution. The pH value influences the solubility. Usually a pH is chosen near the isoelectric point of the macromolecule. Inorganic salts, organic solvents, and commercially available precipitating agents, such as the polymer PEG, can be helpful.

14.9.2.2   Single-Crystal Preparation (Nonmacromolecules)

The purer and more perfect the single crystal, the better the final analysis. The general methods are growth from solutions, sublimation, and solid-state synthesis. Nucleation and growth are competing processes that are usually performed in two stages. First, tiny crystals are quickly precipitated from hot solutions. Then these microcrystals are slowly grown over days or months, sometimes under refrigeration, until the appropriate size is reached.

Crystals that are unaffected by air, moisture, or light are usually mounted directly on a quartz or glass fiber, which is inserted into a goniometer head (Figure 14.3). If the crystal is sensitive to moisture or air, a sealed capillary tube may be used. Suitable apparatus can be used when nonambient temperatures and pressures are needed. The diamond anvil has been developed for high pressure.

ENDNOTES

1. These definitions are adapted from Julian, M. M., *Foundations of Crystallography with Computer Applications* (Boca Raton, FL: CRC Press, 2008), pp. 323–332.
2. Adapted from the library of crystal files in Centre for Innovation & Enterprise, *CrystalMaker Software Limited* (Oxford: Oxford University, 2006).
3. Hahn, T., ed., *International Tables for Crystallography: Space Group Symmetry*, Vol. A (Dordrecht, The Netherlands: International Union of Crystallography, Kluwer Academic Publishers, 2002).

15 Chromatographic Chiral Separation

Nelu Grinberg

Chirality plays a major role in biological processes and enantiomers of a particular molecule can often have different physiological properties. In some cases, enantiomers may have similar pharmacological properties with different potencies; for example, one enantiomer may play a positive pharmacological role, while the other can be toxic. For this reason, advancements in asymmetric synthesis, especially in the pharmaceutical industry and life sciences, has led to the need to assess the enantiomeric purity of drugs. Chromatographic chiral separation plays an important role in this domain. Today, there are a large number of chiral stationary phases on the market that facilitate the assessment of enantiomeric purity.

15.1 TYPES OF MOLECULAR INTERACTIONS

When a compound is synthesized in an achiral environment, the reaction product is obtained as a racemic mixture owing to the fact that in an achiral medium enantiomers are energetically degenerate and interact identically with the environment. Enantiomers can be differentiated only in a chiral environment, provided the proper conditions are offered by the chiral environment. Chiral separation is a very good example of dynamic supramolecular chemistry. Supramolecular chemistry aims at constructing highly complex, functional chemical systems held together by intermolecular forces.[1] Indeed, the interaction between the enantiomeric analytes (selectand) and the chiral phase (selector) can be through hydrogen bonding, inclusion interactions, charge transfer (π-π interactions), ligand exchange, or a combination. The chirality of the selector or the selectand can arise from an asymmetric carbon, the molecular asymmetry, or the helicity of a polymer. Also, the bonds between substituents of the selectand and the selector can involve a single bond, but could also involve multiple bonds or surfaces. Such bonds represent the leading interactions between selectand and selector. Only when the leading interactions take place, and the asymmetric moieties of the two bodies are brought into close proximity, do secondary interactions (e.g., van der Waals, steric hindrance, dipole-dipole) become effectively involved. The secondary interaction can affect the conformation and the energy of the diastereomeric associates. From a chromatographic point of view, the primary interactions affect the retention of the analyte on the chiral column, while the secondary interactions affect the enantioselectivity.[2]

15.2 DIASTEREOMERIC COMPOUNDS AND COMPLEXES

The chromatographic separation of enantiomers involves the formation of diastereomeric complexes between the enantiomers and the chiral environment. These diastereomeric complexes can exist as long-living species, or short-living complexes.

The long-living diastereomeric species are achieved by chemical reaction between a certain pair of enantiomers and a chiral derivatizing reagent. They can be separated in an achiral environment. Their formation energy has no relevance to their chromatographic separation. Their separation is due to the effect that their nonequivalent shape, size, or polarity, etc., has on their solvation energy. Differences in their shape and size are related to the differences in the energy needed to displace solvent molecules to create their nonequivalent solvation cage, while differences in all of the above parameters determine their differential interactions with the solvent molecules in their solvation cage.[3] The formation of diastereomers through chemical reactions has some advantages and disadvantages. The main advantage is that it employs an achiral stationary phase column, which is much cheaper than a chiral stationary phase column. The disadvantage stems from the fact that it relies on the functional groups existent in the molecule, which are capable of being chemically modified. On the other hand, since diastereomers are molecular species with slightly different physical properties, they may have different detector response factors upon elution from the column. As a consequence, a calibration curve is required for each diastereomer when quantitation is needed. The final quantitation results also rely on the purity of the derivatizing reagent.

Short-living diastereomeric species occur through the formation of transient diastereomeric complexes between the enantiomers and the chiral moiety present in the chromatographic column. Such complexes are usually not isolable and may be sufficiently energetically non-degenerate to be used to differentiate between a pair of enantiomers to be separated.[4,5] In the chromatographic system, the chiral agent is added into the mobile phase and constantly pumped through an achiral chromatographic column (the approach is called chiral mobile phases (CMPs)). Alternatively, the chiral agent is chemically bonded on a solid matrix such as silica gel or a synthetic polymer (chiral stationary phases (CSPs)). Each approach has some advantages and some disadvantages.

15.3 CHIRAL MOBILE PHASES

CMP's advantages stem from the fact that it is cheaper, since it uses achiral stationary phases, and the chiral additive can be purchased at a low cost; the approach is flexible, because after using a chiral additive, the chromatographic column can be washed out from the chiral additive and a new additive can be employed. On the other hand, the mechanism is difficult to predict due to the constant presence of a secondary chemical equilibrium in the column. Since the enantiomeric analytes are eluted out of the column as diastereomeric complexes, the detector response may be different for each complex. Also, the sample capacity is relatively small.

15.4 CHIRAL STATIONARY PHASES

The CSP approach also has advantages and disadvantages. The advantages stem from the fact that the mechanism of chiral separation is easier to predict. The enantiomers are eluted out of the column as enantiomeric entities; thus, they have the same detector response. The disadvantages consist of the high price of chiral columns and the fact that, as in the case of CMPs, the sample capacity is relatively small.

15.4.1 CHIRAL SEPARATION BY HYDROGEN BONDING

ChirasilVal is a chiral phase that works through hydrogen bonding interactions between the selectand and the selector, and is well known for its use for gas chromatographic chiral separation of amino acids. This chiral phase consists of a valine diamide incorporated into a polysiloxane. In order to make the amino acid analytes volatile, the amino and the carboxyl groups are blocked through an ester and an amide functional group, respectively. The interactions occur through hydrogen bonding between the amide and ester carbonyl functional groups of the selectand and the amide functional groups of the selector.

15.4.2   Chiral Separation by Inclusion Complexes

Cyclodextrins and chiral crown ethers are chiral phases where the predominant interactions are through inclusion. They are classified as host-guest complexes. These complexes are structured by contacts at multiple sites between the hosts (chiral phase) and the guests (enantiomeric analytes). The host can have a hydrophobic interior (i.e., cyclodextrins) or a hydrophilic interior (i.e., chiral crown ethers). The hydrophilic interior means that the cavity contains heteroatoms such as oxygen, where the lone pair electrons are able to participate in hydrogen bonding with compounds such as organic cations (i.e., ammonium ions). The chromatographic separation on these chiral phases is modulated by the addition of organic modifiers, such as alcohols or acetonitrile in aqueous buffers or mixtures of alcohols.

15.4.3   Chiral Separation by π-π Interactions, Hydrogen Bonding, and Ion Pairing

Another group consists of chiral phases, which work through a combination of π-π interactions with hydrogen bonding or π-π interactions with electrostatic interactions. The first group encompasses Pirckle type phases,[6–8] while the latter includes the Cinchona alkaloids type CSP.[9] The Pirckle type phases are based on derivatized amino acids with an aromatic moiety that can be either a π donor or a π acceptor. These chiral moieties are chemically bounded to silica gel. These CSPs undergo π-π interaction with selectands that have an aromatic moiety. The complex is stabilized through additional interactions such as hydrogen bonding, dipole-dipole interactions, or steric repulsion. An improved chiral stationary phase synthesized by Pirckle's group possesses both dinitrobenzoyl and naphthyl moiety, allowing for simultaneous face-to-face π-π interactions and phase-to-edge interactions. Such chiral phases operate with mobile phases consisting of a mixture of organic solvents such as hexane isopropanol.

The cinchona alkaloid-based stationary phases are chiral stationary phases where quinine/quinidine are chemically bonded to a silica gel matrix. The interaction between the selectand and selector is based on charge transfer π-π interactions as well as ion pairing with the selector. They operate under aqueous-organic mobile phases or mixtures of organic solvents such as hexane-alcohols.

15.4.4   Chiral Separation by Ligand Exchange

Ligand exchange chromatography (LEC) is the typical example of complexation chromatography. Complexes formed during LEC consist of a metal cation associated with ligands (anion or neutral molecules) that is able to donate electron pairs to a vacant orbital of the metal.[10] This technique is applicable for those enantiomers that are able to form metal complexes with the chiral moiety that is anchored to the stationary phase. Enantiomeric analytes such as amino acids and hydroxy acids were successfully separated using LEC. The technique uses aqueous-organic mobile phases containing a transition metal such as copper(*II*).

15.4.5   Chiral Separation by a Combination of Interactions

There are also stationary phases that interact with the selectands through a combination of the interactions, such as hydrogen bonding, π-π interactions, inclusion, hydrophobic interactions, and electrostatic interactions. These stationary phases include polysaccharides (cellulose derivatives, amylose derivatives),[11] protein phases,[12] and macrocyclic antibiotic phases.[13] The polysaccharide phases operate under mobile phase conditions that include aqueous-organic and mixtures of organic solvents such as hexane-alcohols. The protein phases operate under mixtures of aqueous-organic mobile phases, while the macrocycle mobile phases operate under mixtures of aqueous-organic mobile phases, as well as mixtures of acetonitrile-methanol with small amounts of additives (acetic acid and triethyl amine)—polar organic mobile phases.

REFERENCES

1. J.-M. Lehn. From supramolecular chemistry toward constitutional dynamic chemistry and adaptive chemistry. *Chem. Soc. Rev.* 36 (2007) 151.
2. N. Grinberg. Chiral separation in pharmaceutical industry. *Am. Pharm. Rev.* 9 (2006) 65.
3. B. Feibush. Chiral separation via selector/selectand hydrogen bonding. *Chirality* 10 (1998) 382.
4. N. Grinberg, T. Burokowski, and A. M. Stalcup. *HPLC for pharmaceutical scientists*, ed. Y. Cazakevich and R. Lobrutto. Hoboken, NJ: John Wiley & Sons, 2007.
5. W. H. Pirkle and T. C. Pochapsky. Theory and design of chiral stationary phases for direct chromatographic separation. In *Packing and stationary phases in chromatographic techiques*, ed. K. Unger. New York: Marcel Dekker, 1990.
6. W. H. Pirckle, C. J. Welch, and B. Lamm. Design, synthesis and evaluation of an improved enantioselective naproxen selector. *J. Org. Chem.* (1992) 3854.
7. W. H. Pirckle, D. W. House, and J. M. Finn. Broad spectrum resolution of optical isomers using chiral high performance liquid chromatography bonded phases. *J. Chromatogr. A* 192 (1980) 143.
8. W. H. Pirckle and D. L. Sikkenga. Resolution of optical isomers by liquid chromatography. *J. Chromatogr. A* 123 (1976) 400.
9. M. Lammerhofer and W. Lindner. Liquid chromatographic enantiomer separation and chiral recognition by Cinchona alkaloid-derived enantioselective separation materials. In *Advances in Chromatography*, Vol. 46, ed. E. Grushka and N. Grinberg. Boca Raton, FL: CRC Press, Taylor & Francis Group, 2008.
10. V. A. Davankov. Ligand exchange chromatography of chiral compounds. In *Complexation chromatography*, ed. D. Cagniant. New York: Marcel Dekker, 1992.
11. T. Ikai and Y. Okamoto. Structure control of polysaccharide derivatives for efficient separation of enantiomers by chromatography. *Chem. Rev.*, 109 (2009) 6077.
12. S. R. Narayanan. Imobilized proteins as chromatographic support for chiral resolution. *J. Pharm. Biol. Anal.* 10 (1992) 251.
13. I. D'Acquarica, F. Gasparini, D. Misiti, M. Pierini, and C. Villani. HPLC chiral stationary phases containing macrocyclic antibiotics. In *Advances in Chromatography*, Vol. 46, ed. E. Grushka and N. Grinberg. Boca Raton, FL: CRC Press, Taylor & Francis Group, 2008.

16 Laboratory Data and SI Units

16.1 SOLVENTS

16.1.1 POLARITY OF COMMON LABORATORY SOLVENTS

Solvents may be classified according to their polarity into three groups: *apolar aprotic solvents*, *dipolar aprotic solvents*, and (polar) *protic solvents*. Examples of these three classifications for some common laboratory solvents are listed in Table 16.1, in order of increasing polarity (indicated by dielectric constant), together with some other solvent properties. For information on the hazards and toxicity of solvents, see Chapter 11.

TABLE 16.1
Polarity Classifications and Some Properties of Common Laboratory Solvents

Solvent[a]	Bp (°C) (760 mmHg)	Mp (°C)	Dielectric Constant (ε) at 25°C[b]	Density (g/ml) at 20°C[c]	Solubility of Solvent in Water (wt%) at 25°C
Apolar Aprotic Solvents					
Hexane	69	−94	1.9	0.66	0.002
Benzene	80	+6	2.3	0.88	0.18
Toluene	111	−95	2.4	0.87	0.05
Diethyl ether	35	−116	4.3 (20°C)	0.71	6.0
Chloroform	61	−63	4.8 (20°C)	**1.49**	0.82 (20°C)
Ethyl acetate	77	−84	6.0	0.90	8.1
Dipolar Aprotic Solvents					
1,4-Dioxane	101	+12	2.2	**1.03**	Miscible
Tetrahydrofuran	66	−109	7.6	0.89	Miscible
Dichloromethane	40	−95	8.9	**1.33**	1.30
Acetone	56	−94	20.7	0.79	Miscible
Acetonitrile	82	−45	37.5 (20°C)	0.79	Miscible
Dimethylformamide	153	−61	37.0	0.94	Miscible
Dimethyl sulfoxide	189	+19	46.7	**1.10**	25.3
Protic Solvents					
Acetic acid	118	+17	6.2 (20°C)	**1.05**	Miscible
1-Butanol	118	−89	17.5	0.81	7.45
2-Propanol	82	−88	19.9	0.79	Miscible
1-Propanol	97	−126	20.3	0.80	Miscible
Ethanol	78	−117	24.6	0.79	Miscible
Methanol	65	−98	32.7	0.79	Miscible
Formic acid	101	+8	58.5	**1.22**	Miscible
Water	100	0	78.4	1.000	—

(continued on next page)

TABLE 16.1 (continued)
Polarity Classifications and Some Properties of Common Laboratory Solvents

a For more data on solvents, see Riddick, J. A., et al., *Organic Solvents: Physical Properties and Methods of Purification*, 4th ed. (Chichester: Wiley, 1986) and Lide, D. R., *Handbook of Organic Solvents* (Boca Raton, FL: CRC Press, 1995).

b For a detailed discussion of some quantitative indicators of solvent polarity, including dielectric constant, see Reichardt, C., *Solvent Effects in Organic Chemistry* (Weinheim: Verlag Chemie, 1979), pp. 49–51, etc.

c Densities of solvents heavier than water are in bold type.

16.1.2 SOLVENTS USED FOR RECRYSTALLISATION

Many solids may be purified by recrystallisation by dissolving the substance in a minimum quantity of hot solvent, filtering the solution, and then cooling the solution so that crystals of the desired substance form while the impurities remain in solution. A list of solvents commonly used for recrystallisation is given in Table 16.2.

In order to be useful, a solvent should dissolve much of the solid substance at higher temperatures and very little of it at lower temperatures. It should not react with the compound. Solvents with a high boiling point should be avoided if possible. Impurities do not have to be more soluble in the cold solvent than the substance being purified. Since the impurities are present at a lower concentration, they will frequently remain in solution even though less soluble.

In general, polar compounds (e.g., alcohols, thiols, amines, carboxylic acids, amides) tend to dissolve in (polar) protic solvents (e.g., water, alcohols). Nonpolar compounds tend to dissolve in (nonpolar) aprotic solvents (e.g., benzene, petrol, hexane).

Often it is possible to use a mixture of miscible solvents where the substance to be recrystallised is soluble in one of the solvents but relatively insoluble in the other. The solute can be dissolved hot in a suitable solvent mixture, which is then allowed to cool. Alternatively, the solute can be dissolved in the solvent in which it is more soluble either at elevated or at room temperature; the other solvent is then added until crystallisation just begins, and the resulting mixture is cooled to further induce recrystallisation.

TABLE 16.2
Solvents Commonly Used for Recrystallisation (solvents listed in approximate order of decreasing polarity)

Solvent[a]	Bp (°C) (760 mmHg)	Mp (°C)	Flash Point (°C); Flammability Classification	Good for	Second Solvent for Mixture	Comments[b]
Water	100	0	None	Salts, amides, carboxylic acids	Acetone, ethanol, methanol, dioxane	Products dry slowly
Methanol	65	–98	10; highly flammable	Many compounds	Water, diethyl ether, dichloromethane, benzene	

TABLE 16.2 (continued)
Solvents Commonly Used for Recrystallisation (solvents listed in approximate order of decreasing polarity)

Solvent[a]	Bp (°C) (760 mmHg)	Mp (°C)	Flash Point (°C); Flammability Classification	Good for	Second Solvent for Mixture	Comments[b]
Ethanol	78	−117	12; highly flammable	Many compounds	Water, petrol, pentane, hexane, ethyl acetate	
Acetone	56	−94	−17; highly flammable	Many compounds	Water, petrol, pentane, hexane, diethyl ether	Must not be used in combination with chloroform
2-Methoxyethanol	125	−86	43; flammable	Sugars	Water, benzene, diethyl ether	
Pyridine	116	−42	20; flammable	High-melting compounds	Water, methanol, petrol, pentane, hexane	Difficult to remove
Dichloromethane	40	−95	None	Low-melting compounds	Ethanol, methanol, petrol, pentane, hexane	Easily removed
Methyl acetate	56	−98	−9; highly flammable	Many compounds	Water, diethyl ether	
Acetic acid	118	+17	39; flammable	Salts, amides, carboxylic acids	Water	Difficult to remove; pungent odour
Ethyl acetate	77	−84	−4; highly flammable	Many compounds	Diethyl ether, benzene, petrol, pentane, hexane	
Chloroform	61	−63	None	Many compounds	Ethanol, petrol, pentane, hexane	Hepatotoxic and nephrotoxic; must not be used in combination with acetone; traces can affect microanalytical data
Diethyl ether	35	−116	−45; extremely flammable	Low-melting compounds	Acetone, methanol, ethanol, petrol, pentane, hexane	
1,4-Dioxane	101	+12	11; highly flammable	Amides	Water, benzene, petrol, pentane, hexane	Peroxidation hazard

(continued on next page)

TABLE 16.2 (continued)
Solvents Commonly Used for Recrystallisation (solvents listed in approximate order of decreasing polarity)

Solvent[a]	Bp (°C) (760 mmHg)	Mp (°C)	Flash Point (°C); Flammability Classification	Good for	Second Solvent for Mixture	Comments[b]
Tetrachloromethane (carbon tetrachloride)	77	−21	None	Nonpolar compounds	Diethyl ether, benzene, petrol, pentane, hexane	Reacts with some nitrogen bases; hepatotoxic and nephrotoxic; traces can affect microanalytical data
Toluene	111	−95	4; highly flammable	Aromatics, hydrocarbons	Diethyl ether, ethyl acetate, petrol, pentane, hexane	
Benzene	80	+6	−11; highly flammable	Aromatics, hydrocarbons	Diethyl ether, ethyl acetate, petrol, pentane, hexane	Human carcinogen (IARC Group 1)
Petrol	—[c]	—[c]	−40; extremely flammable	Hydrocarbons	Most solvents	
Pentane	36	−129	−49; extremely flammable	Hydrocarbons	Most solvents	
Hexane	69	−94	−23; highly flammable	Hydrocarbons	Most solvents	

Source: Based on information in Gordon, A. J., and Ford, R. A., *The Chemist's Companion* (New York: Wiley-Interscience, 1972), pp. 442–443. Reprinted with permission of John Wiley & Sons, Inc.

[a] For more data on solvents, see Riddick, J. A., et al., *Organic Solvents: Physical Properties and Methods of Purification*, 4th ed. (Chichester: Wiley, 1986) and Lide, D. R., *Handbook of Organic Solvents* (Boca Raton, FL: CRC Press, 1995).

[b] Comments apply to the main solvent.

[c] Petrol refers to a mixture of alkanes obtainable in a number of grades based on boiling ranges, e.g., 40–60°C and 60–80°C.

16.1.3 SOLVENTS USED FOR EXTRACTION OF AQUEOUS SOLUTIONS

A list of some solvents suitable for the extraction of aqueous solutions is given in Table 16.3.

TABLE 16.3
Solvents for Extracting Aqueous Solutions

Solvent	Bp (°C) (760 mmHg)	Density Relative to Water	Solubility of Solvent in Water (wt%)	Solubility of Water in Solvent (wt%)	Comments
Benzene	80	Lighter	0.18	0.06	Tends to form emulsion
2-Butanol	99	Lighter	12.5	44.1	Dries easily; good for highly polar water-soluble materials from buffered solution

TABLE 16.3 (continued)
Solvents for Extracting Aqueous Solutions

Solvent	Bp (°C) (760 mmHg)	Density Relative to Water	Solubility of Solvent in Water (wt%)	Solubility of Water in Solvent (wt%)	Comments
Tetrachloromethane (carbon tetrachloride)	77	Heavier	0.08	0.01	Dries easily; good for nonpolar materials; environmental hazard
Chloroform	61	Heavier	0.82	0.09	May form emulsion; dries easily
Diethyl ether	35	Lighter	6.04	1.47	Absorbs large amounts of water
Diisopropyl ether	69	Lighter	1.2	0.57	Tends to peroxidise on storage
Ethyl acetate	77	Lighter	8.08	2.94	Absorbs large amounts of water; good for polar materials
Dichloromethane	40	Heavier	1.30	0.02	May form emulsions; dries easily
Pentane	36	Lighter	0.004	0.01	Dries easily
Hexane	69	Lighter	0.002	0.01	Dries easily

Source: Based, in part, on information in Gordon, A. J., and Ford, R. A., *The Chemist's Companion* (New York: Wiley-Interscience, 1972), p. 444. Reprinted with permission of John Wiley & Sons, Inc.

16.1.4 COMMERCIAL AND COMMON NAME SOLVENTS

See Table 16.4.

TABLE 16.4
Commercial and Common Name Solvents

Commercial Name	Chemical Name	Molecular Formula	R	R'	Bp (°C) (760 mmHg)
(a) Carbitols. Diethylene Glycol Ethers ($ROCH_2CH_2OCH_2CH_2OR'$)					
Methyl carbitol	2-(2-Methoxyethoxy)ethanol	$C_5H_{12}O_3$	Me	H	193
Carbitol; ethyl carbitol	2-(2-Ethoxyethoxy)ethanol	$C_6H_{14}O_3$	Et	H	195
Diethyl carbitol	1,1'-Oxybis[2-ethoxyethane]; bis(2-ethoxyethyl) ether	$C_8H_{18}O_3$	Et	Et	189
(b) Cellosolves. Ethylene glycol ethers ($ROCH_2CH_2OR'$)					
Cellosolve	2-Ethoxyethanol	$C_4H_{10}O_2$	Et	H	135 (743 mmHg)
Dimethylcellosolve; glyme	1,2-Dimethoxyethane	$C_4H_{10}O_2$	Me	Me	85
Diethylcellosolve	1,2-Diethoxyethane	$C_6H_{14}O$	Et	Et	121
Methylcellosolve	2-Methoxyethanol	$C_3H_8O_2$	Me	H	124
Cellosolve acetate	2-Ethoxyethyl acetate	$C_6H_{12}O_3$	Et	$COCH_3$	156
Butylcellosolve	2-Butoxyethanol	$C_6H_{14}O_2$	Bu	H	171

(c) Glymes. $CH_3O(CH_2CH_2O)_nCH_3$

Commercial Name	Chemical Name	n	Molecular Formula	Bp (°C) (760 mmHg)
Glyme; dimethylcellosolve	1,2-Dimethoxyethane	1	$C_4H_{10}O_2$	83
Diglyme	1,1'-Oxybis[2-methoxyethane], bis(2-methoxyethyl) ether	2	$C_6H_{14}O_3$	161

(continued on next page)

TABLE 16.4 (continued)
Commercial and Common Name Solvents

Commercial Name	Chemical Name	n	Molecular Formula	Bp (°C) (760 mmHg)
Triglyme	1,2-Bis(2-methoxyethoxy)ethane	3	$C_8H_{18}O_4$	216
Tetraglyme	2,5,8,11,14-Pentaoxapentadecane	4	$C_{10}H_{22}O_5$	275–276; 119 (2 mmHg)

(d) Hydrocarbon Petroleum Fractions

Kerosene (also kerosine)	A distillate mixture obtained from crude petroleum, boiling range about 150–300°C.
Naphtha	A generic term for hydrocarbon distillates produced from either petroleum or coal tar. Petroleum naphthas are mixtures of hydrocarbons obtained as distillate fractions from crude petroleum, e.g., with a bp range 175–240°C. The term naphtha is also applied to other (and narrower) bp ranges. Solvent naphtha is a coal-tar distillate consisting mainly of aromatic hydrocarbons.
Petroleum ether (light petroleum)	Fractions of refined petroleum containing mainly short-chain hydrocarbons (pentane, hexane, and heptane isomers) with specified boiling point ranges, e.g., 40–60°C, 60–80°C, 80–100°C, and 100–120°C. The term *ligroin* is sometimes used for higher-boiling-point petroleum ether fractions (typically 130–145°C), but is also associated with lower bp ranges. In the older chemical literature, petroleum ether, petroleum spirits, ligroin, naphtha, and petroleum benzin(e) are synonyms.
Skellysolves	Saturated hydrocarbon mixtures:
Skellysolve A	Mostly pentane, bp range 28–38°C
Skellysolve B	Mostly hexane, bp range 60–71°C
Skellysolve C	Mostly heptane, bp range 88–100°C
Skellysolve D	Mixed heptanes, bp range 80–119°C
Skellysolve E	Mixed octanes, bp range 100–140°C
Skellysolve F	Petroleum ether, bp range 35–60°C
Skellysolve G	Petroleum ether, bp range 40–75°C

16.2   BUFFER SOLUTIONS

A list of buffer solutions that show round values of pH at 25°C is given in Table 16.5. The final volume of all the mixtures is adjusted to 100 ml.

TABLE 16.5
Buffer Solutions[a] Giving Round Values at 25°C

A		B		C		D		E	
pH	x	pH	x	pH	x	pH	x	pH	x
1.00	67.0	2.20	49.5	4.10	1.3	5.80	3.6	7.00	46.6
1.10	52.8	2.30	45.8	4.20	3.0	5.90	4.6	7.10	45.7
1.20	42.5	2.40	42.2	4.30	4.7	6.00	5.6	7.20	44.7
1.30	33.6	2.50	38.8	4.40	6.6	6.10	6.8	7.30	43.4
1.40	26.6	2.60	35.4	4.50	8.7	6.20	8.1	7.40	42.0
1.50	20.7	2.70	32.1	4.60	11.1	6.30	9.7	7.50	40.3
1.60	16.2	2.80	28.9	4.70	13.6	6.40	11.6	7.60	38.5
1.70	13.0	2.90	25.7	4.80	16.5	6.50	13.9	7.70	36.6
1.80	10.2	3.00	22.3	4.90	19.4	6.60	16.4	7.80	34.5
1.90	8.1	3.10	18.8	5.00	22.6	6.70	19.3	7.90	32.0

TABLE 16.5 (continued)
Buffer Solutions[a] Giving Round Values at 25°C

A		B		C		D		E	
pH	x	pH	x	pH	x	pH	x	pH	x
2.00	6.5	3.20	15.7	5.10	25.5	6.80	22.4	8.00	29.2
2.10	5.1	3.30	12.9	5.20	28.8	6.90	25.9	8.10	26.2
2.20	3.9	3.40	10.4	5.30	31.6	7.00	29.1	8.20	22.9
		3.50	8.2	5.40	34.1	7.10	32.1	8.30	19.9
		3.60	6.3	5.50	36.6	7.20	34.7	8.40	17.2
		3.70	4.5	5.60	38.8	7.30	37.0	8.50	14.7
		3.80	2.9	5.70	40.6	7.40	39.1	8.60	12.2
		3.90	1.4	5.80	42.3	7.50	40.9	8.70	10.3
		4.00	0.1	5.90	43.7	7.60	42.4	8.80	8.5
						7.70	43.5	8.90	7.0
						7.80	44.5	9.00	5.7
						7.90	45.3		
						8.00	46.1		

F		G		H		I		J	
pH	x	pH	x	pH	x	pH	x	pH	x
8.00	20.5	9.20	0.9	9.60	5.0	10.90	3.3	12.00	6.0
8.10	19.7	9.30	3.6	9.70	6.2	11.00	4.1	12.10	8.0
8.20	18.8	9.40	6.2	9.80	7.6	11.10	5.1	12.20	12.2
8.30	17.7	9.50	8.8	9.90	9.1	11.20	6.3	12.30	12.8
8.40	16.6	9.60	11.1	10.00	10.7	11.30	7.6	12.40	16.2
8.50	15.2	9.70	13.1	10.10	12.2	11.40	9.1	12.50	20.4
8.60	13.5	9.80	15.0	10.20	13.8	11.50	11.1	12.60	25.6
8.70	11.6	9.90	16.7	10.30	15.2	11.60	13.5	12.70	32.2
8.80	9.6	10.00	18.3	10.40	16.5	11.70	16.2	12.80	41.2
8.90	7.1	10.10	19.5	10.50	17.8	11.80	19.4	12.90	53.0
9.00	4.6	10.20	20.5	10.60	19.1	11.90	23.0	13.00	66.0
9.10	2.0	10.30	21.3	10.70	20.2	12.00	26.9		
		10.40	22.1	10.80	21.2				
		10.50	22.7	10.90	22.0				
		10.60	23.3	11.00	22.7				
		10.70	23.8						
		10.80	24.25						

Source: Reproduced with permission from *CRC Handbook of Chemistry and Physics 2008–2009*, 89th ed., D. R. Lide (Boca Raton, FL: CRC Press, 2008).

[a] The buffer solutions are made up as follows:

   (A) 25 ml of 0.2 molar KCl + x ml of 0.2 molar HCl

   (B) 50 ml of 0.1 molar potassium hydrogen phthalate + x ml of 0.1 molar HCl

   (C) 50 ml of 0.1 molar potassium hydrogen phthalate + x ml of 0.1 molar NaOH

   (D) 50 ml of 0.1 molar potassium dihydrogen phosphate + x ml 0.1 molar NaOH

   (E) 50 ml of 0.1 molar tris(hydroxymethyl)aminomethane + x ml of 0.1 molar HCl

   (F) 50 ml of 0.025 molar borax + x ml of 0.1 molar HCl

   (G) 50 ml of 0.025 molar borax + x ml of 0.1 molar NaOH

   (H) 50 ml of 0.05 molar sodium bicarbonate + x ml of 0.1 molar NaOH

   (I) 50 ml of 0.05 molar disodium hydrogen phosphate + x ml of 0.1 molar NaOH

   (J) 25 ml of 0.2 molar KCl + x ml 0.2 molar NaOH

16.3   ACID AND BASE DISSOCIATION CONSTANTS

16.3.1   First Dissociation Constants of Organic Acids in Aqueous Solution at 298 K

The pK_{a1} values are shown in Table 16.6.

TABLE 16.6
The pK_{a1} Values of Some Organic Acids in Aqueous Solution at 298 K

pK_{a1}	Compound	pK_{a1}	Compound
0.17	1-Naphthalenesulfonic acid	3.12	Iodoacetic acid
0.29	2,4,6-Trinitrophenol	3.13	Citric acid
0.66	Trichloroacetic acid	3.17	2-Furancarboxylic acid
0.70	Benzenesulfonic acid	3.22	Tartaric acid (*meso-*)
1.10	Nitrilotriacetic acid	3.23	2-Aminobenzoic acid
1.25	Oxalic acid	3.33	Ethanethioic acid
1.48	Dichloroacetic acid	3.40	Hydroxybutanedioic acid
1.70	Histidine	3.44	4-Nitrobenzoic acid
1.71	Cysteine	3.46	Glyoxylic acid
1.75	2-Butynedioic acid	3.49	3-Nitrobenzoic acid
1.82	Arginine	3.51	1,4-Benzenedicarboxylic acid
1.83	Maleic acid	3.54	1,3-Benzenedicarboxylic acid
1.95	Proline	3.60	Mercaptoacetic acid
1.99	Aspartic acid (α-COOH)	3.70	1-Naphthalenecarboxylic acid
2.04	Lysine	3.74	Formic acid
2.09	Threonine	3.83	Hydroxyacetic acid
2.14	Asparagine	3.86	2-Hydroxypropanoic acid
2.17	Glutamine	3.91	2-Methylbenzoic acid
2.17	Tyrosine	4.01	2,4,6(1*H*,3*H*,5*H*)-Pyrimidinetrione
2.17	2-Nitrobenzoic acid	4.08	3-Hydroxybenzoic acid
2.19	Serine	4.09	2,4-Dinitrophenol
2.20	Methionine	4.16	Succinic acid
2.23	Glutamic acid (α-COOH)	4.17	2-Naphthalenecarboxylic acid
2.23	Fluoroacetic acid	4.20	Benzoic acid
2.29	Valine	4.26	2-Propenoic acid
2.32	Isoleucine	4.27	3-Methylbenzoic acid
2.32	Leucine	4.30	Ascorbic acid
2.35	Glycine	4.31	Phenylacetic acid
2.35	Tryptophan	4.34	Pentanedioic acid
2.35	Alanine	4.36	4-Methylbenzoic acid
2.49	Pyruvic acid	4.43	Hexanedioic acid
2.69	Bromoacetic acid	4.44	3-Phenyl-2-propenoic acid (*E*-)
2.85	Propanedioic acid	4.48	Heptanedioic acid
2.86	Chloroacetic acid	4.58	4-Hydroxybenzoic acid
2.89	1,2-Benzenedioic acid	4.69	2-Butenoic acid (*E*-)
2.95	Phosphoric acid	4.78	Acetic acid
2.97	2-Hydroxybenzoic acid	4.78	3-Methylbutanoic acid
2.98	Tartaric acid ((±)-)	4.78	3-Aminobenzoic acid
3.05	Fumaric acid	4.83	Butanoic acid

TABLE 16.6 (continued)
The pK_{a1} Values of Some Organic Acids in Aqueous Solution at 298 K

pK_{a1}	Compound	pK_{a1}	Compound
4.84	Pentanoic acid	8.85	3-Chlorophenol
4.84	2-Methylpropanoic acid	9.12	1,2-Benzenediol
4.85	3-Pyridinecarboxylic acid	9.18	4-Chlorophenol
4.87	Propanoic acid	9.34	1-Naphthol
4.88	Hexanoic acid	9.51	2-Naphthol
4.89	Octanoic acid	9.91	1,4-Benzenediol
4.92	4-Aminobenzoic acid	9.99	Phenol
4.96	4-Pyridinecarboxylic acid	10.01	3-Methylphenol
5.03	2,2-Dimethylpropanoic acid	10.17	4-Methylphenol
5.22	3,6-Dinitrophenol	10.20	2-Methylphenol
5.52	2-Pyridinecarboxylic acid	14.15	Glycerol
8.49	2-Chlorophenol		

16.3.2 DISSOCIATION CONSTANTS OF ORGANIC BASES IN AQUEOUS SOLUTION AT 298 K

The pK_a values of some bases are listed in Table 16.7. The dissociation constant of a base B is given in terms of the pK_a value of its conjugate acid BH⁺. The pK_b of a base may be calculated from the pK_a value of its conjugate acid using the equation

$$pK_b = pK_w - pK_a$$

At 298 K this becomes

$$pK_b = 14.00 - pK_a$$

TABLE 16.7
The pK_a Values of Some Organic Bases in Aqueous Solution at 298 K

pK_a	Compound	pK_a	Compound
0.10	Urea	3.12	Nicotine
0.60	1,2-Benzenediamine	3.52	3-Chloroaniline
0.63	Acetamide	3.92	1-Naphthaleneamine
0.65	Pyrazine	4.05	Pteridine
0.79	Diphenylamine	4.12	Adenine
1.00	4-Nitroaniline	4.13	Quinine
2.24	Pyridazine	4.14	4-Chloroaniline
2.30	1,3-Benzenediamine	4.16	2-Naphthaleneamine
2.30	Purine	4.35	2,2'-Bipyridine
2.44	Thiazole	4.45	2-Methylaniline
2.47	3-Nitroaniline	4.60	Aniline
2.48	Pyrazole	4.66	4,4'-Biphenyldiamine
2.61	N,N-Diethylaniline	4.73	3-Methylaniline
2.65	2-Chloroaniline	4.78	2-Aminophenol
2.70	1,4-Benzenediamine	4.85	N-Methylaniline

(continued on next page

TABLE 16.7 (continued)
The pK_a Values of Some Organic Bases in Aqueous Solution at 298 K

pK_a	Compound	pK_a	Compound
4.86	1,10-Phenanthroline	8.88	Diethanolamine
4.88	Quinoline	9.03	1,3-Propanediamine
4.91	8-Hydroxyquinoline	9.11	4-Aminopyridine
5.08	4-Methylaniline	9.35	Benzylamine
5.12	N-Ethylaniline	9.50	2-Aminoethanol
5.15	N,N-Dimethylaniline	9.80	Trimethylamine
5.23	Pyridine	10.41	2-Methylpropylamine
5.33	Piperazine	10.56	2-Butylamine
5.42	Isoquinoline	10.56	Hexylamine
5.58	Acridine	10.60	2-Propylamine
5.68	3-Methylpyridine	10.61	Butylamine
5.96	Hydroxylamine	10.64	Decylamine
5.97	2-Methylpyridine	10.64	Cyclohexylamine
6.02	4-Methylpyridine	10.64	Ethylamine
6.15	3,5-Dimethylpyridine	10.64	Methylamine
6.57	2,3-Dimethylpyridine	10.71	Propylamine
6.61	1,2-Propanediamine	10.72	Triethylamine
6.82	2-Aminopyridine	10.77	Dimethylamine
6.85	1,2-Ethanediamine	10.83	tert-Butylamine
6.99	2,4-Dimethylpyridine	10.93	Diethylamine
6.99	Imidazole	11.12	Piperidine
7.76	Tris(2-hydroxyethyl)amine	11.30	Pyrrolidine
8.01	2-Amino-2-hydroxymethyl-1,3-propanediol	12.34	1,8-Bis(dimethylamino)naphthalene
8.28	Brucine	13.54	Guanidine
8.49	Morpholine		

16.4 RESOLVING AGENTS

In practice, resolution of an organic compound requires a good deal of trial and error. For information on resolution techniques see *Stereochemistry, Fundamentals, and Methods,* ed. H. B. Kagan, Vol. 3 (Stuttgart Georg Thieme Verlag, 1977).

16.4.1 BASES

2-Amino-3-methyl-1-butanol
2-Amino-1-(4-nitrophenyl)-1,3-propanediol
2-Amino-1-phenyl-1-propanol (norephedrine, norpseudoephedrine)
2-Amino-3-phenyl-1-propanol
N-Isopropylphenylalaninol
Brucine
Cinchonidine
Cinchonine
2,2′-Diamino-1,1′-binaphthyl
2-Methyl-2-phenylbutanedioic acid anhydride
1-(1-Naphthyl)ethylamine
1-Phenyl-1-propylamine

1-Phenyl-2-propylamine
Quinine
Sparteine
Strychnine
Plus many suitable derivatives of common protein amino acids

16.4.2 ACIDS

(1,1′-Binaphthalene)-2,2′-dicarboxylic acid
3-Bromo-8-camphorsulfonic acid
Camphor-8-sulfonic acid
Camphor-10-sulfonic acid
7,7-Dimethyl-2-oxobicyclo[2.2.1]heptane-1-carboxylic acid
2,3:4,6-Di-*O*-isopropylidene-*xylo*-hexulosonic acid
4-Hydroxydinaphtho[2,1-*d*:1′,2′-*f*]-1,3,2-dioxaphosphepin 4-oxide
4-Hydroxy-3-phenylbutanoic acid lactone
Mosher's reagent
Lactic acid and many of its derivatives
Mandelic acid and many of its derivatives
3-Menthoxyacetic acid
3-Menthylglycine
2-Methyl-2-phenylbutanedioic acid
Naproxen
5-Oxo-2-pyrrolidinecarboxylic acids
2-[((Phenylamino)carbonyl)oxy]propanoic acid
1-Phenylethanesulfonic acid
Tartaric acid and many of its derivatives
1,2,3,4-Tetrahydro-3-isoquinolinesulfonic acid
(2,4,5,7-Tetranitro-9-fluorenylideneaminoxy)propanoic acid
4-Thiazolidinecarboxylic acid
Plus many suitable derivatives of common protein amino acids

16.4.3 OTHERS

Camphor-10-sulfonyl chloride
Chrysanthemic acid chloride
(1,1′-Binaphthalene)-2,2′-diol
Camphor
2,2′-Dimethoxybutanedioic acid bis(dimethylamide)
3,3-Dimethyl-2-butanol
7,7-Dimethyl-2-oxobicyclo[2.2.1]heptane-1-carbonyl chloride
2,2-Dimethyl-α,α,α′,α′-tetraphenyl-1,3-dioxolane-4,5-dimethanol
α-Methoxy-α-(trifluoromethyl)benzeneacetic acid chloride
1-(1-Isocyanatoethyl)naphthalene
Menthol and its stereoisomers
3-Menthoxyacetyl chloride
N-Methanesulfonylphenylalanyl chloride
Methyl phenyl sulfoximine
2-Phenylpropanoic acid chloride
Tri-*O*-thymotide

16.5   FREEZING MIXTURES

A list of some freezing mixtures and their approximate temperatures is given in Table 16.8.

TABLE 16.8
Freezing Mixtures[a]

Components		Approximate Final Temperature (°C)[b]
100 g water	100 g ice	0
100 g water	30 g ammonium chloride	−5
100 g water	75 g sodium nitrate	−5
100 g water	85 g sodium acetate	−5
100 g water	110 g sodium thiosulfate pentahydrate	−8
100 g water	36 g sodium chloride	−10
100 g ice	30 g potassium chloride	−11
100 g water	133 g ammonium thiocyanate	−18
100 g ice	45 g ammonium nitrate	−17
100 g ice	33 g sodium chloride	−21
100 g ice	81 g calcium chloride hexahydrate	−21
100 g ice	66 g sodium bromide	−28
100 g ice	105 g ethanol	−30
100 g ice	85 g magnesium chloride	−34
100 g ice	123 g calcium chloride hexahydrate	−40
100 g ice	143 g calcium chloride hexahydrate	−55
Ethylene glycol	carbon dioxide (solid)	-11
Aq. calcium chloride (various concentrations)	carbon dioxide (solid)	−30 to −45
Octane	carbon dioxide (solid)	−56
Ethanol	carbon dioxide (solid)	−72
Chloroform	carbon dioxide (solid)	−77
Acetone	carbon dioxide (solid)	−78
2-Propanol	carbon dioxide (solid)	−78
Diethyl ether	carbon dioxide (solid)	−100

Source: Based, in part, on data in Gordon, A. J., and Ford, R. A., *The Chemist's Companion* (New York: Wiley-Interscience, 1972), pp. 451–452. Reprinted with permission of John Wiley & Sons, Inc.

[a] Experimental work with cooling baths and Dewar flasks containing freezing mixtures requires the use of efficient fume hoods and personal protection equipment.

[b] The minimum temperatures reached with salt-ice mixtures depend on the rate of stirring of the mixtures and how finely crushed the ice is.

16.6   MATERIALS USED FOR HEATING BATHS

Some materials that can be used for laboratory heating baths are given in Table 16.9.

TABLE 16.9
Heating Baths[a]

Medium	Mp (°C)	Bp (°C)	Useful Range (°C)	Flash Point (°C)	Comments
Water	0	100	0–80	None	Ideal within a limited range
Silicone oil[b]	−60	—	0–250	~310	Noncorrosive
Triethylene glycol	−4	286	0–250	166	Water soluble, stable
Glycerol	18	290	−20 to +260	160	Water soluble, nontoxic, viscous, supercools
Dibutyl phthalate	−35	340	150–320	157	Viscous at low temperature
Sand	—	—	> About 200	None	Ideal for high-temperature heating
Wood's metal[c]	70	—	73–350	None	Ideal for high-temperature heating

Source: Based on data in Gordon, A. J., and Ford, R. A., *The Chemist's Companion* (New York: Wiley-Interscience, 1972), pp 449–450. Reprinted with permission of John Wiley & Sons, Inc.

[a] Experimental work with heating baths requires the use of efficient fume hoods and personal protection equipment.

[b] Data for Dow Corning 550 silicone oil.

[c] 50% Bi, 25% Pb, 12.5% Sn, 12.5% Cd.

16.7 DRYING AGENTS

Table 16.10 gives a list of drying agents with their uses.

TABLE 16.10
Drying Agents

Drying Agent	Useful for	Comments
Alumina (Al_2O_3)	Hydrocarbons	Very high capacity; very fast; reactivated by heating
Barium oxide (BaO)	Hydrocarbons, amines, alcohols, aldehydes	Slow but efficient; not suitable for compounds sensitive to strong base
Calcium chloride ($CaCl_2$)	Hydrocarbons, alkyl halides, ethers, many esters	Not very efficient; good for predrying; not suitable for most nitrogen and oxygen compounds
Calcium hydride (CaH_2)	Hydrocarbons, ethers, amines, esters, higher alcohols ($>C_4$)	Not suitable for aldehydes and ketones
Calcium oxide (CaO)	Low-boiling alcohols and amines, ethers	Slow but efficient; not suitable for acidic compounds
Calcium sulfate ($CaSO_4$)	Most organic substances	Very fast and very efficient
Lithium aluminium hydride ($LiAlH_4$)	Hydrocarbons, aryl (not alkyl) halides, ethers	Excess may be destroyed by slow addition of ethyl acetate; predrying recommended; reacts with acidic hydrogens and most functional groups
Magnesium sulfate ($MgSO_4$)	Most organic substances	Very fast and very efficient; avoid using with very acid-sensitive compounds
Molecular sieve 4Å	Nonpolar liquids and gases	Very efficient; predrying with a common agent recommended; can be reactivated by heating
Phosphorus pentoxide (P_2O_5)	Hydrocarbons, ethers, halides, esters, nitriles	Fast and efficient; predrying recommended; *not* suitable for alcohols, amines, acids, ketones, etc.
Potassium carbonate (K_2CO_3)	Alcohols, esters, nitriles, ketones	Not suitable for acidic compounds

(continued on next page

TABLE 16.10 (continued)
Drying Agents

Drying Agent	Useful for	Comments
Potassium hydroxide (KOH)	Amines (in inert solvents)	Powerful; not suitable for acidic compounds; pellets can corrode glassware
Silica gel	Hydrocarbons, amines	Very high capacity and very fast; can be reactivated by heating
Sodium sulfate (Na_2SO_4)	Most organic substances	Inefficient and slow; good for gross predrying
Sulfuric acid (H_2SO_4)	Saturated and aromatic hydrocarbons, halides, inert neutral or acidic gases	Very high capacity; very fast, but use limited to saturated or aromatic hydrocarbons

Source: This table is based on data in Gordon, A. J., and Ford, R. A., *The Chemist's Companion* (New York: Wiley-Interscience, 1972), pp. 445–447. Reprinted with permission of John Wiley & Sons, Inc.

16.8   PRESSURE-TEMPERATURE NOMOGRAPH

The pressure-temperature nomograph for correcting boiling points to 760 mmHg (1 atm) is shown in Figure 16.1. It is used as follows. If the boiling point at nonatmospheric pressure (*P* mmHg) is known, line up the values of the boiling point *P* in **A** and the pressure in **C**. The theoretical boiling point at 760 mmHg can then be read off in **B**. Line up this figure in **B** with another pressure in **C** and the approximate corresponding boiling point can be read off in **A**.

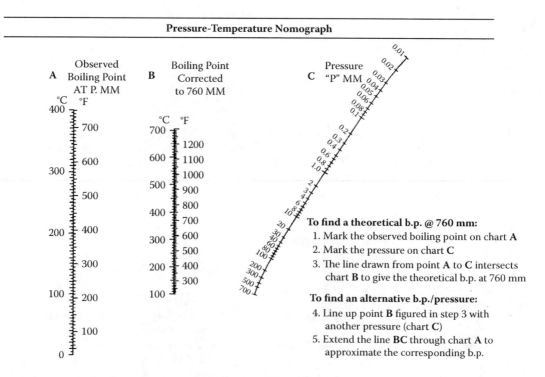

FIGURE 16.1   Pressure-temperature nomograph.

16.9 SI UNITS

16.9.1 SI BASE UNITS

The names and symbols of the seven SI base units are shown in Table 16.11.

TABLE 16.11
SI Base Units

Physical Quantity	Name of SI Base Unit	Symbol for SI Base Unit
Amount of substance	Mole[a]	mol
Electric current	Ampere	A
Length	Metre	m
Luminous intensity	Candela	cd
Mass	Kilogram[b]	kg
Themodynamic temperature	Kelvin	K
Time	Second	s

[a] The mole is the amount of substance of a system that contains as many elementary entities as there are atoms in 0.012 kg of carbon-12. Although it is defined in terms of the number of entities, in practice, 1 mol of atoms, molecules, or specific formula units of a substance is measured by weighing $M \times (1 \text{ mol})$ of the substance, where M is the molar mass, the mass per unit amount of substance. *Molar mass* is synonymous with the terms *atomic weight*, for atoms, and *molecular weight*, for molecules or formula units, respectively, and is reported in grams per mole (g mol^{-1}).

[b] Among the base units of the SI system, the kilogram unit of mass is the only one whose name, for historical reasons, contains a prefix (*kilo-*). Names and symbols for multiples of the unit of mass are formed by attaching prefix names to the unit *gram* and prefix symbols to the unit symbol g. For example, 10^{-6} kg = 1 mg (1 milligram) but *not* 1µkg (1 microkilogram).

16.9.2 SI-DERIVED UNITS

The SI units for derived physical quantities are those coherently derived from the SI base units by multiplication and division. Some of the SI-derived units that have special names and symbols are presented in Table 16.12.

TABLE 16.12
Some SI-Derived Units

Physical Quantity	Name of SI Unit	Symbol for SI Unit	Definition of SI Unit
Electric charge	Coulomb	C	A s
Energy	Joule	J	kg m^2 s^{-2}
Force	Newton	N	kg m s^{-2} = J m^{-1}
Frequency	Hertz	Hz	s^{-1}
Potential difference	Volt	V	kg m^2 s^{-3} A^{-1} = J A^{-1} s^{-1}
Power	Watt	W	kg m^2 s^{-3} = J s^{-1}
Pressure	Pascal	Pa	kg m^{-1} s^{-2} = N m^{-2}

16.9.3 PREFIXES USED WITH SI UNITS

The prefixes listed in Table 16.13 are used to indicate decimal multiples of base and derived SI units.

TABLE 16.13
Multiplying Prefixes for Use with SI Units

Factor	Prefix	Symbol	Factor	Prefix	Symbol
10^{-1}	Deci	d	10	Deca (or deka)	da
10^{-2}	Centi	c	10^2	Hecto	h
10^{-3}	Milli	m	10^2	Kilo	k
10^{-6}	Micro	μ	10^6	Mega	M
10^{-9}	Nano	n	10^9	Giga	G
10^{-12}	Pico	p	10^{12}	Tera	T
10^{-15}	Femto	f	10^{15}	Peta	P
10^{-18}	Atto	a	10^{18}	Exa	E
10^{-21}	Zepto	z	10^{21}	Zetta	Z
10^{-24}	Yocto	y	10^{24}	Yotta	Y

16.9.4 CONVERSION FACTORS FOR NON-SI UNITS

Many non-SI units are now defined exactly in terms of SI; some can only be related to SI units via fundamental constants, and the relationship is therefore restricted by the precision to which the constants are known. Factors for converting some non-SI units into their SI equivalents are listed in Table 16.14. Names of units within the SI are indicated with an asterisk.

TABLE 16.14
Conversion Factors for Non-SI Units

	Unit	Symbol	SI Equivalent		
	Ångström	Å		10^{-10}	m
	Atmosphere	atm	101,325		Pa
	Atomic mass unit (unified)	u	1.661	$\times 10^{-27}$	kg
	Bar	bar		10^5	Pa
*	Becquerel (SI: activity (of a radioactive source))	Bq		1	s^{-1}
	Calorie (thermochemical)	cal_{th}	4.184		J
*	Coulomb (SI: electric charge)	C		1	A s
	Curie (radioactivity)	Ci	3.7	$\times 10^{10}$	Bq
	Debye	D	3.336	$\times 10^{-30}$	C m
	Degree Celsius	°C		1	K
	Degree Fahrenheit	°F	5/9 (0.5556)		K
	Electronvolt	eV	1.602	$\times 10^{-19}$	J
	Hour	h	3,600		s
*	Joule (SI: energy)	J		1	N m
	Kilowatt hour	kW h	3.6	$\times 10^6$	J
	Litre	l, L		10^{-3}	m^3
	Micron	μ		10^{-6}	m
	Millimetre of mercury	mmHg	133.3		Pa
	Minute (time)	min	60		s

(continued on next page)

TABLE 16.14 (continued)
Conversion Factors for Non-SI Units

Unit	Symbol	SI Equivalent		
* Newton (SI: force)	N		1	kg m s^{-2}
* Ohm (SI: resistance)	Ω		1	VA^{-1}
* Pascal (SI: pressure)	Pa		1	N m^{-2}
* Sievert (SI: dose equivalent (of ionizing radiation))	Sv		1	J kg^{-1}
Standard atmosphere	Atm	101 325		Pa
Ton (UK long, 2,240 lb)	Ton	1.016	$\times 10^3$	kg
Tonne (metric ton)	T		10^3	kg
* Volt (SI: electric potential difference)	V		1	J C^{-1}
* Watt (SI: power)	W		1	J s^{-1}

* Names of units within the SI.

16.9.5 Conversion Factors for UK Imperial Units and Other Non-SI Units of Measurement

Length

1 ångström unit (Å) = 10^{-8} cm = 10^{-10} m = 10^{-1} nm
1 micron (μ) = 1 μm = 1^{-4} cm = 10^{-6} m
A wavelength of n microns (n μm) = a wavenumber of $10,000/n$ cm^{-1}
1 inch (in.) = 2.54 cm = 2.54×10^{-2} m
1 metre = 39.3701 in.

Mass

453.592 g = 1 pound (lb)
1 kg = 2.20462 lb

Volume

1 mL (or 1 ml) = 1 cubic centimetre (cm^3)
1 L (or 1 l) = 1 dm^3 = 1×10^{-3} m^3 = 1000 mL (or 1000 ml)
1 litre = 2.12 pints (U.S.) = 1.76 pints (UK)
28.4 ml = 1 fluid ounce

Pressure

1 atm = 1.01325×10^5 pascal (N m^{-2})
　　　 = 101.325 kPa
　　　 = 760 torr = 760 mmHg
　　　 = 1.01325 bar
　　　 = 14.70 lb/in.^{2}
1 mmHg (0°C) = 1 torr = 1/760 atm
　　　　　　　 = 133.322 pascal
　　　　　　　 = 0.0193368 lb/in.^{2}
1 kPa = 7.5006 mmHg
1 lb/in.^{2} = 51.715 mmHg

Temperature
absolute zero (K) = $-273.16°C$
$K = °C + 273.16$
$°F = (9 \times °C)/5 + 32$
$°C = 5 (°F - 32)/9$

Energy
1 joule = 1 watt s = 10^7 erg = 0.737561 ft lb
1 erg = 1 dyne cm = $1 \text{ g cm}^2 \text{ s}^{-2}$
1 calorie = 4.1868 joule
1 electronvolt/molecule = 23.06 kcal mol^{-1}

16.9.6   FURTHER READING ON SI UNITS

Quantities, Units and Symbols in Physical Chemistry, 3rd ed. (Cambridge: IUPAC/Royal Society of Chemistry, 2007).

McGlashan, M. L., *Physicochemical Quantities and Units*, 2nd ed., Royal Institute of Chemistry Monographs for Teachers 15 (London: The Royal Institute of Chemistry, 1971).

Cardarelli, F., *Encyclopaedia of Scientific Units, Weights and Measures: Their SI Equivalences and Origins* (London: Springer, 2003).

16.9.6.1   Websites

Bureau International des Poids et Mesures: http://www.bipm.org/en/home/
National Institute of Standards and Technology (U.S.): http://physics.nist.gov/cuu/Units/units.html
National Physical Laboratory (UK): http://www.npl.co.uk/reference/measurement-units/

17 Languages

The best dictionaries for chemists are:

Patterson, A. M., *German-English Dictionary for Chemists* (Chichester: Wiley).
Patterson, A. M., *French-English Dictionary for Chemists* (Chichester: Wiley).
Dictionary of Chemical Terminology in Five Languages (Amsterdam: Elsevier, 1980) (covers English, German, French, Polish, and Russian).

17.1 A GERMAN-ENGLISH DICTIONARY

Note that the correct form of many German words ending in *ss* is to use the symbol ß, e.g., Blaß, Heiß. Since this symbol is frequently not available on keyboards and complicates indexing, it is becoming less frequent, but will still often be found in books and journals.

For keyboards without an umlaut, or where it is desired to avoid the use of the umlaut, the correct transliteration is to insert a following *e*, e.g., Tröger's base → Troeger's base.

Abbau	decomposition, degradation	Angriff	attack
abdestillieren	to distil off	Anlagerung	addition, approach
aber	but, however	annähernd	approximate
abfiltrieren	to filter off	ansäuern	to acidify
abgeben	to give off	anstelle	instead
abkühlen	to cool down	Anteil	constituent
agnehmend	decreasing	Anwendung	use
Abscheidung	separation	Anwesenheit	presence
abtrennen	to separate	Äpfelsäure	malic acid
Abtrennung	separation	Äthanol	ethanol
Abweichung	deviation, variation	Äther	ether
acht	eight	äthyl	ethyl
ähnlich	similar	auch	also
Alkylierung	alkylation	Aufarbeitung	work up
allgemein	generally	auffangen	to collect
allmählich	gradual(ly)	auflösen	to dissolve
als	as, then	Aufnahme	absorption
alt	old	aus	out of, from
Ameisensäure	formic acid	Ausbeute	yield
ander	other, another	audfällen	to precipitate
ändern	to change	ausführen	to carry out
anders	otherwise, differently	Ausgangsmaterial	starting material
anfänglich	at first	ausgenommen	except
anfangs	at first	ausgescheiden	separated
angesäuert	acidified	Ausscheidung	separation

Ausschluss	exclusion	Brom	bromine
ausser	except, besides	Bromierung	bromination
ausserdem	besides, moreover	Brücke	bridge
		Buttersäure	butyric acid
Bad	bath		
basisch	basic	Chinolin	quinoline
Bedeutung	meaning, significance	Chinon	quinone
behandeln	to treat	Chlor	chlorine
Beispiel	example	Chlorierung	chlorination
bekannt	known	Chlorwasserstoff	hydrogen chloride
Belichtung	exposure to light		
Benzin	petroleum ether	dagegen	on the other hand
Benzol	benzene	Dampf	vapour
beobachten	to observe	danach	after that
Berechnet	calculated	daneben	besides
bereiten	to prepare	darin	therein, in it
bereits	already	Darstellung	preparation
Bernsteinsäure	succinic acid	dass	that
beschleunigen	to accelerate	Dehydratisireung	dehydration
beschreiben	to describe	Dehydrierung	dehydrogenation
besonders	especially	Derivat	derivative
besser	better	desgleichen	likewise
beständig	stable	destillieren	to distil
Bestandteil	constituent	Destillierung	distillation
bestehen	to consist, to exist	deutlich	clear
bestimmen	to determine	dick	thick
Bestimmung	determination	dies	this
Bestrahlung	irradiation	diese	this, these
Beugung	diffraction	digerieren	to digest
beweisen	to prove	doppelt	double
bilden	to form	drei	three
bildung	formation	dreifach	triple
bindung	bond	dreissig	thirty
bis	until	Druck	pressure
blass	pale	dunkel	dark
Blatt	leaf	dünn	thin
Blättchen	leaflet	durch	through, by
blau	blue	durchführen	to carry out
bläulich	bluish		
Blausäure	hydrocyanic acid	ebenfalls	likewise
Blei	lead	Eigenschaft	property
Bor	boron	Ein	one
brauchbar	useful	einbringen	to introduce
Braun	brown	eindampfen	to evaporate
bräunlich	brownish	eindeutig	unequivocal
Brechung	refraction	einengen	to concentrate
Breite	width	einfach	simple
brennen	to burn	einiger	some, several
Brenztraubensäure	pyruvic acid	Einkristall	single crystal

einleiten	to introduce	Feststoff	solid
einmal	once	Feuchtigkeit	moisture
Einschluss	inclusion	Flammpunkt	flash point
einstündig	for one hour	flüchtig	volatile
eintägig	for one day	flüssig	liquid
eintropfen	to add dropwise	Flüssigkeit	liquid
einzig	only	Folge	sequence, series
Eis	ice	folgen	to follow
Eisen	iron	Formel	formula
Eisessig	glacial acetic acid	Fortschritt	progress
elf	eleven	frei	free
eluieren	to elute	frisch	fresh
Enolisierung	enolisation	früher	former(ly)
entfernen	to remove	führen	to lead
entgegen	against	fünf	five
enthalten	to contain		
entsprechend	corresponding	ganz	whole
entstehen	to originate	Gärung	fermentation
Entwässerung	dehydration	gasförmig	gaseous
Entwicklung	evolution	geben	to give
Entzündung	ignition	gebräuchlich	usual
erfolgen	to occur	gebunden	bonded
erforderlich	necessary	geeignet	suitable
ergeben	to yield	gefällt	precipitated
Ergebnis	result	gefärbt	coloured
ergibt	yields	Gefäss	vessel
erhalten	to obtain	gegen	against
erhitzen	to heat	Gegenwart	presence
Erhöhung	increase	Gehalt	contents
erscheinen	to appear	gekocht	boiled
erst	first, only	gekühlt	cooled
Erstarrung	solidification	gelb	yellow
erste	first	gelblich	yellowish
erwärmen	to warm	gelöst	dissolved
erzielen	to obtain	Gemisch	mixture
Essigsäure	acetic acid	gemischt	mixed
		genau	exact
fällen	to precipitate	gepuffert	buffered
falsch	incorrect	gering	small
Farbe	colour	geringer	minor
farbig	coloured	Geruch	odour
farblos	colourless	gerührt	stirred
Farbstoff	dyestuff	gesättigt	saturated
Farbumschlag	colour change	geschmolzen	fused, molten
fast	almost	Geschwindigkeit	rate
fein	fine	getrennt	separated
Feld	field	getrocknet	dried
ferner	further	Gewicht	weight
fest	solid	gewinnen	to obtain

gewiss	certainly
gewogen	weighed
gewöhnlich	usual
gibt	gives
giftig	poisonous, toxic
Gitter	lattice
gleich	equal
gleichfalls	likewise
Gleichgewicht	equilibrium
Gleichung	equation
gleichzeitig	simultaneously
gliedrig	membered
grau	grey
Grenze	limit
gross	great, large
grün	green
Gruppe	group

halb	half
Halogenierung	halogenation
haltbar	stable
Harnstoff	urea
Hauptprodukt	main product
heftig	violently
heiss	hot
hell	light, pale
hemmen	to inhibit
Herkunft	origin
herstellen	to produce
Herstellung	production
Hilfe	help
hingegen	on the contrary
hinzufügen	to add
Hitze	heat
hoch	high
hohe	high
hundert	hundred
Hydratisierung	hydration
Hydrierung	hydrogenation

immer	always
induziert	induced
Inhalt	contents
insgesamt	altogether
Isolierung	isolation

Jahr	year
je nach	according to
jedoch	however

Jod	iodine
Jodierung	iodination
Kalium	potassium
kalt	cold
katalytisch	catalytic
kein	no, not a
Kern	nucleus
Kette	chain
klar	clear
klein	small
kochen	to boil
Kochpunkt (Kp)	boiling point (bp)
Kohlensäure	carbon dioxide, carbonic acid
Kohlenstoff	carbon
Kohlenwasserstoff	hydrocarbon
kondensieren	to condense
konjugiert	conjugated
konzentriert (konz.)	concentrated (conc.)
Kopplung	coupling
Kraft	force
Kühlen	to cool
kühlung	cooling
Kupfer	copper
kurz	short

Ladung	charge
lang	long
langsam	slow(ly)
lassen	to leave
leicht	easy, easily
leiten	to conduct
letzte	last
Licht	light
liefern	to yield
links	left
lösen	to dissolve
löslich	soluble
Löslichkeit	solubility
Lösung	solution
Lösungsmittel	solvent
Luft	air

mässig	moderately
mehr	more
mehrere	several
mehrfach	multiple
mehrmals	several times
mehrstündig	for several hours
meist	most

Menge	amount
Messung	measurement
Milchsäure	lactic acid
mischbar	miscible
Mischbarkeit	miscibility
mischen	to mix
Mischung	mixture
mit	with
mittels	by means of
möglich	possible
Molverhältnis	molar ratio
müssen	must
Mutterlauge	mother liquor
nach	after
nachfolgend	subsequent
nachstehend	following
Nacht	night
Nachweis	proof, detection
Nadel	needle
nahe	near
nämlich	namely
Natrium	sodium
neben	beside, in addition to
Nebenprodukt	by-product
neun	nine
Niederschlag	precipitate
niedrig	low
niemals	never
Nitrierung	nitration
noch	still, yet
nochmalig	repeated
notwendig	necessary
nunmehr	now
nur	only
oben	above
Oberfläche	surface
oberhalb	above
oder	or
offen	open
offenbar	obvious
ohne	without
Öl	oil
ölig	oily
Ölsäure	oleic acid
Phosphor	phosphorus
primär	primary

protoniert	protonated
Puffer	buffer
Pulver	powder
Punkt	point
Quecksilber	mercury
rasch	rapid
Raum	space, room
rechts	right
Reihe	series
rein	pure
Reinheit	purity
Reinigung	purification
restlich	residual
richtig	correct
Rohprodukt	crude product
rosa	pink
rot	red
rötlich	reddish
Rückfluss	reflux
Rückgewinnung	recovery
Rückstand	residue
rühren	to stir
Salpetersäure	nitric acid
Salz	salt
Salzsäure	hydrochloride acid
sättigen	to saturate
sauer	acidic
Sauerstoff	oxygen
Säure	acid
Schall	sound
scheiden	to separate
scheinbar	apparently
schlecht	poor
schliessen	to close
schliesslich	finally
schmelzen	to melt
Schmelzpunkt (Schmp)	melting point (mp)
schnell	fast, quickly
schon	already
schütteln	to shake
Schutzgas	inert gas
schwach	weak
schwarz	black
Schwefel	sulfur
Schwefelsäure	sulfuric acid
schwer	heavy, difficult

Schwingung	vibration	Überschluss	excess
sechs	six	überwiegend	predominantly
sehr	very	üblich	usual
Seitenkette	side chain	übrig	remaining
sieben	seven	Umesterung	transesterification
sieden	to boil	Umkristallisierung	recrystallisation
siedend	boiling	Umlagerung	rearrangement
Siedepunkt	boiling point	Umsatz	exchange
Silizium	silicon	Umsetzung	reaction
sofort	immediately	Umwandlung	conversion
sonst	otherwise, else	unbeständig	unstable
sorgfältig	carefully	unkorrigiert	uncorrected
Spaltung	cleavage, scission	unlöslich	insoluble
Spiegel	mirror	unrein	impure
Stäbchen	small rod	unten	below, underneath
stark	strong	unter	under
starr	rigid	Untersuchung	investigation
statt	instead of	ursprünglich	original
stattfinden	to take place		
stehen	to stand	Verbindung	compound
stehen lassen	to leave standing	Verbrennung	combustion
Stellung	position	Verdampfung	evaporation, vaporisation
Stickstoff	nitrogen	verdünnt (verd.)	dilute (dil.)
Stoff	substance	vereinigen	to combine
Stoffwechsel	metabolism	Veresterung	esterification
Stoss	substance	Verfahren	procedure
Strahlung	radiation	verfärben	to change colour
streuen	to scatter	Vergärung	fermentation
Stufe	step, stage	Vergleich	comparison
Stunde	hour	vergleichen	to compare
substituiert	substituted	Verhalten	behaviour
		Verhältnis	proportion, ratio
Tafel	plate	Verlauf	course, progress
Täfelchen	platelet	vermindern	to diminish, to reduce
Tag	day	vermischen	to mix
Teil	part	verrühren	to stir up
Teilchen	particle	Verschiebung	shift
teilweise	partially	Verseifung	saponification
tief	deep	versetzen	to add, mix
toluol	toluene	Versuch	experiment
trennen	to separate	verwandt	related
Trennung	separation	Verwendung	use
trocken	dry	verzweigt	branched
trocknen	to dry	viel	much, many
Tropfen	drop	vieleicht	perhaps, possibly
		vier	four
über	over, above	voll	full
Übergang	transition	vom	of the, from the

vor allem	above all
Vorbehandlung	pretreatment
Vorkommen	occurrence
Vorsicht	caution, care
vorsichtig	cautious(ly)
vorwiegend	predominant
wahrscheinlich	probable, probably
waschen	to wash
Wasser	water
Wasserdampf	water vapour, steam
wasserfrei	anhydrous
wasserhaltig	hydrated or wet
wässerig	aqueous
Wasserstoff	hydrogen
wässrig	aqueous
Weg	route
wegen	on account of
Weinsäure	tartaric acid
weiss	white
weiter	additional
Welle	wave
Wellenlänge	wavelength
wenig	little, few
werden	to become
Wertigkeit	valency
wesentlich	essential
wichtig	important
wiederholt	repeated(ly)
Winkel	angle
wird	becomes, is
Wirkung	action, effect
Wismut	bismuth
Woche	week

zehn	ten
Zeit	time
Zeitschrift	periodical, journal
zerfliesslich	deliquescent
zersetzen	to decompose
zersetzlich	unstable
Zersetsung (Zers.)	decomposition (dec.)
ziegelrot	brick red
Zimmer	room
Zimtsäure	cinnamic acid
Zinn	tin
Zucker	sugar
zuerst	at first
zufügen	to add
Zugabe	addition
zugebeu	to add
zugleich	at the same time, together
zuletzt	at last, finally
zum Beispiel (z.B.)	for example (e.g.)
Zunahme	increase
zur	to the
zurückbleiben	to remain behind
zusammen	together
zusäzlich	additional
Zustand	state, condition
zutropfen	to add drop by drop
zuvor	before, previously
zwanzig	twenty
zwecks	for the purpose of
zwei	two
zweimal	twice
zwischen	between
Zwischenprodukt	intermediate
zwölf	twelve

17.2 RUSSIAN AND GREEK ALPHABETS

The Russian and Greek alphabets, with their capitals, small letters, and English equivalents, are shown in Table 17.1.

Most chemical names in Russian are very similar to their Western equivalents, once transliteration from the Cyrillic alphabet has been applied.

For example:

Пиридин	Pyridine
Тестостерон	Testosterone
2-Аллил-2-метил-1,3-циклопентандиол	2 Allyl-2 methyl-1,3-cyclopentanediol
6-метокси-2-пропионилнафталин	6-Methoxy-2-propionylnaphthalene

TABLE 17.1

Greek			Russian	
A α	alpha	a	А а	a
B β	beta	b	Б б	b
Γ γ	gamma	g, n	В в	v
Δ δ	delta	d	Г г	g
E ε	epsilon	e	Д д	d
Z ζ	zeta	z	Е е	e
H η	eta	ē	Ж ж	zh
Θ θ	theta	th	З з	z
I ι	iota	i	И и Й й	i, ĭ
K κ	kappa	k	К к	k
Λ λ	lambda	l	Л л	l
M μ	mu	m	М м	m
N ν	nu	n	Н н	n
Ξ ξ	xi	x	О о	o
O o	omicron	o	П п	p
Π π	pi	p	Р р	r
P ρ	rho	r, rh	С с	s
Σ σ ς	sigma	s	Т т	t
T τ	tau	t	У у	u
Υ υ	upsilon	y, u	Ф ф	f
Φ φ	phi	ph	Х х	kj
X χ	chi	ch	Ц ц	ts
Ψ ψ	psi	ps	Ч ч	ch
Ω ω	omega	ō	Ш ш	sh
			Щ щ	shch
			*Ъ ъ	
			Ы ы	y
			*Ь ь	
			Э э	e
			Ю ю	yu
			Я я	ya

* Characters that have no sound themselves but alter the pro-
nunciation of the preceding consonant.

Index

9CI nomenclature, 44

A

Abbreviations and acronyms, 103–127, 224
Abstracting services, 1–2, *See also Chemical Abstracts*;
    Chemical Abstracts Service
    patent literature, 21
    Web of Science, 10
Acids
    class I, 69
    dissociation constants, 244–245
    resolving agents, 247
Additive names, 48
Alcohols, class I, 69
Alditols, 87–88
Aldose nomenclature, 81–84
Alkaloids dictionary, 12
Alkene NMR chemical shifts, 203
Allene stereochemistry, 150
American Conference of Governmental Industrial
    Hygienists (ACGIH), 170
Amino acids, 90–92
    D,L- system, 152
Anteiso acids, 95
Aqueous extraction solvents, 240–241
Aromatic compound representation, 160
Arsenic compounds, 98–100
Atomic weight of nuclear particles, 222
Attached proton test (APT), 206
Author Index, 5
Available Chemicals Directory, 22
Azo compounds, 100
Azoxy compounds, 100

B

Base pK_a values, 245–246
Bases, resolving agents, 246–247
Beilsteins Handbuch der Organischen Chemie, 12–14, 167
Biaryl stereochemistry, 150
Bicyclo nomenclature, 74
Boiling point correction nomograph, 250
Boron compounds, 98
Boughton system, 100
Bragg's law, 230
Bridged ring systems, 74–75
Buffer solutions, 242–243

C

Cage structures, 75
Cahn-Ingold-Prelog (CIP) system, 146
CAplus^{SM}, 8, 9
Carbohydrate nomenclature, 81–87

    cyclic forms, 85
    D,L- system, 45, 81–83, 151–152
    disaccharides, 86
    fundamental aldoses, 81–83
    fundamental ketoses, 84
    glycosides, 85–86
    graphical representation, 81
    higher sugars, 84
    modified aldoses and ketoses, 84
    oligosaccharides, 86–87
    suffixes, 84
    trivially named sugars, 86–87
Carbohydrates dictionary, 12, 81
Carcinogenic risk, 178
Carcinogens, 171, 173
Carotenoids, 95–96
CA Selects, 8
CASREACT®, 8, 9
CAS Registry database, 8, 9
CAS registry numbers, 3, 163–165
    asterisks, 164
    check digit, 163
    chronology, 164
    racemates, 164–165
    Reaxys database and, 15
CAS *Ring Systems Handbook*, 16
CASSI, 6, 23, 39
CD-ROM resources, 7, 11, 12
Chain numbering, 42
Chapman & Hall/CRC chemical database, 11–12
Characteristic group, 53, *See also* Functional groups
Chemaxon, 22
CHEMCATS®, 8, 9
Chemical Abstracts (CA), 1
    abstracts, 2
    Author Index, 5
    Collective Indexes, 3–5
    current awareness bulletins, 8
    electronic products, 7–10
    Formula Index, 3, 5
    Hill system order, 167
    Index Guide, 3, 5–6
    molecular formula conventions, 167
    patent information resources, 2, 5, 21
    printed products, 1–7
    publication schedule and contents, 1–2
    Volume Indexes, 2–3
    web edition, 1, 7
Chemical Abstracts Service (CAS), 1
    nomenclature systems, 44–48
    online databases, 8
    peptide nomenclature revisions, 93
    Registry Handbook: Number Section, 6–7
    registry numbers, 3, 15, 163–165

Multiples of element weights

C	12.01	H_5	5.040	H_{60}	60.48	$(OCH_3)_7$	217.24
C_2	24.02	H_6	6.048	H_{61}	61.49	$(OCH_3)_8$	248.27
C_3	36.03	H_7	7.056	H_{62}	62.50		
C_4	48.04	H_8	8.064	H_{63}	63.50	OC_2H_5	45.06
C_5	60.05	H_9	9.072	H_{64}	64.51	$(OC_2H_5)_2$	90.12
C_6	72.06	H_{10}	10.08	H_{65}	65.52	$(OC_2H_5)_3$	135.18
C_7	84.07	H_{11}	11.09			$(OC_2H_5)_4$	180.24
C_8	96.08	H_{12}	12.10	O	16	$(OC_2H_5)_5$	225.30
C_9	108.09	H_{13}	13.10	O_2	32		
C_{10}	120.10	H_{14}	14.11	O_3	48	$OCOCH_3$	59.04
C_{11}	132.11	H_{15}	15.12	O_4	64	$(OCOCH_3)_2$	118.09
C_{12}	144.12	H_{16}	16.13	O_5	80	$(OCOCH_3)_3$	177.13
C_{13}	156.13	H_{17}	17.14	O_6	96	$(OCOCH_3)_4$	236.18
C_{14}	168.14	H_{18}	18.14	O_7	112	$(OCOCH_3)_5$	295.22
C_{15}	180.15	H_{19}	19.15	O_8	128	$(OCOCH_3)_6$	354.26
C_{16}	192.16	H_{20}	20.16	O_9	144	$(OCOCH_3)_7$	413.31
C_{17}	204.17	H_{21}	21.17	O_{10}	160	$(OCOCH_3)_8$	472.35
C_{18}	216.18	H_{22}	22.18			$(OCOCH_3)_9$	531.40
C_{19}	228.19	H_{23}	23.18	N	14.007	$(OCOCH_3)_{10}$	590.44
C_{20}	240.20	H_{24}	24.19	N_2	28.02		
C_{21}	252.21	H_{25}	25.20	N_3	42.02	$(H_2O)_{0.5}$	9.01
C_{22}	264.22	H_{26}	26.21	N_4	56.03	H_2O	18.02
C_{23}	276.23	H_{27}	27.22	N_5	70.04		
C_{24}	288.24	H_{28}	28.22	N_6	84.05	$(H_2O)_{1.5}$	27.02
C_{25}	300.25	H_{29}	29.23			$(H_2O)_2$	36.03
C_{26}	312.26	H_{30}	30.24	S	32.064	$(H_2O)_3$	54.05
C_{27}	324.27	H_{31}	31.25	S_2	61.12	$(H_2O)_4$	72.06
C_{28}	336.28	H_{32}	32.26	S_3	96.19	$(H_2O)_5$	90.08
C_{29}	348.29	H_{33}	33.26	S_4	128.26	$(H_2O)_6$	108.10
C_{30}	360.30	H_{34}	34.27				
C_{31}	372.31	H_{35}	35.28	F	19.00	P	30.974
C_{32}	384.32	H_{36}	36.29	F_2	38.00	P_2	61.948
C_{33}	396.33	H_{37}	37.30	F_3	57.00	P_3	92.922
C_{34}	408.34	H_{38}	38.30			P_4	123.90
C_{35}	420.35	H_{39}	39.31	Cl	35.453		
C_{36}	432.36	H_{40}	40.32	Cl_2	70.91	Na	22.990
C_{37}	444.37	H_{41}	41.33	Cl_3	106.37	Na_2	45.98
C_{38}	456.38	H_{42}	42.34	Cl_4	141.83	Na_3	68.97
C_{39}	468.39	H_{43}	43.34	Cl_5	177.28		
C_{40}	480.40	H_{44}	44.35			K	39.10
C_{41}	492.41	H_{45}	45.36	Br	79.909	K_2	78.20
C_{42}	504.42	H_{46}	46.37	Br_2	159.82	K_3	117.30
C_{43}	516.43	H_{47}	47.38	Br_3	239.73		
C_{44}	528.44	H_{48}	48.38	Br_4	319.64	Ag	107.87
C_{45}	540.45	H_{49}	49.39			Ag_2	215.74
C_{46}	552.46	H_{50}	50.40	I	126.90	Cu	63.54
C_{47}	564.47	H_{51}	51.41	I_2	253.80	Cu_2	127.08
C_{48}	576.48	H_{52}	52.42	I_2	380.70	Cr	52.00
C_{49}	588.49	H_{53}	53.42			Hg	200.59
C_{50}	600.50	H_{54}	54.43	OCH_3	31.03	Pb	207.19
		H_{55}	55.44	$(OCH_3)_2$	62.07	Pt	195.09
H	1.008	H_{56}	56.45	$(OCH_3)_3$	93.10	Se	78.96
H_2	2.016	H_{57}	57.46	$(OCH_3)_4$	124.14		
H_3	3.024	H_{58}	58.46	$(OCH_3)_5$	155.17		
H_4	4.032	H_{59}	59.47	$(OCH_3)_6$	186.20		

Periodic Table of the Elements

New Notation →
Previous IUPAC Form →
CAS Version →

Key to Chart

Atomic Number →	50
Symbol →	Sn
2001 Atomic Weight →	118.710
Oxidation States →	+2 +4
Electron Configuration →	-18-18-4

Legend — each cell lists: atomic number, oxidation states, symbol, atomic weight, electron configuration (shell).

Group header notation (New / Previous IUPAC Form / CAS Version):

| 1 (IA / IA) | 2 (IIA / IIA) | 3 (IIIA / IIIB) | 4 (IVA / IVB) | 5 (VA / VB) | 6 (VIA / VIB) | 7 (VIIA / VIIB) | 8–10 (VIIIA / VIII) | 11 (IB / IB) | 12 (IIB / IIB) | 13 (IIIB / IIIA) | 14 (IVB / IVA) | 15 (VB / VA) | 16 (VIB / VIA) | 17 (VIIB / VIIA) | 18 (VIIIA) |

Main Table (cells: Z Sym — atomic weight — ox. states — electron configuration; Shell series noted at right)

Grp 1	Grp 2	Grp 3	Grp 4	Grp 5	Grp 6	Grp 7	Grp 8	Grp 9	Grp 10	Grp 11	Grp 12	Grp 13	Grp 14	Grp 15	Grp 16	Grp 17	Grp 18	Shell
1 H 1.00794 +1 -1 / 1																	2 He 4.002602 0 / 2	K
3 Li 6.941 +1 / 2-1	4 Be 9.012182 +2 / 2-2											5 B 10.811 +3 / 2-3	6 C 12.0107 +2+4-4 / 2-4	7 N 14.0067 +1+2+3+4+5-2-3 / 2-5	8 O 15.9994 -2 / 2-6	9 F 18.9984032 -1 / 2-7	10 Ne 20.1797 0 / 2-8	K-L
11 Na 22.989770 +1 / 2-8-1	12 Mg 24.3050 +2 / 2-8-2											13 Al 26.981538 +3 / 2-8-3	14 Si 28.0855 +2+4 / 2-8-4	15 P 30.973761 +3+5-3 / 2-8-5	16 S 32.065 +4+6-2 / 2-8-6	17 Cl 35.453 +1+5+7-1 / 2-8-7	18 Ar 39.948 0 / 2-8-8	K-L-M
19 K 39.0983 +1 / -8-8-1	20 Ca 40.078 +2 / -8-8-2	21 Sc 44.955910 +3 / -8-9-2	22 Ti 47.867 +2+3+4 / -8-10-2	23 V 50.9415 +2+3+4+5 / -8-11-2	24 Cr 51.9961 +2+3+6 / -8-13-1	25 Mn 54.938049 +2+3+4+7 / -8-13-2	26 Fe 55.845 +2+3 / -8-14-2	27 Co 58.933200 +2+3 / -8-15-2	28 Ni 58.6934 +2+3 / -8-16-2	29 Cu 63.546 +1+2 / -18-1	30 Zn 65.409 +2 / -18-8-2	31 Ga 69.723 +3 / -8-18-3	32 Ge 72.64 +2+4 / -8-18-4	33 As 74.92160 +3+5-3 / -8-18-5	34 Se 78.96 +4+6-2 / -8-18-6	35 Br 79.904 +5-1 / -8-18-7	36 Kr 83.798 0 / -8-18-8	-L-M-N
37 Rb 85.4678 +1 / -18-8-1	38 Sr 87.62 +2 / -18-8-2	39 Y 88.90585 +3 / -18-9-2	40 Zr 91.224 +4 / -18-10-2	41 Nb 92.90638 +3+5 / -18-12-1	42 Mo 95.94 +6 / -18-13-1	43 Tc (98) +7 / -18-13-2	44 Ru 101.07 +3 / -18-15-1	45 Rh 102.90550 +3 / -18-16-1	46 Pd 106.42 +2+4 / -18-18-0	47 Ag 107.8682 +1 / -18-18-1	48 Cd 112.411 +2 / -18-18-2	49 In 114.818 +3 / -18-18-3	50 Sn 118.710 +2+4 / -18-18-4	51 Sb 121.760 +3+5-3 / -18-18-5	52 Te 127.60 +4+6-2 / -18-18-6	53 I 126.90447 +1+5+7-1 / -18-18-7	54 Xe 131.293 0 / -18-18-8	-M-N-O
55 Cs 132.90545 +1 / -18-8-1	56 Ba 137.327 +2 / -18-8-2	57* La 138.9055 +3 / -18-9-2	72 Hf 178.49 +4 / -32-10-2	73 Ta 180.9479 +5 / -32-11-2	74 W 183.84 +6 / -32-12-2	75 Re 186.207 +4+6+7 / -32-13-2	76 Os 190.23 +3+4+6+8 / -32-14-2	77 Ir 192.217 +3+4 / -32-15-2	78 Pt 195.078 +2+4 / -32-17-1	79 Au 196.96655 +1+3 / -32-18-1	80 Hg 200.59 +1+2 / -32-18-2	81 Tl 204.3833 +1+3 / -32-18-3	82 Pb 207.2 +2+4 / -32-18-4	83 Bi 208.98038 +3+5 / -32-18-5	84 Po (209) +2+4 / -32-18-6	85 At (210) / -32-18-7	86 Rn (222) 0 / -32-18-8	-N-O-P
87 Fr (223) +1 / -18-8-1	88 Ra (226) +2 / -18-8-2	89** Ac (227) +3 / -18-9-2	104 Rf (261) +4 / -32-10-2	105 Db (262) / -32-11-2	106 Sg (266) / -32-12-2	107 Bh (264) / -32-13-2	108 Hs (277) / -32-14-2	109 Mt (268) / -32-15-2	110 Ds (271) / -32-16-2	111 Rg (272) / -32-17-1	112 Uub (285)		114 Uuq (289)		116 Uuh (289)			-O-P-Q

* Lanthanides

58 Ce 140.116 +3+4 / -19-9-2	59 Pr 140.90765 +3+4 / -21-8-2	60 Nd 144.24 +3 / -22-8-2	61 Pm (145) +3 / -23-8-2	62 Sm 150.36 +2+3 / -24-8-2	63 Eu 151.964 +2+3 / -25-8-2	64 Gd 157.25 +3 / -25-9-2	65 Tb 158.92534 +3 / -27-8-2	66 Dy 162.500 +3 / -28-8-2	67 Ho 164.93032 +3 / -29-8-2	68 Er 167.259 +3 / -30-8-2	69 Tm 168.93421 +3 / -31-8-2	70 Yb 173.04 +3 / -32-8-2	71 Lu 174.967 +3 / -32-9-2

Shell: -N-O-P

** Actinides

90 Th 232.0381 +4 / -18-10-2	91 Pa 231.03588 +4+5 / -20-9-2	92 U 238.02891 +3+4+5+6 / -21-9-2	93 Np (237) +3+4+5+6 / -22-9-2	94 Pu (244) +3+4+5+6 / -24-8-2	95 Am (243) +3+4+5+6 / -25-8-2	96 Cm (247) +3 / -25-9-2	97 Bk (247) +3+4 / -27-8-2	98 Cf (251) +3 / -28-8-2	99 Es (252) / -29-8-2	100 Fm (257) / -30-8-2	101 Md (258) / -31-8-2	102 No (259) / -32-8-2	103 Lr (262) +3 / -32-8-3

Shell: -O-P-Q

Legend (states of matter / categories):
- Gases
- Liquids
- Metallic solids
- Non-metallic solids

The new IUPAC format numbers the groups from 1 to 18. The previous IUPAC numbering system and the system used by Chemical Abstracts Service (CAS) are also shown. For radioactive elements that do not occur in nature, the mass number of the most stable isotope is given in parentheses. Elements 112, 114, and 116 have been reported but not confirmed.

References
1. G. J. Leigh, Editor, *Nomenclature of Inorganic Chemistry*, Blackwell Scientific Publications, Oxford, 1990.
2. *Chemical and Engineering News*, 63(5), 27, 1985.
3. Atomic Weights of the Elements, 2001, *Pure & Appl. Chem.*, 75, 1107, 2003.

STANDARD ATOMIC WEIGHTS (2007)

Z	Element	Symbol	Atomic Weight	Z	Element	Symbol	Atomic Weight	Z	Element	Symbol	Atomic Weight
1	Hydrogen	H	1.00794(7)	39	Yttrium	Y	88.90585(2)	77	Iridium	Ir	192.217(3)
2	Helium	He	4.002602(2)	40	Zirconium	Zr	91.224(2)	78	Platinum	Pt	195.084(9)
3	Lithium	Li	6.941(2)	41	Niobium	Nb	92.90638(2)	79	Gold	Au	196.966569(4)
4	Beryllium	Be	9.012182(3)	42	Molybdenum	Mo	95.96(2)	80	Mercury	Hg	200.59(2)
5	Boron	B	10.811(7)	43	Technetium	Tc	[97.9072]	81	Thallium	Tl	204.3833(2)
6	Carbon	C	12.0107(8)	44	Ruthenium	Ru	101.07(2)	82	Lead	Pb	207.2(1)
7	Nitrogen	N	14.0067(2)	45	Rhodium	Rh	102.90550(2)	83	Bismuth	Bi	208.98040(1)
8	Oxygen	O	15.9994(3)	46	Palladium	Pd	106.42(1)	84	Polonium	Po	[208.9824]
9	Fluorine	F	18.9984032(5)	47	Silver	Ag	107.8682(2)	85	Astatine	At	[209.9871]
10	Neon	Ne	20.1797(6)	48	Cadmium	Cd	112.411(8)	86	Radon	Rn	[222.0176]
11	Sodium	Na	22.98976928(2)	49	Indium	In	114.818(3)	87	Francium	Fr	[223.0197]
12	Magnesium	Mg	24.3050(6)	50	Tin	Sn	118.710(7)	88	Radium	Ra	[226.0254]
13	Aluminum	Al	26.9815386(8)	51	Antimony	Sb	121.760(1)	89	Actinium	Ac	[227.0277]
14	Silicon	Si	28.0855(3)	52	Tellurium	Te	127.60(3)	90	Thorium	Th	232.03806(2)
15	Phosphorus	P	30.973762(2)	53	Iodine	I	126.90447(3)	91	Protactinium	Pa	231.03588(2)
16	Sulfur	S	32.065(5)	54	Xenon	Xe	131.293(6)	92	Uranium	U	238.02891(3)
17	Chlorine	Cl	35.453(2)	55	Cesium	Cs	132.9054519(2)	93	Neptunium	Np	[237.0482]
18	Argon	Ar	39.948(1)	56	Barium	Ba	137.327(7)	94	Plutonium	Pu	[244.0642]
19	Potassium	K	39.0983(1)	57	Lanthanum	La	138.90547(7)	95	Americium	Am	[243.0614]
20	Calcium	Ca	40.078(4)	58	Cerium	Ce	140.116(1)	96	Curium	Cm	[247.0704]
21	Scandium	Sc	44.955912(6)	59	Praseodymium	Pr	140.90765(2)	97	Berkelium	Bk	[247.0703]
22	Titanium	Ti	47.867(1)	60	Neodymium	Nd	144.242(3)	98	Californium	Cf	[251.0796]
23	Vanadium	V	50.9415(1)	61	Promethium	Pm	[144.9127]	99	Einsteinium	Es	[252.0830]
24	Chromium	Cr	51.9961(6)	62	Samarium	Sm	150.36(2)	100	Fermium	Fm	[257.0951]
25	Manganese	Mn	54.938045(5)	63	Europium	Eu	151.964(1)	101	Mendelevium	Md	[258.0984]
26	Iron	Fe	55.845(2)	64	Gadolinium	Gd	157.25(3)	102	Nobelium	No	[259.1010]
27	Cobalt	Co	58.933195(5)	65	Terbium	Tb	158.92535(2)	103	Lawrencium	Lr	[262.1097]
28	Nickel	Ni	58.6934(4)	66	Dysprosium	Dy	162.500(1)	104	Rutherfordium	Rf	[261.1088]
29	Copper	Cu	63.546(3)	67	Holmium	Ho	164.93032(2)	105	Dubnium	Db	[262.1141]
30	Zinc	Zn	65.38(2)	68	Erbium	Er	167.259(3)	106	Seaborgium	Sg	[266.1219]
31	Gallium	Ga	69.723(1)	69	Thulium	Tm	168.93421(2)	107	Bohrium	Bh	[264.12]
32	Germanium	Ge	72.64(1)	70	Ytterbium	Yb	173.054(5)	108	Hassium	Hs	[277]
33	Arsenic	As	74.92160(2)	71	Lutetium	Lu	174.9668(1)	109	Meitnerium	Mt	[268.1388]
34	Selenium	Se	78.96(3)	72	Hafnium	Hf	178.49(2)	110	Darmstadtium	Ds	[271]
35	Bromine	Br	79.904(1)	73	Tantalum	Ta	180.94788(2)	111	Roentgenium	Rg	[272.1535]
36	Krypton	Kr	83.798(2)	74	Tungsten	W	183.84(1)	112	Ununbium	Uub	[285]
37	Rubidium	Rb	85.4678(3)	75	Rhenium	Re	186.207(1)	114	Ununquadium	Uuq	[289]
38	Strontium	Sr	87.62(1)	76	Osmium	Os	190.23(3)	116	Ununhexium	Uuh	[289]